theclinics.com

OTOLARYNGOLOGIC CLINICS OF NORTH AMERICA

Skull Base Medical and Surgical Issues Commonly Encountered in the Practice of Otolaryngology

GUEST EDITORS
Douglas D. Backous, MD, FACS
and Carlos R. Esquivel, MD, FACS

August 2005 • Volume 38 • Number 4

SAUNDERS

An Imprint of Elsevier, Inc.
PHILADELPHIA LONDON TORONTO MONTREAL SYDNEY TOKYO

W.B. SAUNDERS COMPANY
A Division of Elsevier Inc.

1600 John F. Kennedy Boulevard, Suite 1800, Philadelphia, PA 19103–2822

http://www.theclinics.com

THE OTOLARYNGOLOGIC CLINICS OF NORTH AMERICA
August 2005
Editor: Molly Jay

Volume 38, Number 4
ISSN 0030–6665
ISBN 1-4160-2863-3

The Otolaryngologic Clinics of North America (ISSN 0030–6665) is published bimonthly by W.B. Saunders Company. Corporate and editorial offices: Elsevier, Inc., 1600 John F. Kennedy Boulevard, Suite 1800, Philadelphia, PA 19103-2822. Accounting and circulation offices: 6277 Sea Harbor Drive, Orlando, FL 32887–4800. Periodicals postage paid at Orlando, FL 32862, and additional mailing offices. Subscription price is $199.00 per year (US individuals), $350.00 per year (US institutions), $100.00 per year (US student/resident), $269.00 per year (Canadian individuals), $430.00 per year (Canadian institutions), $280.00 per year (international individuals), $430.00 per year (international institutions), $140.00 per year (international & Canadian student/resident). Foreign air speed delivery is included in all *Clinics'* subscription prices. All prices are subject to change without notice. POSTMASTER: Send address changes to *The Otolaryngologic Clinics of North America*, W.B. Saunders Company, Periodicals Fulfillment, Orlando, FL 32887–4800. **Customer Service: 1-800-654-2452 (US). From outside the US, call 407-345-4000.**

The Otolaryngologic Clinics of North America is also published in Spanish by McGraw-Hill Interamericana Editores S.A., P.O. Box 5-237, 06500 Mexico D.F., Mexico.

The Otolaryngologic Clinics of North America is covered in *Index Medicus, Current Contents/Clinical Medicine, Excerpta Medica, BIOSIS, Science Citation Index,* and *ISI/BIOMED.*

Printed in the United States of America.

GUEST EDITORS

DOUGLAS D. BACKOUS, MD, FACS, Director, Otology, Neurotology and Skull Base Surgery; and Medical Director, The Listen for Life Center at Virginia Mason, Virginia Mason Medical Center, Seattle, Washington

CARLOS R. ESQUIVEL, MD, FACS, Madigan Army Medical Center, United States Army-Ft. Lewis, Tacoma, Washington

CONTRIBUTORS

DOUGLAS D. BACKOUS, MD, FACS, Director, Otology, Neurotology and Skull Base Surgery; and Medical Director, The Listen for Life Center at Virginia Mason, Virginia Mason Medical Center, Seattle, Washington

STEPHEN W. BAYLES, MD, Department of Otolaryngology/Head and Neck Surgery, Virgina Mason Medical Center, Seattle, Washington

DAVID C. BLOOM, MD, Clinical Instructor, Department of Otolaryngology–Head and Neck Surgery, University of Washington; and Division of Pediatric Otolaryngology, Children's Hospital and Regional Medical Center, Seattle, Washington

FELIX W.K. CHU, MD, Department of Otolaryngology/Head and Neck Surgery, Virginia Mason Medical Center, Seattle, Washington

JOHNNY B. DELASHAW JR., MD, Vice-Chairman and Professor of Neurological Surgery, Division of Skull Base Neurosurgery, Department of Neurological Surgery; and Professor of Otolaryngology, Division of Otology and Neurotology, Department of Otolaryngology/Head and Neck Surgery, Oregon Health & Science University, Portland, Oregon

BRUCE M. EDWARDS, AuD, Senior Audiologist, Division of Audiology and Electrophysiology, Department of Otolaryngology–Head and Neck Surgery, University of Michigan Health System, Ann Arbor, Michigan

JOANNE FENN, CCC-SLP, Voice and Swallowing Clinic, Department of Otolaryngology/Head and Neck Surgery, Virginia Mason Medical Center, Seattle, Washington

LUCY W. GLENN, MD, Chief, Department of Radiology, Virginia Mason Medical Center, Seattle, Washington

JOSEPH S. GRUSS, MD, Professor, Department of Plastic and Reconstructive Surgery, University of Washington; and Division of Pediatric Plastic and Reconstructive Surgery, Children's Hospital and Regional Medical Center, Seattle, Washington

CHANG YONG HAN, MD, Department of Otolaryngology/Head and Neck Surgery, Maryknoll General Hospital, Pusan, Korea

GADY HAR-EL, MD, FACS, Professor of Otolaryngology and Neurosurgery, State University of New York-Downstate Medical Center; Department of Otolaryngology, Long Island College Hospital; and Othmer Cancer Centers, Brooklyn, New York

WAYNE J. HARSHA, MD, Resident, Otolaryngology–Head & Neck Surgery Service, Madigan Army Medical Center, Tacoma, Washington

DAVID H. HILTZIK, MD, Resident Physician, Department of Otolaryngology, Weill Medical College of Cornell University, New York, New York

ANDREW INGLIS, MD, Associate Professor, Department of Otolaryngology–Head and Neck Surgery, University of Washington; and Division of Pediatric Otolaryngology, Children's Hospital and Regional Medical Center, Seattle, Washington

JULIE T. KERR, MD, Department of Otolaryngology–Head and Neck Surgery, Madigan Army Medical Center, Tacoma, Washington

PAUL R. KILENY, PhD, Director, Division of Audiology and Electrophysiology, Department of Otolaryngology–Head and Neck Surgery, University of Michigan Health System; and Professor, University of Michigan Medical School, Ann Arbor, Michigan

SCOTT C. MANNING, MD, Professor, Department of Otolaryngology–Head and Neck Surgery, University of Washington; and Division of Pediatric Otolaryngology, Children's Hospital and Regional Medical Center, Seattle, Washington

BECKY L. MASSEY, MD, Chief Resident, Division of Otolaryngology–Head and Neck Surgery, Department of Surgery, University of Utah, Salt Lake City, Utah

SEAN O. McMENOMEY, MD, Associate Professor of Otolaryngology, Division of Otology and Neurotology, Department of Otolaryngology/Head and Neck Surgery; and Associate Professor of Neurological Surgery, Division of Skull Base Neurosurgery, Department of Neurological Surgery, Oregon Health & Science University, Portland, Oregon

KAPIL MOZA, MD, Instructor of Neurological Surgery, Division of Skull Base Neurosurgery, Department of Neurological Surgery, Oregon Health & Science University, Portland, Oregon

BRIAN A. NEFF, MD, Department of Otolaryngology, Mayo Clinic, Rochester, Minnesota

NOOSHIN PARHIZKAR, MD, Resident Physician, Department of Otolaryngology, Weill Medical College of Cornell University, New York, New York

JONATHAN A. PERKINS, DO, Associate Professor, Department of Otolaryngology–Head and Neck Surgery, University of Washington; and Division of Pediatric Otolaryngology, Children's Hospital and Regional Medical Center, Seattle, Washington

K. LINNEA PETERSON, MD, FACS, Voice and Swallowing Clinic, Department of Otolaryngology/Head and Neck Surgery, Virginia Mason Medical Center, Seattle, Washington

CHRISTOPHER RAINE, ChM, FRCS, Department of Otorhinolaryngology, Bradford Royal Infirmary, Bradford, United Kingdom

DAVID H. ROBINSON, MD, Director of the Vascular Center and Section Head of Interventional Radiology, Department of Radiology, Virginia Mason Medical Center Seattle, Washington

SAMUEL H. SELESNICK, MD, Professor and Vice Chair, Department of Otolaryngology, Weill Medical College of Cornell University, New York, New York

PRAMOD K. SHARMA, MD. FACS, Assistant Professor, Division of Otolaryngology–Head and Neck Surgery, Department of Surgery; and Director, Multidisciplinary Head and Neck Oncology Program, Huntsman Cancer Institute, University of Utah, Salt Lake City, Utah

P. ASHLEY WACKYM, MD, FACS, FAAP, John C. Koss Professor and Chairman, Department of Otolaryngology and Communication Sciences, Medical College of Wisconsin, Milwaukee, Wisconsin

PETER C. WEBER, MD, MBA, Professor and Program Director, Implantable Hearing Devices, The Cleveland Clinic Foundation, Cleveland, Ohio.

D. BRADLEY WELLING, MD, PhD, Professor and Chair, Department of Otolaryngology–Head and Neck Surgery, The Ohio State University College of Medicine, Columbus, Ohio

CONTENTS

FORTHCOMING ISSUES

October 2005

Oculofacial Surgery
Stephen Bosniak, MD, *Guest Editor*

December 2005

Chronic Rhinosinusitis
Berrylin J. Ferguson, MD
and Allen Seiden, MD, *Guest Editors*

RECENT ISSUES

June 2005

Image-Guided Surgery of the Paranasal Sinuses
Raj Sindwani, MD, FRCS, *Guest Editor*

April 2005

Bioengineering in Otolaryngology
Arlen D. Meyers, MD, MBA, *Guest Editor*

February 2005

Contemporary Diagnosis and Management of Head and Neck Cancer
Jeffrey H. Spiegel, MD, FACS and
Scharuk Jalisi, MD, *Guest Editors*

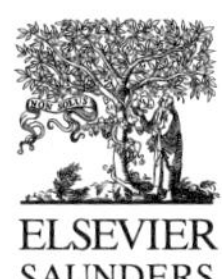
ELSEVIER
SAUNDERS

Otolaryngol Clin N Am
38 (2005) xiii–xiv

OTOLARYNGOLOGIC
CLINICS
OF NORTH AMERICA

Preface

Skull Base Medical and Surgical Issues Commonly Encountered in the Practice of Otolaryngology

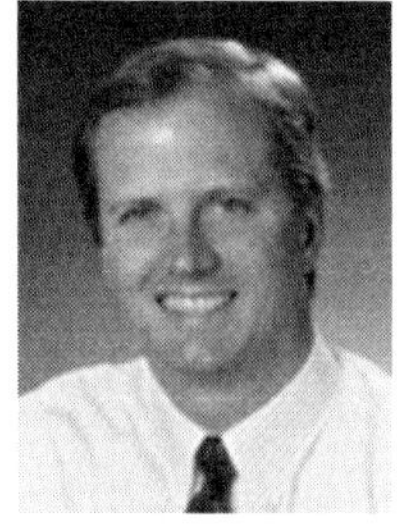

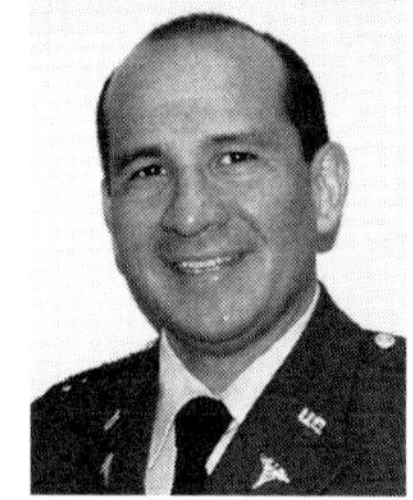

Douglas D. Backous, MD, FACS   Carlos R. Esquivel, MD, FACS
Guest Editors

Advances in neuroimaging, surgical instrumentation, and operative techniques have made the management of complex diseases of the ear, paranasal sinuses, and head/neck commonplace in the practice of general otolaryngology. The anterior and lateral skull base, once considered an area reserved for subspecialty trained surgeons, is now being approached endoscopically and through open procedures as part of operations performed in hospitals and in ambulatory surgery centers. A thorough understanding of head and neck anatomy complemented by knowledge of acute management of complications in the skull base interface is critical to avoid diagnostic and surgical pitfalls while providing safe and effective patient care.

This issue of the *Otolaryngologic Clinics of North America* begins with an overview of cerebrospinal fluid metabolism as it relates to intracranial pressure homeostasis followed by three articles addressing the management of cerebrospinal fluid leakage. New developments in neuroimaging and a review of cranial nerve monitoring are presented with an emphasis on applications important to common head and neck procedures.

Although vestibular schwannomas (acoustic neuromas) and pediatric skull base tumors are not commonly encountered by general otolaryngologists, an updated understanding of current treatment options is offered to foster effective initial diagnosis, counseling, and appropriate subspecialty

doi:10.1016/j.otc.2005.03.010

patient referral. Contributions describing endovascular intervention options and management of common surgical complications complete this issue.

Please enjoy the basic principles, clinical pearls, and interventional techniques presented in this issue of the *Clinics*. We hope this issue will become a resource to you as you practice otolaryngology for years to come.

Douglas D. Backous, MD, FACS
Virginia Mason Medical Center
1100 Ninth Avenue, X10-ON
Seattle, WA 98111, USA

E-mail address: otoddb@vmmc.org

Carlos R. Esquivel, MD, FACS
Madigan Army Medical Center
9040 Jackson Avenue
MCJH-SET
Tacoma, WA 98431, USA

E-mail address: Carlos.Esquivel@nw.amedd.army.mil

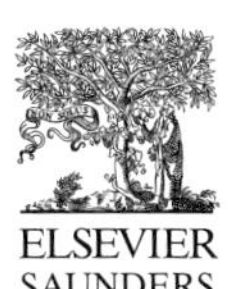
ELSEVIER
SAUNDERS

Otolaryngol Clin N Am
38 (2005) 569–576

OTOLARYNGOLOGIC
CLINICS
OF NORTH AMERICA

Basic Principles of Cerebrospinal Fluid Metabolism and Intracranial Pressure Homeostasis

Chang Yong Han, MD[a],
Douglas D. Backous, MD, FACS[b,*]

[a]*Department of Otolaryngology/Head and Neck Surgery, Maryknoll General Hospital, 12 4-Ga Daechung Joong-Ku, Pusan, Korea*
[b]*Department of Otolaryngology/Head and Neck Surgery, Virginia Mason Medical Center, 1100 Ninth Avenue, X10-ON, Seattle, WA 98111, USA*

Cerebrospinal fluid (CSF) is continually produced, absorbed, and circulated in the ventricles and around the surface of the brain and spinal cord. There are four functions of CSF in the human nervous system. The most obvious function of CSF is the provision of physical support and buoyancy for the brain. This "water jacket" is also protective, because CSF volume fluctuates reciprocally with changes in intracranial blood volume to contribute to a safe intracranial pressure (ICP). Because the brain is devoid of a lymphatic system, by-products of metabolism are principally removed by the capillary circulation or directly by transfer through the CSF. The direct CSF route is particularly important when increased amounts of lactic acid are produced in the brain. Finally, the CSF functions to regulate the chemical environment of the brain [1].

According to the Monro-Kellie hypothesis, the skull is a rigid sphere occupied by noncompressible liquid/gel tissues [2]. Blood (75 mL), CSF (150 mL,), and brain tissue (1400 mL) are the three principle components of the cranial vault. Acute changes in ICP result in shifting or compression of the fixed brain liquid/gel mass within the intracranial cavity. Compression of brain against the falx cerebri or tentorium cerebelli, herniation through the foramen magnum, or leakage of CSF from sites in the skull or spinal canal can occur when ICP remains high or when there has been spontaneous, traumatic, or iatrogenic violation of the dura.

* Corresponding author.
E-mail address: otoddb@vmmc.org (D.D. Backous).

doi:10.1016/j.otc.2005.01.005 **oto.theclinics.com**

This article reviews the physiology of CSF and the basic mechanisms leading to changes in ICP and CSF leakage pertinent to the otolaryngologist.

Anatomy and physiology of CSF flow

CSF is located in the cerebral ventricles and the subarachnoid spaces, including the spinal canal. In the normal physiologic state, the ventricles of the brain account for roughly 30 cm^3 of the total CSF volume of 140 to 50 cm^3. The choroid plexus, found in the lateral, third, and fourth ventricles, secretes approximately 60% of the CSF. The choroid plexus is formed from invaginations of ependyma into the ventricular cavities by the blood vessels of the pia mater. The blood–CSF barrier at the choroid plexus is composed of the tight junction (zonula occludens) between secretory cells. Extrachoroidal formation of CSF, constituting the remaining 40% of production, occurs across parenchymal capillaries, by the ependyma, and from intracellular water generated metabolically through the complete oxidation of glucose. CSF is formed in humans at a rate of 0.35 mL/min or 500 mL/d [3–5]. Production of CSF varies with a circadian rhythm with a 3.5-fold difference between the maximal production period at 2:00 AM and the nadir at 6:00 PM [6].

CSF flows from its production sites in the two lateral ventricles through the foramina of Monro into the third ventricle and then to the fourth ventricle through the aqueduct of Sylvius. Flow continues through the fourth ventricle, located in the brain stem, and communicates with the cisterna magna through the midline foramen of Magendie and the two lateral foramina of Luschka. From the cisterna magna, CSF flows dorsally into the subarachnoid space of the cerebellum, caudally into the spinal subarachnoid space, and rostrally into several subarachnoid cisterns of the brain (pontis, interpeduncularis, ambiens, and the suprasellar). From these cisterns, the CSF reaches the subarachnoid space of the cerebral hemispheres. The major branches of the circle of Willis traverse the major cisterns in the subarachnoid space at the base of the brain, giving rise to the vascular pulsations in the CSF (Fig. 1) [1,3].

The secretion of CSF by choroid plexus epithelium results from the active transport of sodium. The current human model (Fig. 2) is incomplete and somewhat speculative [4]. Multiple ion exchangers in the luminal and adluminal surfaces of epithelial cells secrete sodium, chloride, and bicarbonate from plasma to CSF. A Na^+-K^+ pump located on the apical membrane pumps Na^+ out of the choroid cells, driving down the intracellular Na^+ concentration. The subsequent Na^+ gradient generated on the basolateral membrane secondarily activates the active transport of Na^+ into the cell through a Na^+-H^+ exchange and a Na^+-Cl^- co-transport. Inhibitors of the Na^+-K^+ pump, such as the cardiac glycoside ouabain, decrease CSF production [7].

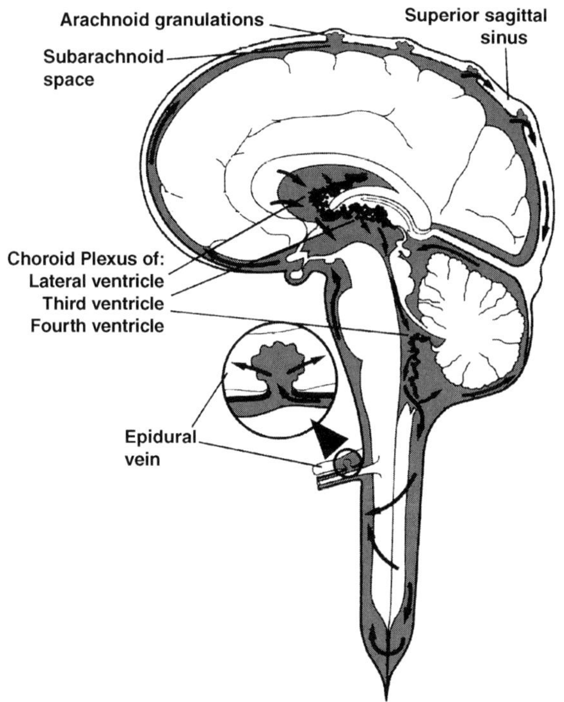

Fig. 1. The sites of formation, circulation, and absorption of the CSF. The circulation of the CSF to the subarachnoid space and its absorption into the venous system through the arachnoid villi are shown. The presence of arachnoid villi adjacent to the spinal roots supplements the absorption that takes place into the intracranial venous sinuses.

The main function of the basolateral Na^+-H^+ antiport and Cl^--HCO_3^- pump is to regulate intracellular pH. Intracellular HCO_3^- is generated from the hydration of carbon dioxide by carbonic anhydrase [8]. The carbonic anhydrase inhibitor acetazolamide reduces CSF sodium exchange to 35% to 60% of control value and is regarded as the most effective pharmacologic agent for reducing choroidal secretion [9]. The choroid plexus contributes to the clearance of CSF, neurotransmitters, and various metabolites, although the quantitative importance is unknown. Additional lipophilic solutes such as carbon dioxide, lactate, hydrogen ions, and ammonia are cleared by simple diffusion from the CSF into the adjacent brain and capillaries [4].

CSF is resorbed into the cerebral venous system through the pacchionian granulations and arachnoid villi, the major sites for bulk flow absorption of CSF. The macroscopic granulations, composed of multiple microscopic arachnoid villi, are herniations of the arachnoid membrane into the lumen of the superior sagittal sinus and adjacent to the emerging spinal nerve roots, penetrating the dura of the root sleeves and extending into small spinal veins [3].

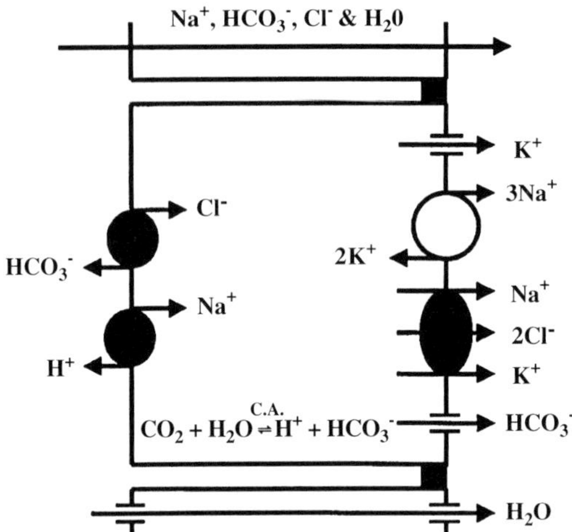

Fig. 2. CSF secretion by the mammalian choroid plexus. The model includes recently obtained immunocytochemical and patch clamp data on the expression of ion transport proteins and ion channels in choroids plexus epithelial cells. CA, carbonic anhydrase.

The amount of resorption at the arachnoid villi is primarily determined by the venous pressure and the hydrostatic pressure within the subarachnoid space. By using ventriculo-lumbar perfusion, Cutler [10] determined that CSF absorption begins at an average CSF pressure of 68 mm H_2O and increases linearly with pressure up to 250 mm H_2O, maintaining an absorption rate of 1.5 mL/min. Formation and absorption are equal at a pressure of 112 mm H_2O. CSF absorption may begin at a pressure of about 40 mm, as noted in Fig. 3. The reduction in CSF absorption below the null point of the ICP and the increase in CSF absorption that occurs with increased ICP are homeostatic responses to maintain normal ICP and CSF volume.

According to the hyperdynamic model of CSF circulation, the main absorption of the CSF and its constituents occurs through the capillaries of the central nervous system (Fig. 4). Because of the blood–brain barrier, water, most ions, and lipids pass freely from blood into cerebral extracellular fluids, whereas proteins and polar molecules are excluded. The major anatomic sites of the blood–brain barrier are at the choroid plexus epithelium and at the cerebral microvascular endothelial cells, where tight junctions restrict the passage of all substances with a diameter greater than 10 to 15 A. The very low content in intracytoplasmic pinocytotic vesicles of cerebral endothelial cells allows a low rate of transcellular transport of various substances [11]. Although blood–brain barrier is impermeable for blood-to-brain passage, it may not be impermeable for brain-to-blood passage: albumin and radiographic contrast media appear in the blood within minutes after administration into the subarachnoid space [12,13].

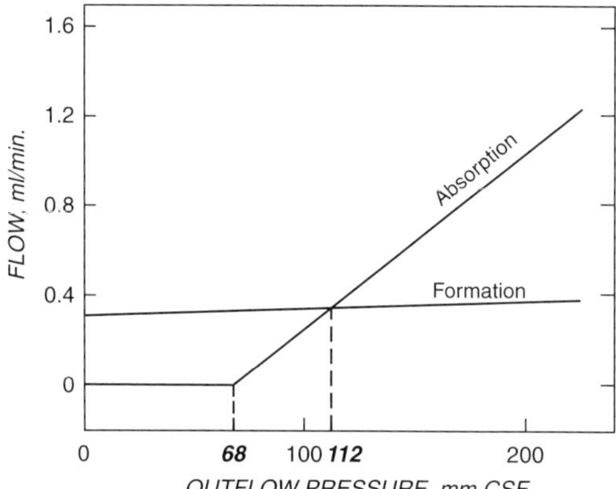

Fig. 3. Superimposed regression lines for CSF formation and absorption as a function of outflow pressure. The null point (112 mm H_2O or CSF) indicates the pressure at which formation and absorption are equal. The pressure at which absorption is zero is also indicated.

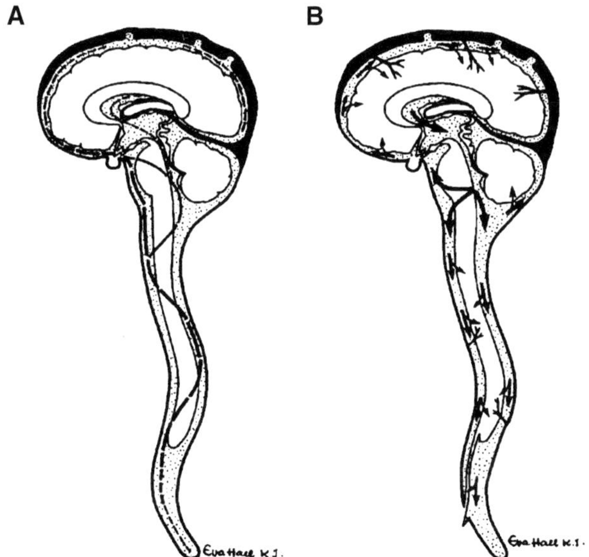

Fig. 4. The two proposed pathways of cerebrospinal fluid circulation. (*A*) There is a dominant pulsatile flow with a fast-velocity compartment in the brain stem-cord area and slow velocities at the upper and lower ends of the subarachnoid spaces. The amplitude and velocity are indicated by the length of the segments of the dashed line. The systolic and diastolic flows in the spinal canal follow one main channel, which is located toward the convexities showing a meandering S-shaped route caused by centrifugal forces and lower resistance in wider subarachnoid spaces. (*B*) The minute bulk flows are exaggerated for clearer illustration. The thickness of the arrows is related to the magnitude of the bulk flow, which decreases in both directions from the foramen magnum. The CSF is resorbed everywhere in the central nervous system by the circulating blood. The spinal nerves, including the cauda equina, are represented by one caudal root in this schematic drawing.

The bidirectional oscillatory movement of CSF results from cardiac cycle–related variations in cerebral blood volume. The simultaneous egress of venous blood and the cranio-caudal displacement of CSF into the spinal canal compensate for the net inflow of arterial blood during systole [14]. In addition, intraventricular movement of CSF is caused by the centripetal motion of the cerebral hemispheres during systole [15]. Lateral ventricular volume varies by as much as 20% [16]. Transient retrograde CSF flow through the cerebral aqueduct and anterograde flow out the foramen of Magendie occurs at the beginning of systole. Caudal movement, by piston action of the entire brain, and a posterior movement of the basal ganglia occur during mid-systole and reverse at end systole. Both CSF flows are retrograde during diastole [15].

In the closed cranial cavity, the systolic arterial pressure peak is instantaneously transmitted to the subarachnoid spaces and hence to the cortical veins. The compression of the venous outlets and the ensuing increase in their outlet resistance sufficiently distends the intracerebral veins to accommodate the high normal cerebral blood flow. In diastole, the ensuing increase in pressure in the spinal canal causes an inflow to the cranial cavity. ICP is maintained in the subarachnoid space during the entire cardiac cycle. Once the fontanelles have closed, the compressible pacchionian granulations act as Starling resistors to maintain stable blood flow and to regulate the intracranial pulse pressure [17].

Physiology of intracranial pressure

Factors controlling ICP have been modeled by Marmarou [18] as follows:

$$ICP = I_f \times R_{out} + P_{ss}$$

when I_f is the CSF formation rate, R_{out} is the resistance to outflow of CSF, and P_{ss} is the sagittal sinus pressure.

Normal ICP ranges from 5 to 15 mm Hg or 5 to 195 mm H_2O. A very large increase in the rate of CSF formation would be required to create an elevated CSF pressure (eg, in the rare instance of a choroid plexus papilloma). The effect of increased protein concentration in the CSF or inflammatory changes in the dura caused by meningitis, subarachnoid hemorrhage, or iatrogenic entry of blood into the subarachnoid space may create resistance to outflow by impairing CSF absorption at the arachnoid villi. Pressure changes in the sagittal sinus reduce the gradient for flow from the subarachnoid space to the cerebral venous outflow. Such conditions as superior vena cava syndrome, jugular venous occlusion, surgical removal of a dominant jugular vein, and acute thrombosis of the sagittal sinus secondarily decrease flow through the arachnoid granulations. Because of the phenomenon of autoregulation, the brain is able to regulate arterial blood flow in accord with metabolic demand. Constant arterial blood flow is maintained over a range of perfusion pressures from 60 to 150 mm Hg. With loss of autoregulation, most commonly seen in end-stage intracranial hypertension, cerebral blood flow and blood volume fluctuate passively with changes in systolic pressure. The valveless central venous system has no autoregulation, so fluctuations in systemic venous pressures directly affect CSF pressure.

Summary

Significant progress has been made in understanding the production, circulation, and absorption of CSF. In part because of autoregulation, rapid changes in arterial pressure produce parallel but significantly dampened changes in CSF pressure. Chronic arterial hypertension rarely affects ICP, but changes in venous pressure are transmitted directly into the CSF, taking precedence over arterial effects. An understanding of basic CSF physiology, particularly in relation to ICP homeostasis, is important for surgeons treating intracranial hypertension, low ICP pressure, and spontaneous, traumatic, or iatrogenic CSF leakages. The principles discussed in this article are valuable to remember when planning surgical procedures in the head and neck, both to prevent and to treat potential complications related to increased or decreased CSF pressure.

References

[1] Milhorat TH. The third circulation revisited. J Neurosurg 1975;42:628–45.
[2] Davson H, Welch K, Segal MB. The physiology and pathology of the cerebrospinal fluid. New York: Churchill Livingstone; 1987. p. 1013.
[3] Johanson CE. Ventricles and cerebrospinal fluid. In: Conn PM, editor. Neuroscience in Medicine. Philadelphia: JB Lippincott; 1995. p. 171–96.
[4] Speake T, Whitwell C, Kajita H, et al. Mechanisms of CSF secretion by the choroid plexus. Microsc Res Tech 2001;52:49–59.
[5] Pollay M, Curl F. Secretion of cerebrospinal fluid by the ventricular ependyma of the rabbit. Am J Physiol 1967;213:1031–8.
[6] Nilsson C, Stahlberg F, Thomsen C, et al. Circadian variation in human cerebrospinal fluid production measured by magnetic resonance imaging. Am J Physiol 1992;262:20–4.
[7] Davison H, Segal MB. The effects of some inhibitors and accelerators of sodium transport on the turnover of 22Na in the cerebrospinal fluid and the brain. J Physiol 1970;209:139–53.
[8] Baudrie V, Roullet JB, Goureau Y, et al. Determination of cerebrospinal fluid production rate using a push-pull perfusion procedure in the conscious rat. Fundam Clin Pharmacol 1990;4:269–74.
[9] Faraci FM, Mayhan WG, Heistad DD. Vascular effects of acetazolamide on the choroid plexus. J Pharmacol Exp Ther 1990;254:23–7.
[10] Cutler RWP, Page L, Galicich J, et al. Formation and absorption of cerebrospinal fluid in man. Brain 1968;91:707–20.
[11] Janzer RC. The blood-brain barrier: cellular basis. J Inherit Metab Dis 1993;16:639–47.
[12] Reed DJ, Woodbury DM. Kinetics of iodide, sucrose, inulin and radio-iodinated serum albumin in the central nervous system and cerebrospinal fluid of the rat. J Physiol 1963;169: 816–50.

[13] Golman K. Absorption of metrizamide from cerebrospinal fluid to blood: pharmacokinetics in humans. J Pharm Sci 1975;64:405–7.
[14] Bhadlia RA, Bogdan AR, Kaplan RF, et al. Cerebrospinal fluid pulsation amplitude and its quantitative relationship to cerebral blood flow pulsations: a phase-contrast MR flow imaging study. Neuroradiology 1997;39:258–64.
[15] Greitz D. Cerebrospinal fluid circulation and associated intracranial dynamics: a radiologic investigation using MR imaging and radionuclide cisternography. Acta Radiol Suppl 1993; 386:1–23.
[16] Lee E, Wang JZ, Mezrich R. Variation of lateral ventricular volume during the cardiac cycle observed by MR imaging. Am J Neuroradiol 1989;10:1145–9.
[17] Greitz D, Hannerz J, Bellander B-M, et al. Restricted arterial expansion as a universal causative factor in communication hydrocephalus. Neuroradiology Suppl 1995;37:14–8.
[18] Marmarou A, Shulman K, Rosende RM. A nonlinear analysis of the cerebrospinal fluid system and intracranial pressure dynamics. J Neurosurg 1978;48:332–44.

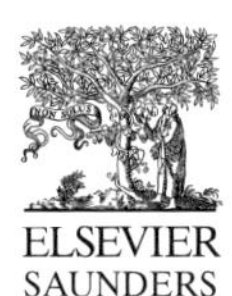
ELSEVIER
SAUNDERS

Otolaryngol Clin N Am
38 (2005) 577–582

OTOLARYNGOLOGIC
CLINICS
OF NORTH AMERICA

Indications for Cerebrospinal Fluid Drainage and Avoidance of Complications

Kapil Moza, MD[a], Sean O. McMenomey, MD[a,b], Johnny B. Delashaw Jr., MD[a,b,*]

[a]*Division of Skull Base Neurosurgery, Department of Neurological Surgery, Oregon Health & Science University, 3181 Southwest Sam Jackson Park Road, Portland, OR 97239, USA*

[b]*Division of Otology and Neurotology, Department of Otolaryngology/Head and Neck Surgery, Oregon Health & Science University, 3181 Southwest Sam Jackson Park Road, Portland, OR 97239, USA*

Cerebrospinal fistulae result from an aberrant communication between the sinonasal area and the subarachnoid space. Based on cause, these fistulae may be divided into four categories: (1) traumatic, (2) nontraumatic, (3) spontaneous, and (4) iatrogenic. The diagnosis and management of cerebrospinal leakage remains a challenge, and recent reports display an evolution from intracranial repair to endoscope-assisted extracranial repair techniques. This article describes the management of cerebrospinal fluid (CSF) fistulae using different diversion techniques including external lumbar drainage, lumboperitoneal (LP) shunts, and ventriculoperitoneal (VP) shunts. The potential complications associated with each system are also discussed. A brief review of normal CSF physiology is helpful in understanding treatment paradigms.

Physiology of cerebrospinal fluid

Seventy percent of CSF is produced by the choroid plexus located in the fourth, third, and lateral ventricles, at a rate of 0.2 to 0.4 cm^3/min or 300 to 500 cm^3/d. Approximately 20% of CSF is produced by capillary

* Corresponding author. Neurological Surgery, L-472, Oregon Health & Science University, 3181 Southwest Sam Jackson Park Road, Portland, OR 97239.

E-mail address: delashaw@ohsu.edu (J.B. Delashaw).

doi:10.1016/j.otc.2005.01.001 **oto.theclinics.com**

ultrafiltrate, and 10% is produced by water metabolism. In adults the average CSF volume is 90 to 150 cm^3, with 40 cm^3 in the lateral ventricles. CSF flows from the choroid plexus in the lateral ventricles to the third ventricle through the foramen of Monroe. From the third ventricle, fluid travels through the sylvian aqueduct to the fourth ventricle and then to the subarachnoid space by way of the foramina of Luschka and Magendie. Fluid absorption occurs at the arachnoid villi, which are essentially one-way valves. A gradient of 1.5 to 7 cm H_2O is required to drive fluid through the villi.

Normal intracranial pressure (ICP) lies in the range of 5 to 15 cm H_2O in the prone position and increases to 40 cm H_2O with movement into the sitting position. The cardiac cycle and respiratory phase cause the ICP to vary. Valsalva maneuvers, coughing, and sneezing increase ICP, thereby reducing venous outflow from the intracranial compartment. This reduced outflow in turn leads to an elevation in the ICP. ICP is considered increased when a pressure higher than 20 cm H_2O is sustained, and symptoms may develop at levels as low as 15 cm H_2O.

Hydrocephalus is an imbalance in CSF production and absorption resulting in a net increase in the fluid volume of the ventricles. Hydrocephalus may arise as a result of increased CSF production (a rare event), impaired venous drainage, or anatomic obstruction of the CSF pathway [1]. Dilatation commonly occurs proximal to the site of obstruction. In communicating hydrocephalus, when the point of obstruction is at the arachnoid villi, all ventricles are enlarged. Sustained ICP in turn exerts force on certain weak anatomic locations, such as the cribiform plate and sella turcica. These areas behave as release valves; as a result, fistulae are created.

Historical overview of cerebrospinal fluid drainage and shunting

After the elucidation of normal CSF physiology, a number of drainage techniques were devised [2]. In 1881, Wernicke [3] introduced an open drainage technique, followed by Henle [4], who in 1896 devised a procedure connecting the ventricles to the subgaleal space. In 1914, Dandy [5] classified hydrocephalus as obstructive or nonobstructive (communicating), and in 1939 Torkildsen [6] developed a ventriculocisternostomy technique using rubber tubing. This technique involved cannulization of the occipital horn of the lateral ventricle and passing the distal portion of the tube into the cisterna magna; a craniectomy was performed to gain access to the foramen magnum. As extracranial sites and one-way valves were introduced, this technique became outdated, and in 1952 Nulsen and Spitz [7] used a unidirectional valve in a shunt system. In addition to the ureter, pleura, and peritoneum, the atrium was used in shunt systems, as first described by Pudenz [8] in the 1950s. This technique became less popular because the ventriculoatrial shunt posed the risk of introducing a foreign body into the vascular system. Recently, VP shunts have become the treatment of choice in pediatric hydrocephalus patients. LP shunting plays an important role in adults with nonobstructive hydrocephalus and postoperative CSF leaks, such as those occurring after skull base procedures or transsphenoidal surgeries.

External lumbar drainage

External lumbar drainage is a common modality used in the setting of CSF leaks occurring after cranial trauma, preoperatively for brain relaxation, and postoperatively for prevention or treatment of CSF fistulae. These systems are prone to infection if left in place more than 10 days; therefore, diversions of longer duration require internal drainage techniques.

The placement of an external lumbar drainage system involves wide prepping of the lumbar region with iodine antiseptic solution and, should a higher level of entry be required, prepping of the thoracolumbar region. Local anesthetic is injected subcutaneously at the L4–L5 level with a large needle affixed for deeper tissue injection. Following the injection of local anesthesia, a 14-gauge Touhy needle is inserted into the interspace. Care must be taken to keep the bevel of the needle up, to proceed slowly, and to appreciate the resistance of the dura as it is punctured. After entry into the thecal sac, the needle is rotated 90° so the bevel points cephalad, and the inner stylet is removed. Following egress of CSF, a catheter is introduced through a needle (over a wire), and the needle is removed carefully, taking care not to lacerate the catheter. The inner wire is then withdrawn while the catheter is stabilized, and a sterile cap is applied to the distal end. This cap is connected to a closed reservoir system, and the chamber is kept at a level that drains approximately 10 to 20 cm^3/h (slightly less than the amount normally produced). Extreme caution must be exercised regarding the amount drained; overdrainage can result in headaches and, more importantly, subdural bleeding, especially in the posterior fossa from tethering and disruption of the precentral cerebellar vein. To rule out obstructive hydrocephalus or a posterior fossa lesion impinging the fourth ventricle, a CT scan of the brain should be performed before placement.

The authors do not advocate the use of prophylactic antibiotics during drainage. If meningitis is suspected, CSF may be sent for laboratory analysis, with prompt initiation of empiric antimicrobial therapy until the laboratory results are available. External lumbar drainage is an effective modality, but the duration of application is restricted because prolonged drainage carries an increased risk of meningitis.

Lumboperitoneal shunts

LP shunts are valuable therapy modality for CSF leaks in the setting of communicating hydrocephalus. Introduced by Jackson and Snodgrass [9] in

1955, LP shunts avoid the risks of ventricular catheterization (including intracranial hematoma and ventriculitis). LP shunts are used for treating pseudomeningoceles in patients who have undergone retrosigmoid and far lateral approaches in which dural repair is difficult or not feasible. The authors use LP shunts in cases of refractory CSF fistulae following transsphenoidal and translabyrinthine approaches for tumors and other lesions. The LP shunt system has a single-chamber reservoir and two distal slit valves. The perforated end of the catheter is introduced into the subarachnoid space as described for external lumbar drainage. The end of the catheter with the slit valves is tunneled subcutaneously to the abdominal region and inserted into the peritoneum. No reservoir or flush chamber is available for CSF withdrawal or fluid injection.

Complications associated with LP shunts include bowel injury, wound infection, obstruction, spinal epidural hematoma, and overdrainage headaches. In rare cases, ascites may result when the peritoneum cannot absorb CSF. Anteroposterior and lateral plain abdominal tomograms are used to identify the radiopaque Silastic catheter and verify the intraperitoneal location. An abdominal CT scan is performed when it is unclear if the abdominal end is truly intraperitoneal. Meticulous dissection and identification of various tissue layers helps reduce the possibility of catheter misplacement. In cases of overdrainage headaches, the shunt is either ligated with a suture or clip or, in some cases, removed. These patients may require the placement of a VP shunt with a programmable valve that allows adjustment of the drainage volume.

Ventriculoperitoneal shunts

VP shunt systems involve three components: (1) a ventricular catheter, (2) a valve-reservoir, and (3) a peritoneal catheter. The ventricular catheter is placed intracranially through a burr hole, 11 cm posterior to the nasion and 3 cm lateral to midline, approximating the mid-pupillary line. A trajectory aiming for the ipsilateral medial canthus is followed, and care is taken to avoid passing more than 6 cm of catheter. The stylet is removed, and the end is connected to a unidirectional valve. The peritoneal catheter is passed up from the abdominal region and attached to the distal part of the valve. The valve is pulled distally to occupy a subgaleal pocket, and the distal catheter is buried in the peritoneum. A number of ventricular catheter designs are available, including a right-angled catheter, flanged-tip catheters, and straight catheters with tip perforation. The authors use straight catheters with tip perforation. Because of the development of arachnoidal and ependymal adhesions, many no longer use flanged-tip catheters. Various valve designs are available, such as low (20–40 mm H_2O), medium (40–70 mm H_2O), or high pressure (80–120 mm H_2O). Programmable differential-pressure valves are being used increasingly, especially in patients with normal-pressure hydrocephalus. These valves allow modulation of the closing pressure at the bedside with the use of a handheld magnet. Final verification of valve settings is performed by skull radiograph or by bedside interrogation with a device. Aside from these designs, an on–off valve can be used to provide intermittent shunting, but these devices carry the risk of the patient's unknowingly deactivating the shunt by mistakenly depressing the valve.

Complications with VP shunts include insertion problems, obstruction, wound infections, and over- and underdrainage. Insertion of the ventricular catheter carries a small but significant risk of intracerebral bleeding. Ventriculitis is another possible complication. Bowel perforation, preperitoneal placement, and injuries during subcutaneous tunneling of the catheter are other risks of surgical placement. Preoperative use of antimicrobial prophylactic agents against *Staphylococcus epidermidis* and *Staphylococcus aureus* and meticulous intraoperative handling of shunt hardware reduce infection rates. Use of intraoperative radiography and careful attention to anatomic landmarks may help reduce insertion-related complication rates. Postoperatively, underdrainage may present as a persistent leakage or signs and symptoms of hydrocephalus including headache, somnolence, papilledema, persistent pseudomeningocele, or engorgement of scalp veins in neonates. Overdrainage may manifest in positional headaches, vomiting, and malaise. Another important potential sequela of overdrainage is subdural hematoma formation, which must be suspected in an individual with altered mental status or a new focal deficit postoperatively. In such cases, a brain CT should be obtained immediately. These complications may be avoided by using a manometer to measure the opening pressure at surgery, followed by the placement of a programmable valve set appropriately.

Summary

An understanding of normal CSF physiology is a prerequisite to treating problems such as CSF fistulae and pseudomeningoceles. CSF diversion techniques fall into two categories, external and internal. External lumbar drainage is useful when temporary CSF diversion is necessary (eg, in cases necessitating manipulation and retraction of the brain to gain access to deep lesions) and in treating otorrhea or rhinorrhea following traumatic or iatrogenic insults to the cranial base. Drawbacks include insertion discomfort and limited duration of therapy. LP and VP shunts came into widespread use in the 1970s [2], and both systems share risks of bowel perforation, obstruction, overdrainage and wound-related complications. In addition, VP shunts add the risks of intracerebral hematoma and ventriculitis. New valve technology has made it possible to alter the volume drained, thus alleviating problems of over- and underdrainage.

References

[1] Millhorat T. Hydrocephalus: pathophysiology and clinical features. In: Wilkins R, Rengachary S, editors. Neurosurgery, vol. III. 2nd edition. New York: McGraw-Hill; 1996. p. 3625–31.
[2] Post EM. Shunt systems. In: Wilkins R, Rengachary S, editors. Neurosurgery, vol. III. 2nd edition. New York: McGraw-Hill; 1996. p. 3645–53.
[3] Wernicke C. Lehrbuch der Gehirnkrankheiten fur Aertze und Studirende, vol. 3. Kassel (Germany): Theodor Fischer; 1881. p. 253–572.
[4] Henle A. Beitrag zur Pathologie und Therapie des Hydrocephalus. Mitteilungen aus dem Grenzgebieten der Medizin und Chirurgie 1896;1:264–301.
[5] Dandy W, Blackfan K. Internal hydrocephalus: an experimental clinical and pathological study. Am J Dis Child 1914;8:406–82.
[6] Torkildsen A. A new palliative operation in cases of inoperable occlusion of the sylvian aqueduct. Acta Chir Scand 1939;82:117–24.
[7] Nulsen F, Spitz E. Treatment of hydrocephalus by direct shunt from ventricles to jugular vein. Surg Forum 1952;2:399–403.
[8] Pudenz R, Russell F, Hurd A, et al. Ventriculoauriculostomy. A technique for shunting cerebrospinal fluid from the right auricle. Preliminary report. J Neurosurg 1957;14:171–9.
[9] Jackson I, Snodgrass R. Peritoneal shunts in the treatment of hydrocephalus and increased intracranial pressure: a 4-year survey of 62 patients. J Neurosurg 1955;12:216–22.

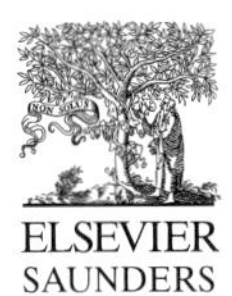
ELSEVIER
SAUNDERS

Otolaryngol Clin N Am
38 (2005) 583–595

OTOLARYNGOLOGIC
CLINICS
OF NORTH AMERICA

Diagnosis and Management of Otologic Cerebrospinal Fluid Leak

Christopher Raine, ChM, FRCS

Department of Otorhinolaryngology, Bradford Royal Infirmary, Duckworth Lane, Bradford, BD9 6RJ, UK

Cerebrospinal fluid (CSF) leakage is a rare but potentially life-threatening condition that requires thorough and timely intervention. It occurs when the barriers retaining CSF around the brain are breached. Otorrhea occurs only when there is violation of these barriers within the temporal bone. Thus, there is breach of the arachnoid membrane, dura mater, bone, and mucosal lining of the mastoid and middle ear. To complete the route of egress there must be a defect in the external auditory canal or perforation of the tympanic membrane. If this defect is not present, CSF, once in the middle ear cleft, can flow down the eustachian tube and present as otorhinorrhea. A physician therefore must remember that rhinorrhea does not always come from the anterior skull base and must be vigilant for an otologic cause.

In this article, CSF leaks are categorized as either nontraumatic or traumatic. The article explains the physiology of the milieu of CSF that surrounds the brain and spinal cord. It then discusses the detection, assessment, causes, clinical presentation, and management related to clinical pathologies.

Physiology

The bulk of the CSF is formed in the choroid plexuses of the lateral and, to a lesser extent, in the third and fourth ventricles. The remainder of the intracranial production occurs in the interstitial space. Extrachoroidal production occurs in the ventricular ependyma, and some CSF may be derived from the capillaries on the surface of the brain and spinal medulla.

E-mail address: CHRaine@aol.com

0030-6665/05/$ - see front matter
doi:10.1016/j.otc.2005.03.009 **oto.theclinics.com**

CSF is normally a clear, colorless fluid with a specific gravity of 1.007 contained within the ventricles and subarachnoid space. Its function is to cushion the brain and spinal cord from trauma. It is also a vehicle for supplying nourishment to neural tissues and removing waste products.

In the adult, the rate of production is relatively constant at approximately 0.3 mL/min. With an average CSF volume of 150 mL, the CSF is turned over about three times a day. The rate of production is independent of intracranial pressure [1] except when the intracranial pressure is high enough to reduce cerebral blood flow [2].

CSF reabsorption occurs passively, primarily by the arachnoid granulations, which extend into the dural venous sinuses. It is dependent on the hydrostatic gradient between the subarachnoid space and the venous sinuses [3].

Various factors influence CSF pressure, which is maintained between 70 to 150 mm H_2O (as recorded from the lumbar subarachnoid space, with the patient in a relaxed, lateral decubitus position). CSF pressure varies with age and position. Significant increase occurs during coughing, straining, and Valsalva's maneuver.

Detection of cerebrospinal fluid

In most situations, taking a detailed clinical history and performing a full otorhinolarygologic and neurologic examination may alert the physician to the presence of otorrhea or otorhinorrhea.

Leakage may be intermittent, because raising the intracranial pressure by straining may provoke leakage. Leaning forward with the nose pointing down while performing the Valsalva's maneuver usually induces fluid from the nostril and tends to correlate with the side of otologic pathology (Dandy maneuver).

Halo sign, ring sign, doughnut sign, and target sign are descriptive terms that have been given to the blood and CSF stains seen on pillows and sheets. The blood remains in the center of the stain, and the less dense CSF migrates outwards. This process can be demonstrated by collecting the fluid on to filter paper.

Ancillary tests used to aid diagnosis include biochemical evaluation of the liquorrhea, intrathecal dye studies, and a gamut of imaging techniques.

Although the concentrations of glucose and protein differ in CSF and plasma, their chemical identification has poor sensitivity and specificity and is not a reliable diagnostic tool, especially when the fluid is contaminated with blood, tears, and saliva. Their use is generally obsolete, especially for subclinical liquorrhea [4–6].

For many years, β_2-transferrin has been used to detect CSF. This protein is produced by neuraminidase activity in the brain and is unique to CSF, perilymph, and aqueous humor. It is not found in blood, nasal secretions, tears, or saliva. It is detected by immunofixation and silver staining [7] or by immunoblotting [8]. Immunofixation, although labor-intensive and time-consuming, requires only small quantities of fluid for analysis (< 100 μL). Also, moderate contamination with other body fluids does not invalidate the method [9]. Skedros et al [10] reported that only a couple of drops of fluid are necessary. Samples can be extracted from carrier materials such as Gelfoam tissue or bed sheets. Warnecke et al [11] recommend the use of the β_2-transferrin test as a primary screening procedure in all cases of suspected CSF leakage. They also recommended that serial testing be performed to exclude the possibility of sampling errors that may occur with intermittent leaks.

The presence of β-trace protein (β-TP) in CSF was first reported by Clausen [12] in 1961. It is synthesized mainly in the epithelial cells of the choroid plexus and is found in the CSF in concentrations 33-fold higher than in plasma [13]. Aside from prealbumin, albumin, and IgG, β-TP is the most abundant protein in human CSF. It has been found in perilymph, urine, aqueous humor, and other body fluids, which in normal circumstances would not interfere with analysis of CSF. Hence, it is an ideal marker for CSF fluid traces. In a study using immunoelectrophoresis in 98 individuals, β-TP showed a sensitivity of 91.17% and a specificity of 100% [14]. In a later, retrospective study, β-TP was analyzed using laser nephelometry [15]. This method provides quantitative data and is much faster than traditional semiquantitative immunoelectrophoretic assays. A sample was considered positive for CSF when the β-TP concentration was more than 6 mg/L. In correlation with clinical course, surgical findings, intraoperative visualization with sodium fluorescein, high-resolution CT, CT cisternography, MRI, and radionuclide cisternography, Bachmann et al [15] found the overall accuracy of the β-TP test was 0.974. They found the β-TP had a negative predictive value of 0.971 and a positive predictive value of 1.0. Meco et al [16] similarly concluded that the β-TP test can diagnose CSF rhinorrhea reliably and is even slightly better than β_2-transferrin. Disadvantages of assessment using β-TP must be considered, however. β-TP should not be used in patients with renal insufficiency and bacterial meningitis, because in these conditions the β-TP serum values are substantially increased, and CSF values are decreased. It is the high concentration of β-TP in CSF that makes it useful in the diagnosis of CSF leakages. Contamination and dilution may give rise to misleading results.

Schnabel et al [17] report that nephelometric quantification of β-trace protein is preferable to electrophoretic quantification because of better sensitivity and specificity and also is less time-consuming.

Although not commercially available for this purpose, intrathecal sodium fluorescein has been used for a number of years to detect and localize CSF leaks pre- and perioperatively. In a recent review, Keerl et al [18] point out that side effects seem to be dose dependent, and a dose of 50 mg or less is unlikely to be associated with a serious reaction.

Radiologic imaging is discussed in appropriate sections.

Etiology

CSF otorrhea can be categorized as either nontraumatic or traumatic (Box 1). The logic for this categorization is related primarily to the main modality of treatment. Nontraumatic otorrhea usually requires surgical intervention, whereas many traumatically induced leaks can be managed conservatively or by medical means.

Nontraumatic cerebrospinal fluid leaks

Spontaneous leaks

Primarily presenting during childhood, spontaneous CSF fistulas are usually caused by developmental anomalies of the labyrinth such as Mondini-type defect or widely patent vestibular and cochlear aqueducts that allow outflow through the oval or round window [19,20]. Variable degrees of sensorineural hearing loss are associated with defects of the otic capsule. Similarly, microdehiscences of the temporal bone are seen with patent Fallopian canal, defects in the tympanomeningeal fissure of Hyrtl, and petromastoid canal related to the subarcuate artery [21–24].

CSF within the middle ear produces a conductive hearing loss mimicking features of otitis media with effusion. It may detected as only a persistent clear watery discharge following the insertion of ventilation tubes or as rhinorrhea. Clinical presentations also include recurrent meningitis, temporal lobe seizures, and features of space-occupying lesions. A child with recurrent meningitis of unknown cause should have complete otologic and audiologic evaluation, CT of temporal bones, skull base, and paranasal sinuses, and immunologic appraisal [25].

Box 1. Classification of cerebral spinal fluid otorrhea

Nontraumatic
Spontaneous otorrhea
Middle ear disease ± cholesteatoma
Neoplastic otorrhea
Miscellaneous causes

Traumatic
Trauma (blunt or penetrating)
Iatrogenic otorrhea
Postirradiation otorrhea

Presentation during adulthood is related primarily to bony defects in the tegmental plate of the tympani or mastoideum (Fig. 1) or posterior fossa. Some arachnoid granulations do not find venous terminations and, after penetrating the dura mater, over time may produce pits in the bone surface. Common sites for aberrant granulations are lateral to the cribriform plate and along the floor of the middle fossa from the tegmen tympani to the lateral surface of the sella turcica [26].

Åhrén and Thulin's study [27] showed that 15% of temporal bones had fewer than five perforations, 6% had between 5 and 10 perforations, and 16% had very thin cortical bone of the tegmen tympani. Although such bone defects may be common, the occurrence of symptoms is rare. There are theories to explain possible delay in presentation:

- Focal atrophy caused by normal CSF pressure pulse causing bony erosion [28,29]
- Thinning of dura with age [29,30]
- Erosion by enlargement or presence of aberrant arachnoid granulations [21,23] in individuals with idiopathic intracranial hypertension and central obesity [31]

Clinical presentation usually consists of a conductive hearing loss and a sensation of fullness in the ear suggestive of secretory otitis media.

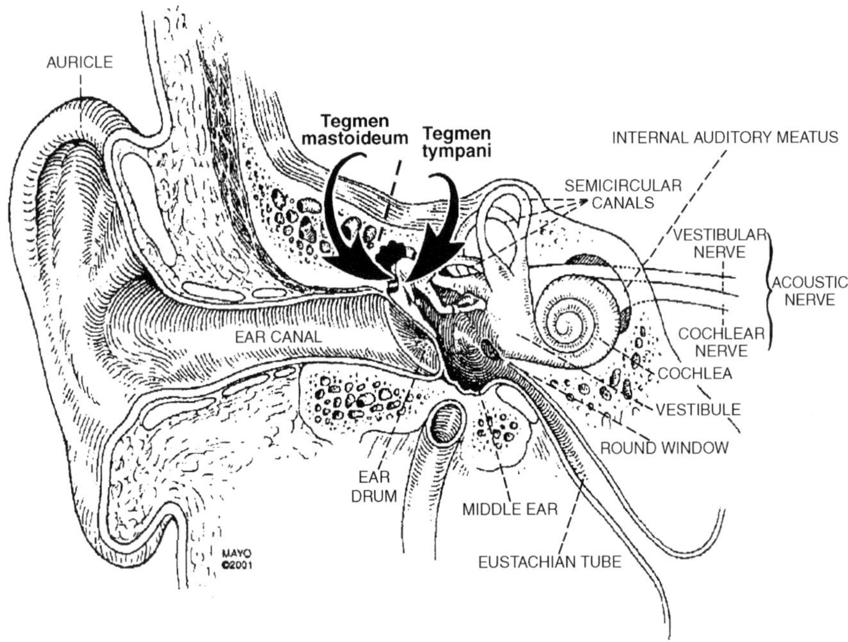

Fig. 1. Routes of CSF leaks from tegmen defects. (*By permission of* Mayo Foundation for Medical Education Research. All rights reserved)

Continuous pressure over the years results in herniation and formation of meningocele or encephalocele. An avascular, firm, but soft and pulsatile mass appearing in the mesotympanum, in the external auditory canal, or in a mastoid cavity is a characteristic finding. Such a mass may be an incidental finding during mastoid surgery (Fig. 2). Herniation into the epitympanum could impair movement of the ossicles (Fig. 3).

Almost one quarter of adult-onset CSF leaks present with acute meningitis [32]. Loss of dural integrity also predisposes to pneumocephalus, extradural abscess, and subsequent neurologic sequelae similar to those seen in children.

In addition to clinical examination and biochemical testing, radiologic studies aid in the localization of defects.

High-resolution CT with thin coronal axial images of the temporal bone demonstrates the bony anatomy and morphology of the otic capsule. Multidetector CT scanners can acquire thin, overlapping axial scans and thereby obtain an image of a block of temporal bone that can be reconstructed in any orthogonal plane. A bone algorithm is the best used to display the images.

Water-soluble contrast CT cisternography using non-ionic, iso-osmolar, iodinated organic compounds, preferably a dimmer injected by lumbar or cervical puncture, is reserved for patients in whom

- No site is identified on plain coronal CT
- Multiple bony defects are noted, and it is essential to determine which site is actively leaking
- A bony defect is seen on plain CT, but there is no enhancement of adjacent brain parenchyma

MRI is useful in confirming the presence and site of leak and is even more useful in evaluating the herniation of meninges or brain tissue through tegmen defects. In the right clinical context, the presence of high signal within the middle ear cavity on T2-weighted images and low signal on T1-weighted spin echo images indicates the presence of CSF leak.

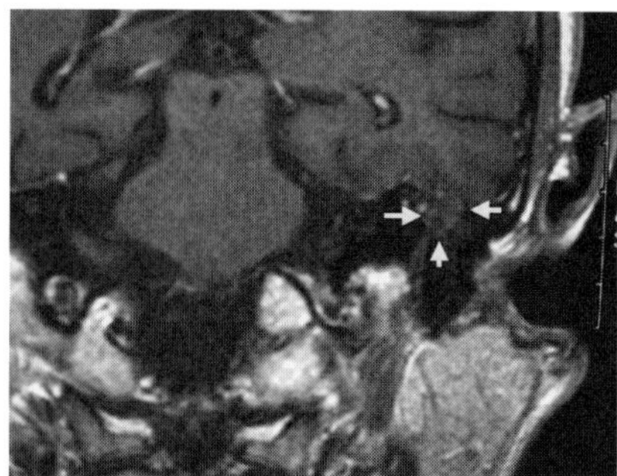

Fig. 2. T1 coronal MRI with gadolinium contrast illustrating a temporal lobe encephalocele herniating through the tegmen (arrows).

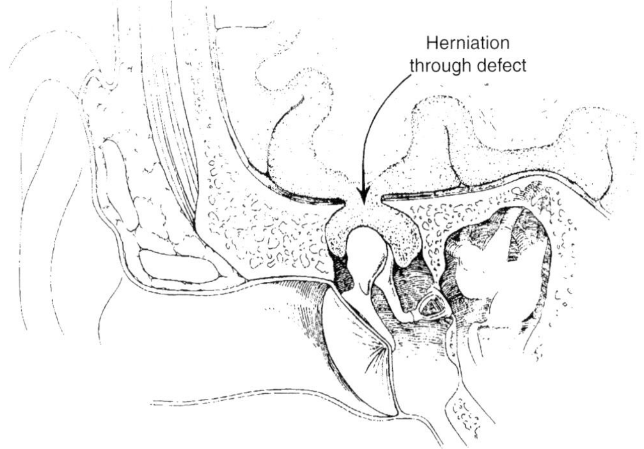

Fig. 3. Dural herniation (*arrow*) impinging on ossicles. (*From* Lundy LB, Graham MD, Kartush JM, et al. Temporal bone encephalocele and cerebrospinal fluid leaks. Am J Otol 1996; 17(3):461–9; with permission.)

Herniation of the dura (low signal) through the tegmen defect is clearly depicted on coronal and sagittal T2-weighted images, because it is bordered by high-signal CSF on either side.

The presence of an encephalocele is well demonstrated on gadolinium-enhanced T1-weighted spin echo coronal scans by enhancement of the meninges and the brain in and around the site of herniation. Herniated tissue may not be normal and hence may not be clearly defined, however. T2 sequences may identify spinal fluid entering the middle ear. Inflammatory tissue associated with herniation may also be enhanced with gadolinium. On nonenhanced T1-weighted images, hypointense material may be indicative of cholesteatoma.

Previous lumbar puncture may conceal an active CSF fistula by reducing CSF pressure.

Surgical intervention is the primary treatment for congenital and spontaneous CSF leaks. In children, deformities of the otic capsule such as Mondini-type defect can be repaired with a transcanal approach with obliteration of the cochlea with soft tissue [28]. CSF leaks are encountered after cochlear implant surgery and, again, are controlled with temporalis muscle plugs or fascia [33].

The transmastoid approach offers access to the posterior fossa and posterior tegmental defects with low risks and complications [34]. Leaks from the posterior fossa related to the basal cistern can be profuse. Obliteration of the mastoid with fat is required.

Defects that are large, multiple, or recurrent are best addressed by a combined transmastoid and middle fossa approach. The middle fossa approach optimizes access to all of the tegmen plate [22,35–37], allowing accurate placement of grafts without disturbing the middle ear and ossicles. A combined approach is logical in cases of large brain herniations. Herniated material that is devitalized or shows signs of infection should be resected to prevent intracranial infection.

The main disadvantage of a middle fossa approach is the related morbidity. Adkins and Osguthorpe [38] advocated a minicraniotomy with lower complications, and May et al [22] have described a keyhole craniotomy. They believe space is adequate for the retraction of the temporal lobe and have not reported any complications or recurrences with this technique.

Multilayer repair with autologous or allogenic materials offers the best results [39]. Autologous material, such as temporalis fascia, temporalis muscle, fascia lata, cortical bone, cartilage, and fat, is widely available. Calvarial bone harvested from the craniotomy and sandwiched between fascia offers robust support (Fig. 4) [40]. As part of the multilayer repair, the bony defect should be covered with rigid material such as bone or cartilage that is capable of supporting the brain. Fibrin glue helps secure material in place during healing but should not be used alone to seal a defect. It does create a seal but does not reduce subsequent leakage [41].

Bone plate mixed with fibrin glue, as described by the Cambridge group [36], produces an excellent, malleable graft that can be insinuated into every defect. Various synthetic materials are commercially available. Biocompatible materials become integrated with host tissue [42]. Inert materials generally are not used because of higher infection rates and potential extrusion than seen with native tissues [43,44].

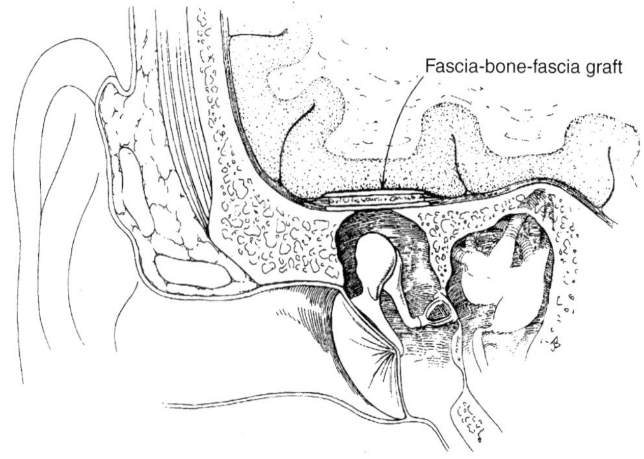

Fig. 4. Placement of fascia–bone–fascia graft (*arrow*). (*From* Lundy LB, Graham MD, Kartush JM, et al. Temporal bone encephalocele and cerebrospinal fluid leaks. Am J Otol 1996;17(3): 461–9; with permission.)

Chronic middle ear disease, neoplasia, and irradiation

A prerequisite for developing brain herniation is erosion of the bone vault and degradation of the dura, which is inherently robust. Bony erosion can be caused by the chronic inflammatory process of otitis media, with or without the presence of cholesteatoma [36]. CSF otorrhea, together with a soft, pulsatile mass in the middle ear or external auditory canal, may be present.

When chronic disease and brain herniation are detected, a two-stage procedure is required. Primary mastoid surgery to remove and eradicate infection is followed a few months later by a middle fossa approach. Alternatively, Aristegui et al [45] advocate a primary middle fossa approach with extradural division of the hernia and reconstruction of the defect with subsequent surgery to remove the herniated tissue and diseased tissue from the mastoid.

Reliable dural closure is not always possible when margins are surrounded by friable dura or when dura has been resected for tumor. In cases of osteoradionecrosis, radical removal of bone and obliterative procedures are necessary [46].

Traumatic cerebrospinal fluid leak

Traumatic CSF leaks occur because of blunt or penetrating trauma or as a consequence to surgery.

Blunt or penetrating trauma

CSF otorrhea may occur after fracture of the temporal bone. In a series of 820 proven fractured temporal bones, Brodie and Thompson [47] reported a 15% incidence of CSF leak. Dahiya et al [48] reported an incidence of 20%. In addition to a clinical history of trauma, typically related to automobile accidents and falls [48,49], there may be evidence of postauricular bruising (Battle's sign; Fig. 5), hemotympanum, bloody otorrhea, facial nerve palsies, hearing loss, vestibular disturbance, and features of intracranial pathology.

Penetrating trauma from gunshot creates a cone of damage, which can create various areas of leakage [50]. As in nontraumatic leaks, imaging, especially high-resolution CT, is important in the assessment and management. Classification of fractures as otic capsule–sparing and otic capsule–violating is clinically relevant. Otic-violating fractures are four times more likely to develop CSF leak and are several times more likely to be associated with severe sensorineural hearing loss [48].

In most cases, traumatic CSF otorrhea abates spontaneously. Medical management includes bed rest with head elevation and avoidance of straining and nose blowing. Antiemetics, antitussives, and stool softeners may help. Occasionally a lumbar drain for 4 or 5 days can prove effective.

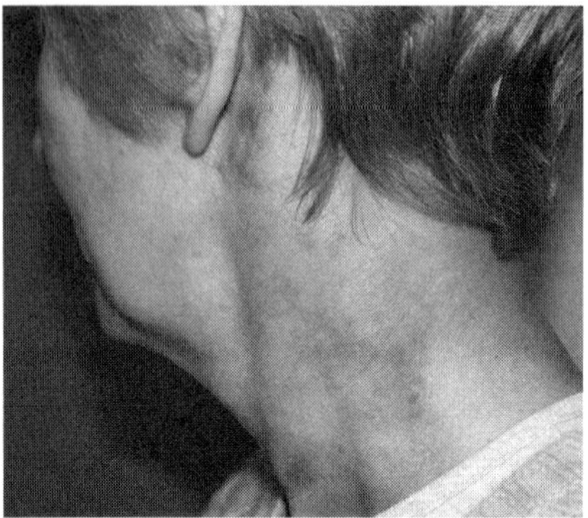

Fig. 5. Battle's sign showing postauricular bruising.

Persistence of otorrhea for more than 7 days is associated with a significantly increased risk of meningitis, especially if there is concurrent infection. The use of prophylactic antibiotics is controversial [51] but would be considered appropriate when patients are immunocompromised, when there is obvious contamination of the CSF, or when lumbar drain is in situ. Otherwise, the patient should be monitored closely for signs of meningitis or development of pneumocephalus.

In the rare event that CSF leakage does not abate, it is necessary to explore and repair the site of the leak.

Postsurgical trauma

Removal of vestibular schwannoma is the temporal bone surgery associated with CSF leak. On review, Becker and colleagues [52] reported that overall incidence of postoperative CSF leak for translabyrinthine, retrosigmoid, and middle fossa approaches was between 11% and 12%. CSF leaks can present through the wound, as rhinorrhea and, very rarely, as otorrhea. Onset may be delayed [53].

Wound leak

Initial treatment is additional suturing of the incision, head bandaging, and medical measures as previously described. A continuous lumbar drain typically is used after a few days if not already in situ following surgery. Most wound leaks settle after a few days [53,54].

Rhinorrhea

For minor sniffles, Becker et al [52] advocate restriction of fluid and activity and prescribe acetazolamide. For more copious rhinorrhea occurring within the first 10 days of surgery, a lumbar drain is used for about 5 days. All patients with lumbar drains require close monitoring. Beware of pneumocephalus and increased intracranial pressure.

If there is no resolution, re-exploration with obliteration of the middle ear, eustachian tube, external auditory canal, and blind-end closure is necessary. Re-exploration is usually required when onset is delayed.

Recalcitrant leaks may require ventriculo-peritoneal shunts or lumboperitoneal shunts.

Although a rare event following mastoid surgery [55], formation of brain hernias is probably under-recognized. Mosnier et al [36] comment that using a cutting burr near the tegmen and monopolar electrocautery on the surface of the dura may contribute to this process. Clinical symptoms may present many years after mastoid surgery. A meningoencephalocele or encephalocele presents as a soft, pulsatile mass. Chronic mastoid disease may mask the herniated brain, which may be recognized only during revision surgery. Surgical repair is usually required.

In conclusion, whilst CSF leak may be anticipated after trauma or surgery, the clinician must be vigilant to detect nontraumatic leaks to have the best chance of avoiding neurologic complications.

References

[1] Lorenzo AV, Page LK, Walters GV. Relationship between cerebrospinal fluid formation, absorption and pressure in human hydrocephalus. Brain 1970;93(4):679–92.

[2] Bering EA, Sato O. Hydrocephalous: changes in formation and absorption of cerebrospinal fluid within the cerebral ventricles. J Neurosurg 1963;20:1050–63.

[3] Griffith HB, Jamjoom AB. The treatment of childhood hydrocephalus by choroid plexus coagulation and artificial cerebrospinal fluid perfusion. Br J Neurosurg 1990;4(2):95–100.

[4] Oberascher G, Arrer E. Efficiency of various methods of identifying cerebrospinal fluid. ORL J Otorhinolaryngol Relat Spec 1986;48(6):320–5.

[5] Steedman DJ. CSF rhinorrhea: significance of glucose oxidase strip test. Injury 1985;18(5): 327–8.

[6] Jones NS, Becker DG. Advances in the management of CSF leaks. BMJ 2001;322(7279): 122–3.

[7] Ritchie RF, Smith R. Immunofixation 1: general principles and applications to agarose gel electrophoresis. Clin Chem 1976;22(4):497–9.

[8] Delaroche O, Bordure P, Lippert E, et al. Perilymph detection by beta2-transferrin immunoblotting assay. Application to the diagnosis of perilymphatic fistulae. Clin Chim Acta 1996;245(1):93–104.

[9] Irjala K, Suonpää J, Laurent B. Identification of CSF leak by immunofixation. Arch Otolaryngol 1979;105(8):447–8.

[10] Skedros DG, Cass SP, Hirsch BE, et al. Beta-2 transferrin assay in clinical management of cerebral spinal fluid and perilymphatic fluid leaks. J Otolaryngol 1993;22(5):341–4.

[11] Warnecke A, Averbeck T, Wurster U, et al. Diagnostic relevance of beta2-transferrin for the detection of cerebrospinal fluid fistulas. Arch Otolaryngol Head Neck Surg 2004;130(10): 1178–84.

[12] Clausen J. Proteins in normal cerebrospinal fluid not found in serum. Proc Soc Exp Biol Med 1961;107:170–2.

[13] Melegos DN, Freedman MS, Diamandis EP. Prostaglandin D synthase concentration in cerebrospinal fluid and serum of patients with neurological disorders. Prostaglandins 1997; 54(1):463–74.

[14] Bachmann G, Nekic M, Michel O. Clinical experience with beta-trace protein as a marker for cerebrospinal fluid. Ann Otol Rhinol Laryngol 2000;109(12):1099–102.

[15] Bachmann G, Petereit H, Djenabi U, et al. Predictive values of beta-trace protein (prostaglandin D synthase) by use of laser-nephelometry assay for the identification of cerebrospinal fluid. Neurosurgery 2002;50(3):571–6.
[16] Meco C, Oberascher G, Arrer E, et al. Beta-trace protein test: new guidelines for the reliable diagnosis of cerebrospinal fluid fistula. Otolaryngol Head Neck Surg 2003;129(5):508–17.
[17] Schnabel C, Di Martino E, Gilsbach JM, et al. Comparison of beta2-transferrin and beta-trace protein for detection of cerebrospinal fluid in nasal and ear fluids. Clin Chem 2004; 50(3):661–3.
[18] Keerl R, Weber RK, Draf W, et al. Use of sodium fluorescein solution for detection of cerebrospinal fluid fistulas: an analysis of 420 administrations and reported complications in Europe and the United States. Laryngoscope 2004;114(2):266–72.
[19] Quiney RE, Mitchell DB, Djazeri B, et al. Recurrent meningitis in children due to inner ear abnormalities. J Laryngol Otol 1989;103(5):473–80.
[20] MacRae DL, Ruby RF. Recurrent meningitis secondary to perilymph fistula in young children. J Otolaryngol 1990;19(3):222–5.
[21] Gacek RR, Leipzig B. Congenital cerebrospinal otorrhea. Ann Otol Rhinol Laryngol 1979; 88(3 Pt 1):358–65.
[22] May JS, Mikus JL, Matthews BL, et al. Spontaneous cerebrospinal fluid otorrhea from defects of the temporal bone: a rare entity? Am J Otol 1995;16(6):765–71.
[23] Gacek RR, Gacek MR, Tart R. Adult spontaneous cerebrospinal fluid otorrhea: diagnosis and management. Am J Otol 1999;20(6):770–6.
[24] Foyt D, Brackmann DE. Cerebrospinal fluid otorrhea through a congenitally patent fallopian canal. Arch Otolaryngol Head Neck Surg 2000;126(4):540–2.
[25] Drummond DS, de Jong AL, Giannoni C, et al. Recurrent meningitis in the pediatric patient—the otolaryngologist's role. Int J Pediatr Otorhinolaryngol 1999;48(3):199–208.
[26] Brunner H. Intracranial complications of ear nose and throat infections. Chicago: The year book publishers; 1946. p. 32–3.
[27] Åhrén C, Thulin CA. Lethal intracranial complications following inflation of the external auditory canal in treatment of serous otitis media and due to defects in the petrous bone. Acta Otolaryngol 1965;60:407–21.
[28] Wetmore SJ, Herrmann P, Fisch U. Spontaneous cerebrospinal fluid otorrhea. Am J Otol 1987;8(2):96–102.
[29] Ommaya AK. Cerebrospinal fluid rhinorrhea. Neurology 1964;15:106–13.
[30] Kaufman B, Yonas H, White RJ, et al. Acquired middle cranial fossa fistulas: normal pressure and nontraumatic in origin. Neurosurgery 1979;5(4):466–72.
[31] Sugerman HJ, DeMaria EJ, Felton WL, et al. Increased intra-abdominal pressure and cardiac filling pressures in obesity-associated pseudotumor cerebri. Neurology 1997;49(2): 507–11.
[32] Pappas DG Jr, Hoffman RA, Cohen NL, et al. Spontaneous temporal bone cerebrospinal fluid leak. Am J Otol 1992;13(6):534–9.
[33] Wooley AL, Jenison V, Stroer BS, et al. Cochlear implantation in children with inner ear malformations. Ann Otol Rhinol Laryngol 1998;107(6):492–500.
[34] Jackson CG, Pappas DG Jr, Manolidis S, et al. Brain herniation into the middle ear and mastoid: concepts in diagnosis and surgical management. Am J Otol 1997;18(2):198–205.
[35] Moffat DA, da Cruz MJ, Batten A, et al. Use of autologous osteocyte containing bone pate for closure of tegmental bone defects. Am J Otol 1998;19(6):819–23.
[36] Mosnier I, Fiky LEL, Shahidi A, et al. Brain herniation and chronic otitis media: diagnosis and surgical management. Clin Otolaryngol 2000;25(5):385–91.
[37] Dutt SN, Mirza S, Irving RM. Middle cranial fossa approach for the repair of spontaneous cerebrospinal fluid otorrhea using autologous bone pate. Clin Otolaryngol 2001;26(2): 117–23.
[38] Adkins WY, Osguthorpe JD. Mini-craniotomy for management of CSF otorrhea from tegmen defects. Laryngoscope 1983;93(8):1038–40.

[39] Savva A, Taylor MJ, Beatty CW. Management of cerebrospinal fluid leaks involving the temporal bone: report on 92 patients. Laryngoscope 2003;113(1):50–6.
[40] Lundy LB, Graham MD, Kartush JM, et al. Temporal bone encephalocele and cerebrospinal fluid leaks. Am J Otol 1996;17(3):461–9.
[41] Lebowitz RA, Hoffman RA, Roland JT, et al. Autologous fibrin glue in the prevention of cerebrospinal fluid leak following acoustic neuroma surgery. Am J Otol 1995;16(2):172–4.
[42] Verheggen R, Schulte-Baumann WJ, Hahm G, Lang J, et al. A new technique of dural closure—experience with a Vicryl mesh. Acta Neurochir (Wien) 1997;139(11):1074–9.
[43] Glasscock ME III, Dickins JRE, Jackson CG, et al. Surgical management of brain tissue herniation into the middle ear and mastoid. Laryngoscope 1979;89(11):1743–54.
[44] Ramsden RT, Latif A, Lye RH, et al. Endaural cerebral hernia. J Laryngol Otol 1985;99(7): 643–51.
[45] Aristegui M, Falcioni M, Saleh E, et al. Meningoencephalic herniation into the middle ear: a report of 27 cases. Laryngoscope 1995;105(5 Pt1):513–8.
[46] Sharma RR, Keogh AJ, Small M, et al. Osteoradionecrosis of the petrous bone and recurrent cerebrospinal fluid otorrhea. Br J Neurosurg 1993;7(3):303–6.
[47] Brodie HA, Thompson TC. Management of complications from 820 temporal bone fractures. Am J Otol 1997;18(2):188–97.
[48] Dahiya R, Keller JD, Litofsky NS, et al. Temporal bone fractures: otic capsule sparing versus otic capsule violating clinical and radiographic considerations. J Trauma 1999;47(6): 1079–83.
[49] Lee D, Honrado C, Har-El G, et al. Pediatric temporal bone fractures. Laryngoscope 1998; 108(6):816–21.
[50] Backous DD, Jenkins HA, Coker NJ. Gunshot injuries to the intratemporal facial nerve. Eur Arch Otorhinolaryngol 1994;(Suppl):S287–9.
[51] Brodie HA. Prophylactic antibiotics for posttraumatic cerebrospinal fluid fistulae. A meta-analysis. Arch Otolaryngol Head Neck Surg 1997;123(7):749–52.
[52] Becker SS, Jackler RK, Pitts LH. Cerebrospinal fluid leak after acoustic neuroma surgery: a comparison of the translabyrinthine, middle fossa, and retrosigmoid approaches. Otol Neurotol 2003;24(1):107–12.
[53] Bani A, Gilsbach JM. Incidence of cerebrospinal fluid leak after microsurgical removal of vestibular schwannomas. Acta Neurochir (Wien) 2002;144(10):979–82.
[54] Fishman AJ, Marrinan MS, Golfinos JG, et al. Prevention and management of cerebrospinal fluid leak following vestibular schwannoma surgery. Laryngoscope 2004;114(3):501–5.
[55] Neely JG, Kuhn JR. Diagnosis and treatment of iatrogenic cerebrospinal fluid leak and brain herniation during or following mastoidectomy. Laryngoscope 1985;95(11):1299–300.

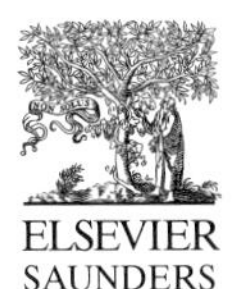
ELSEVIER
SAUNDERS

Otolaryngol Clin N Am
38 (2005) 597–611

OTOLARYNGOLOGIC
CLINICS
OF NORTH AMERICA

Cerebrospinal Fluid Rhinorrhea: Diagnosis and Management

Julie T. Kerr, MD[a], Felix W.K. Chu, MD[b,*], Stephen W. Bayles, MD[b]

[a]*Department of Otolaryngology–Head and Neck Surgery, Madigan Army Medical Center, Tacoma, WA, USA*
[b]*Department of Otolaryngology/Head and Neck Surgery, Virginia Mason Medical Center, 1100 Ninth Avenue, Seattle, WA 98101, USA*

Elucidating the cause to a cerebrospinal fluid (CSF) leak is central to its management. CSF rhinorrhea is commonly classified as (1) traumatic, (2) nontraumatic, (3) spontaneous, and (4) iatrogenic [1,2]. The diagnostic localization and management of CSF leak, although challenging, have improved over the years with the evolution of diagnostic tests and improved surgical techniques.

Cause

Traumatic leaks are subdivided as surgical (whether planned or unplanned) or nonsurgical (whether blunt or penetrating). Seventy percent to 80% of CSF rhinorrhea is caused by accidental trauma [3]; 2% to 4% of acute head injuries result in CSF rhinorrhea [4].

Nontraumatic CSF rhinorrhea includes high-pressure and normal-pressure leaks. High-pressure CSF rhinorrhea comprises 45% of nontraumatic CSF rhinorrhea, and 84% of these leaks result from tumor obstruction. The remainder is caused by either benign intracranial hypertension or hydrocephalus. Normal-pressure leaks may result from bony erosion by tumor, tumor treatment with radiation therapy, arachnoid granulations, infection, empty sella syndrome, or congenital defects such as preformed pathways, fistulas, meningoceles, meningoencephaloceles, or encephaloceles.

* Corresponding author.
E-mail address: otofwc@vmmc.org (F.W.K. Chu).

doi:10.1016/j.otc.2005.03.011 ***oto.theclinics.com***

The term spontaneous cerebrospinal fluid leak is controversial. Har-El [2], Ommaya [3], and Rice [5] categorize spontaneous CSF leaks as idiopathic or unknown in origin, with the understanding that most, if not all, eventually have a specific diagnosis.

Signs and symptoms

The presence of a halo sign on tissue or linens should arouse suspicion of CSF rhinorrhea. Although not generally used now, components of CSF, such as glucose, protein and electrolytes, have been measured. The sensitivity and specificity of these tests remain quite poor [5,6].

Beta-2 transferrin is highly specific and sensitive in identifying fluid as CSF [7]. Beta-2 transferrin is produced by desialization (carbohydrate-free form) of normal beta-1 transferrin in CSF through cerebral neuraminidase [8]. It is found only in perilymph, vitreous humor, and CSF. Only 0.5 cm^3 of fluid is required for diagnosis. The test can be performed and completed in less than 3 hours by immunofixation electrophoresis. Negative testing, however, does not exclude the diagnosis of CSF leak, particularly if a high mucus content of the secretions results in difficulty concentrating fluids [9–11]. False-positive results are possible in patients with chronic liver disease, inborn errors of glycoprotein metabolism, or genetic variants of transferrin [12]. When these pathologic conditions are suspected, sampling f venous blood should be sampled for comparison.

Patients with CSF rhinorrhea may complain of a salty taste or even a sweet taste, because CSF has two thirds the sugar content of blood. A low-pressure headache may result from an acute or chronic leak. The drainage may be continuous, may be elicited with Valsalva's maneuver, or may gush with change in position because the sphenoid and frontal sinus may act as reservoirs. Unfortunately, some leaks may be intermittent and not easily diagnosable.

The most common cause of rhinorrhea from surgical trauma is transphenoidal management of pituitary tumors (0.5–15%) [13–18]. Seven percent to 11% of surgeries for acoustic neuromas have been found to result in CSF rhinorrhea [17,18]. The risk of CSF leak secondary to functional endoscopic sinus surgery varies from 0.5 to 3% [19,20].

In comparison with accidental trauma, postsurgical traumatic CSF rhinorrhea may present immediately postoperatively in 50% of patients. The remainder of leaks ensue 7 days to 1 month later secondary to progressive maturation and contraction of wounds, devascularization, necrosis of the soft tissue or bony edges, slow resolution of edema, or increased CSF pressure [21].

An association has been found between empty sella syndrome, meningoencephaloceles, and CSF leaks. Patients with an empty sella commonly present with pressure-type headaches, pulsatile tinnitus, or visual disturbances. Idiopathic or acquired intracranial hypertension results in hydrostatic pressure at anatomically weakened sites of the skull. The dura then herniates into the sella turcica and fills with CSF. This fluid-filled sac compresses the pituitary gland and results in the radiographic appearance of an empty sella. The appearance of an empty sella can also occur with necrosis of a pituitary tumor. These patients have the potential of developing benign intracranial hypertension, have the highest failure rate with closure of a CSF leak, and have the greatest likelihood for developing a meningoencephalocele [22].

Of utmost concern with a CSF leak is the potential for meningitis. There seems to be a higher risk in cases of CSF rhinorrhea occurring after accidental trauma and in patients whose CSF leak does not close spontaneously. Mincy's [5] series of 54 patients with traumatic CSF rhinorrhea demonstrated that meningitis developed in 11% of patients in whom draining stopped spontaneously in 7 days, compared with 88% of patients in whom drainage lasted longer than 7 days. Authors recommend surgical closure of CSF leaks if drainage has not ceased within 1 to 2 weeks. Surgical closure earlier than 1 to 2 weeks is unlikely to prevent meningitis.

Immunologically competent individuals presenting with meningitis should be investigated for CSF fistula [6]. Thirty-five percent of individuals presenting with recurrent meningitis have a CSF fistula caused by head trauma. Accidental head trauma and basilar skull fracture can result in recurrent meningitis any time from 2 months to 21 years after the initial incident [23].

A dural defect may also result in pneumocephalus. Trauma is the most common cause of pneumocephalus (74%), followed by tumor, infection, surgery, and idiopathic causes. Eighty-five percent of these cases heal within the first week, whether or not they are complicated by meningitis [24]. More commonly, pneumocephalus results if there is a large dural tear, because air columns in the frontal or ethmoid sinuses transmit respiratory pressures with straining, coughing, or sneezing. These tears do not heal spontaneously and are at higher risk for meningitis; thus, more aggressive surgical management is warranted [21].

Localization

Key in management of CSF leakage is localization of the dural defect, which can originate from the anterior, middle, or posterior cranial fossas. The most common site of accidental traumatic fracture seems to be at the cribiform plate where the bone is thick, the area adjacent is thin, and the dura is very adherent [25]. Congenital defects most commonly arise from the superior or lateral walls of the sphenoid sinus or from the cribriform niche adjacent to the middle turbinate vertical attachment.

Multiple imaging studies are available to help localize sites of dural defects. The sensitivities and specificities of these studies vary with patient population, defect size, operator interpretation, and leak flow rate.

High-resolution coronal and axial CT

High-resolution CT is the primary imaging modality for localization of cranial vault defects. It often is the only test needed for diagnosis [26]; however, it is limited to identifying defects in bone. High-resolution CT scan in conjunction with an intrathecal fluorescein study accurately localizes active leaks and supersedes other studies [27]. One- to 2-mm sections in coronal and axial planes are recommended to evaluate fully all walls of the sinuses. Partial volume averaging can cause both false-positive and false-negative findings. Plain CT scans have a 9.5% false-positive identification of a bony defect in inactive CSF fistulas [28].

CT cisternograms

CT cisternography (CTC) is complementary in both false-positive and false-negative cases of high-resolution CT imaging. With active leaks, CTC demonstrates movement of contrast through the defect with a success rate of 85% [29,30].

Weaknesses of this technique include its inability to detect an inactive leak at the time of study, yielding sensitivities from 48% to 96% [31]. It is also invasive, cumbersome, and increases exposure to radiation. This exposure is an important factor in pediatric patients and in patients requiring multiple imaging studies. CTC is of particular use when the frontal and sphenoid sinuses act as reservoirs.

Today's contrast agents include low-osmolarity nonionic substances such as iohexol and iopamidol. These agents have a low incidence of the side effects seen with older compounds such as metrizamide [32]. Compounds such as indigo carmine and Evans blue dye are no longer used because of their neurotoxicity [29].

Radionuclide cisternograms

Radionuclide cisternography is similar to CTC in that the radiopharmaceutical agent, most commonly Technetium 99m, is administered intrathecally, followed by gamma camera imaging. It also entails the endoscopic placement of nasal pledgets. This method is particularly useful in low-volume or intermittent leaks because, depending on the half-life of the agent used, the imaging and measurement of uptake can be completed hours to days (54 hours) after injection of the agent [33].

Radionuclide cisternography, however, has a high number of false-positive findings (33%) and sensitivities ranging from 62% to 76% [31]. It is also invasive, has less spatial resolution and localizing ability, and shows less fine anatomic detail and specificity than CTC [33].

Intrathecal fluorescein

Fluorescein is most commonly used as an adjunct to intraoperative localization of a skull based defect. The process involves a standard lumbar puncture followed by withdrawal of 10 cm^3 of CSF, which is then mixed with 0.2 to 0.25 cm^3 of 5% fluorescein (40–60 kg/0.2 cm^3; >60 kg/0.25 cm^3). This mixture is injected at a rate of 1 cm^3/minute. Thirty minutes is required for the mixture to diffuse within the CSF. A brilliant yellow fluid leaking in the nose is visualized in the vicinity of the defect. Use of a blue-light filter makes the test sensitive to dilutions up to 1 in 10 million [34].

Protocols for appropriate administration have been described, because side effects can be significant, including lower extremity weakness, numbness, generalized seizures, opisthotonos, and cranial nerve deficits [35–37]. If complications do ensue, CSF should be diluted and the head elevated. Informed consent is required before use.

MRI and MR cisternography

MRI and MR cisternography are noninvasive alternatives to intrathecal contrast-enhanced high-resolution CT. These modalities are able to distinguish inflammatory tissue from meningoencephaloceles but cannot define bony details, as with CT scanning. T2 images highlight the CSF leak on MRI. A fast spin echo sequence with fat suppression and image reversal on MR cisternography highlights the fistula, because CSF appears stark black among faded surrounding tissues [38]. This study is reported to be 85% to 92% sensitive and 100% specific [39].

As with CT and radionuclide cisternography, there must be active leakage at the time of the study; however, serial MR studies can be done without ill effect. These studies have roughly the same cost as CT cisternography but are more time efficient and subject patients to less radiation.

Conservative management

Most CSF leaks resulting from accidental and surgical trauma heal with conservative measures over the course of 7 to 10 days. Less likely to heal spontaneously are leaks in which CSF rhinorrhea develops days or weeks after surgical or accidental trauma, massive leaks that develop immediately after surgery, leaks caused by sustain gunshot wounds, or normal-pressure CSF leaks. CSF fistulae found at the time of endoscopic sinus surgery require repair at the time of initial surgery [4]. Leaks noted 5 to 7 days after surgery may close spontaneously; if there is not resolution in 1 to 2 weeks, surgery is indicated.

First-line treatment includes bed rest with head elevation, avoidance of straining activity such as nose blowing, sneezing, and coughing, and the use of stool softeners.

Antibiotic prophylaxis remains controversial. Most authors avoid antibiotics to reduce development of resistant organisms [40,41]. Friedman [42] found the incidence of meningitis after accidental trauma to be 10% in those treated with antibiotics versus 21% in those not treated. Pappas [6] found that, given the greater incidence of resistant organisms with use of prophylactic antibiotics, surgical management is the only definitive treatment. If there is gross contamination along a fluid pathway, such as with a comminuted fracture of the paranasal sinus resulting from acute trauma, antibiotic prophylaxis does have a role.

A nontraumatic, high-pressure CSF leak caused by increased intracranial pressure will probably resolve if the intracranial pressure is normalized. The intracranial pressure can be normalized by use of diuretics such as acetazolamide or with ventriculoperitoneal shunting. Leaks that do not resolve with normalization of intracranial pressures warrant surgical management [43].

Surgical management

Numerous factors are involved in the surgical management of CSF leaks. These factors include use of a lumbar drain, the approach for repair, the type of graft or flap and its placement, and the use of sealant and nasal packing.

Lumbar drain

Controversy surrounds use of a lumbar drain [44–48]. Use of a subarachnoid lumbar drain or serial lumbar punctures is controversial, as well. If resolution has not occurred after 72 hours in a patient managed conservatively, draining 150 cm^3/day of CSF for 4 additional days before entertaining surgical options may be beneficial [49]. Lumbar drainage is not without risk, however. Overdrainage may create a siphon effect with resultant pneumocephalus. Additional complications include headache, nausea, vomiting, vocal cord paralysis, occlusion of the posterior cerebral artery, and lumbar radiculopathy. Hegazy's [46] meta-analysis documents that lumbar drainage does not affect success rates. Casiano [44] reports a 97% success rate in more than 30 patients without use of lumbar drain. Sixty-seven percent of otolaryngologists use lumbar drainage routinely and drain for an average of 4 days [48].

Komisar et al [50] recommend drainage if there is suspicion for increased intracranial pressure. In long-term or congenital leaks, a lumbar drain may offset the initial rise in intracranial pressure. Suspicion for increased intracranial pressure is warranted with leak recurrence [51]. Preoperative intracranial pressure reading will be inaccurate because of the leak, but an accurate reading can be taken postoperatively.

Surgical approach

Transcranial

Dandy [52], in 1929, was the first to document successful repair of a CSF leak using an intracranial approach. Success rates ranging from 60% to

95% have been reported [53–55]. Spetzler et al [56] experienced a failure rate of 27% on initial operation and a 10% overall failure rate with multiple procedures.

Advantages of this approach include improved exposure, ability to identify multiple defects, and ability to tamponade a leak in a high-pressure situation. Drawbacks include the inherent increased morbidity, increased length of hospitalization, and permanent anosmia.

Extracranial

Dohlman [57] was the first to document a successful extracranial repair of a CSF leak in 1948. Success rates of 86% on initial operation with a 97% success rate overall have been documented [58,59].

Extracranial repair results in decreased morbidity, no anosmia, improved endonasal exposure of the sphenoid, parasellar and posterior ethmoids, cribriform plate, fovea ethmoidalis, and the posterior wall of the frontal sinus. Inherent to this procedure is a facial scar, risk for facial numbness, and orbital complications. The procedure can be quite cumbersome. Cerebral damage and the lateral extensions of the frontal and sphenoid sinuses cannot be assessed.

Transnasal

A transnasal approach for closure of CSF rhinorrhea was first described by Hirsch [60] in 1952. Lehrer and Deutsch [61] improved visualization with use of the microscope, but visualization of the lateral and superior walls of the sphenoid sinus is limited. Transnasal approaches risk facial numbness as well as septal perforation. With use of endoscopes, these approaches are rarely used today.

Endoscopic

In 1981 Wigand described closure of a cerebrospinal fistula using an endoscopic approach. Endoscopic intranasal fistula repair is now the preferred approach, with higher success rates and less morbidity than intracranial surgical repair [62,63].

Multiple studies have documented high success rates with a wide variety of grafting materials and adjuncts to closure such as lumbar drain, tissue sealant, and nasal packing. Regardless of materials used, success rates of 92% to 96% have been documented [38,62,64,65]. Hegazy's [46] meta-analysis of 575 cases demonstrates a 90% success rate on first attempt and a 96% success rate on second attempt.

Generally, a small defect can be closed with an overlay free mucosal graft or a free fascial graft. The free mucosal grafts can be acquired from the inferior turbinate or the septum. Fascia can be obtained from the temporalis region or fascia lata. It is important that, after identification of the bony defect, mucosa surrounding the perimeter of the defect be removed to stimulate osteogenesis, thus thickening bone around defect and improving graft incorporation.

References

[1] Har-El G. What is "spontaneous" cerebrospinal fluid rhinorrhea? Classification of cerebrospinal fluid leaks. Ann Otol Rhinol Laryngol 1999;108:323–6.
[2] Ommaya AK, Di Chiro G, Baldwin M, et al. Non-traumatic cerebrospinal fluid rhinorrhea. J Neurol Neurosurg Psychiatry 1968;31:214–55.
[3] Bernal-Sprekelsen M, Bleda-Vazquez C, Carrau RL. Ascending meningitis secondary to traumatic cerebrospinal fluid leaks. Am J Rhinol 2000;14:257–9.
[4] Mincy J. Post-traumatic spinal fluid fistulas of the frontal fossa. J Trauma 1966;6:618–22.
[5] Rice DH. Cerebrospinal fluid rhinorrhea: diagnosis and treatment. Curr Opin Otolaryngol Head Neck Surg 2003;11:19–22.
[6] Pappas DG, Hammerschlag PE, Hammerschlag M. Cerebrospinal fluid rhinorrhea and recurrent meningitis. Clin Infect Dis 1993;17:364–8.
[7] Sibler H. The normal cerebrospinal fluid proteins identified by means of thin-layer isoelectric focusing and crossed immnunoelectrofocusing. J Neurol Sci 1978;36:273–88.
[8] Ridley F. The intraocular pressure and drainage of the aqueous humor. Br J Exp Pathol 1930;11:215–40.
[9] Skedros DG, Cass SP, Hisrch BE, et al. Sources of error in use of beta-2 transferrin analysis for diagnosing perilymphatic and cerebral spinal fluid leaks. Otolaryngol Head Neck Surg 1993;109:861–4.
[10] Oberashcer G. A modern concept of cerebrospinal fluid diagnosis in oto and rhinorrhea. Rhinology 1988;26:89–103.
[11] Ryell RG, Peacock MK, Simpson DA. Usefulness of beta 2-transferrin assay in the detection of cerebrospinal fluid leaks following head injury. J Neurosurg 1992;77:737–9.
[12] Roelandse FWC, Van de Zwart AZJ, Didden JH, et al. Detection of CSF leakage by isoelectric focusing on polyacrimide gel, direct immunofixation of transferrins and silver staining. Clin Chem 1998;44:351–3.
[13] Seiler RW, Mariani L. Sellar reconstruction with resorbable Vicryl patches, gelatin foam, and fibrin glue in transphenoidal surgery: a 10 year experience with 376 patients. J Neurosurg 2000;93:762–5.
[14] Ciric I, Ragin A, Baumgartner C, et al. Complications of transsphenoidal surgery: results of a national survey, review of literature and personal experience. Neurosurgery 1997;40: 225–36.
[15] Black PM, Zervas NT, Candia GL. Incidence and management of complications of transphenoidal operation for pituitary adenomas. Neurosurgery 1987;20:920–4.
[16] Koltai PJ, Goufman DB, Parnes SM, et al. Transphenoidal hyophysectomy through the external rhinoplasty approach. Otolaryngol Head Neck Surg 1994;111:197–200.
[17] Jane JA, Laws ER. The surgical management of pituitary adenomas in a series of 3093 patients. J Am Coll Surg 2001;193:651–9.
[18] Jho H. Endoscopic transphenoidal surgery. J Neurooncol 2001;54:187–95.
[19] Lawson W. The intranasal ethmoidectomy: evolution and assessment of the procedure. Laryngoscope 1994;104(Suppl 64):1–25.
[20] May M, Levine HL, Mester SJ, et al. Complications of endoscopic sinus surgery: analysis of 2108 patients—incidence and prevention. Laryngoscope 1994;1040:1080–3.
[21] Park JI, Strelzow VV, Friedman WH. Current management of cerebrospinal fluid rhinorrhea. Laryngoscope 1983;93:1294–300.
[22] Schlosser RJ, Bolger WE. Spontaneous nasal cerebrospinal fluid leaks and empty sella syndrome: a clinical association. Am J Rhinol 2003;17:91–6.
[23] Levin S, Nelson KE, Spies HW, et al. Pneumococcal meningitis: the problem of the unseen cerebrospinal fluid leak. Am J Med Sci 1972;264:319–27.
[24] Jacob JB, Persky MS. Traumatic pneumocephalus. Laryngoscope 1980;90:515–20.
[25] Som ML, Kramer R. Cerebrospinal rhinorrhea pathological findings. Laryngoscope 1940; 50:1167.

[26] Lloyd MNH, Kimber PM, Burrows EH. Post traumatic cerebrospinal fluid rhinorrhea: modern high definition computed tomography is all that is required for the effective demonstrated of the site of leakage. Clin Radiol 1994;49:100–3.
[27] Bateman N, Jones NS. Rhinorrhoea feigning cerebrospinal fluid leak: nine illustrative cases. J Laryngol Otol 2000;114:462–4.
[28] El Gammal T, Brooks BS. MR cisternography: initial experience in 41 cases. AJNR 1994;15: 1647–56.
[29] Chow JM, Goodman D, Mafee MF. Evaluation of CSF rhinorrhea by computerized tomography with metrizamide. Otolaryngol Head Neck Surg 1989;100:99–105.
[30] Manelfe C, Cellerier P, Sobel D, et al. Cerebrospinal fluid rhinorrhea: evaluation with metrizamide cisternography. AJR Am J Roentgenol 1982;138:471–6.
[31] Stone JA, Castillo M, Neelon B, et al. Evaluation of CSF leaks: high resolution CT compared with contrast enhanced CT and radionuclide cisternography. AJNR Am J Neuroradiol 1999;20:706–12.
[32] Manelfe C, Guirand B, Tremoulet M. Diagnosis of CSF rhinorrhea by computerized cisternography using metrizamide. Lancet 1997;2:1073.
[33] Flynn BM, Butler SP, Quinn RJ, et al. Radionuclide cisternography in the diagnosis and management of cerebrospinal fluid leaks: the test of choice. Med J Aust 1987;146:82–4.
[34] Stammberger H. Endoscopic sinus surgery. Philadelphia: BC Decker; 1991.
[35] Lund VJ, Savy G, Lloyd GAS. Optimum imaging and diagnosis of cerebrospinal fluid rhinorrhea. J Laryngol Otol 2000;114:395–7.
[36] Stammberger H. Special problems in functional endoscopic sinus surgery. Philadelphia: B Dekker; 1991. p. 437–40.
[37] Keerl R, Weber RK, Draf W, et al. Use of sodium fluorescein solution for detection of cerebrospinal fluid fistulas: analysis of 420 administrations and reported complications in Europe and the United States. Laryngoscope 2004;114:266–72.
[38] Zweig JL, Carrau RI, Celin SE, et al. Endoscopic repair of CSF leaks to the sinonasal tract: predictors of success. Otolaryngol Head Neck Surg 2000;123:195–201.
[39] Sillers MJ, Morgan E, El Gammal T. Magnetic resonance cisternography and thin coronal computerized tomography in the evaluation of cerebrospinal fluid rhinorrhea. Am J Rhinol 1997;11:387–92.
[40] Rathor MH. Do prophylactic antibiotics prevent meningitis after basilar skull fracture? Pediatr Infect Dis J 1991;10:87–8.
[41] Stankiewicz JA. Cerebrospinal fluid fistula and endoscopic sinus surgery. Laryngoscope 1991;101:250–6.
[42] Friedman JA, Ebersold MJ, Quast LM. Post traumatic cerebrospinal fluid leakage. World J Surg 2001;25:1062–6.
[43] Briant TDR, Bird R. Extracranial repair of cerebrospinal fluid fistulae. J Otolaryngol 1982; 11:191.
[44] Casiano RR, Jassir D. Endoscopic cerebrospinal fluid rhinorrhea repair: is a lumbar drain necessary? Otolaryngol Head Neck Surg 1999;37:33–6.
[45] Marshall AN, Jones NS, Robertson IJA. An algorithm for the management of CSF rhinorrhea illustrated by 36 cases. Rhinology 1999;37:182–5.
[46] Hegazy HM, Carrau RL, Snyderman CH, et al. Transnasal endoscopic repair of cerebrospinal fluid rhinorrhea: a meta analysis. Laryngoscope 2000;110:1166–72.
[47] Chin G, Rice D. Transnasal endoscopic closure of cerebrospinal fluid leaks. Laryngoscope 2003;113:136–8.
[48] Senior BA, Jafri K, Benninger M. Safety and efficacy of endoscopic repair of CSF leaks: a survey of the members of the American rhinologic society. Am J Rhinol 2001;15:21–5.
[49] Cooper PR. Skull fracture and traumatic cerebro-spinal fluid fistulas in head injury. In: Cooper PR, editor. Head injury. Baltimore (MD): Williams and Wilkins; 1982.
[50] Komisar A, Weitz S, Ruben RJ. Cerebrospinal fluid dynamics and rhinorrhea: the role of shunting in repair. Otolaryngol Head Neck Surg 1983;91:399–403.

[51] Lund V. Endoscopic management of cerebrospinal fluid leaks. Am J Rhinol 2002;16:17–23.
[52] Dandy W. Pneumocephalus (intracranial pneumatocele or aerocele). Arch Surg 1926;12: 949–82.
[53] Dagi TF, George ED. The management of cerebrospinal fluid leaks. In: Schmidek HH, Sweet WH, editors. Operative neurosurgical techniques. New York: Grune and Stratton; 1988. p. 57–69.
[54] White DR, Dubin MG, Senior BA. Endoscopic repair of cerebrospinal fluid leaks after neurosurgical procedures. Am J Otolaryngol 2003;24:213–6.
[55] Calcaterra TC, Moseley JI, Rand RW. Cerebrospinal rhinorrhea, extracranial surgical repair. West J Med 1977;127:279.
[56] Spetzler RF, Wilson CB. Management of recurrent CSF rhinorrhea of the middle and posterior fossa. J Neurosurg 1978;49:593.
[57] Dohlman G. Spontaneous cerebrospinal fluid rhinorrhea. Acta Otolaryngol (Stockh) 1948; 67(Suppl):20–3.
[58] McCormack B, Cooper PR, Persky M, et al. Extracranial repair of cerebrospinal fluid fistulas: technique and results in 37 patients. Neurosurgery 1990;27:412–7.
[59] Persky MS, Rothstein SG, Breda SD, et al. Extracranial repair of cerebrospinal fluid otorhinorrhea. Laryngoscope 1991;101:134–6.
[60] Hirsch O. Successful closure of cerebrospinal fluid rhinorrhea by endonasal surgery. Arch Otolaryngol 1952;80:218–29.
[61] Lehrer J, Deutsch H. Intranasal surgery for cerebrospinal fluid rhinorrhea. Mt Sinai J Med 1970;37:113–38.
[62] Lanza DC, O'Brien DA, Kennedy DW. Endoscopic repair of cerebrospinal fluid fistulae and encephaloceles. Laryngoscope 1996;106:1119–25.
[63] Mattox DE, Kennedy DW. Endoscopic management of CSF leaks and cephaloceles. Laryngoscope 1990;100:857–62.
[64] Luund VJ. Endoscopic management of cerebrospinal fluid leaks. Am J Rhinol 2002;16: 17–23.
[65] Schick B, Ibing R, Brors D, et al. Long term study of endonasal duraplasty and review of the literature. Ann Otol Rhinol Laryngol 2001;110:142–7.
[66] Bolger WE, McLaughlin K. Cranial bone grafts in cerebrospinal fluid leak and encephalocele repair: a preliminary report. Am J Rhinol 2003;17:153–8.
[67] Lorenz RR, Dean RL, Hurley DB, et al. Endoscopic reconstruction of anterior and middle cranial fossa defects using acellular dermal allograft. Laryngoscope 2003;113:496–501.
[68] Verheggen R, Schulte-WJ, Hahm G, et al. A new technique for dural closure–experience with a Vicryl mesh. Acta Neurochir (Wien) 1997;139:1074–9.
[69] Stankiewicz JA, Vaidya AM, Chow JM, Petruzzelli G. Complications of hydroxyapatite use for transnasal closure of cerebrospinal fluid leaks. Am J Rhinol 2002;16:337–41.
[70] Wormald P, McDonogh M. The bath-plug closure of anterior skull base cerebrospinal fluid leaks. Am J Rhinol 2003;17:299–305.
[71] Hosemann W, Goede U, Sauer M. Wound healing of mucosal autografts for frontal cerebrospinal fluid leaks: clinical experience and experimental investigations. Rhinology 1999;37:108–12.
[72] Chana JS, Chen HC, Sharma R, et al. Use of the free vastus lateralis flap in skull base reconstruction. Plast Reconstr Surg 2003;111:568–74.
[73] Burkey BB, Gerek M, Day T. Repair of the persistent cerebrospinal fluid leak with the radial forearm free flap. Laryngoscope 1999;109:1003–6.
[74] Spinelli HM, Persing JA, Walser B. Reconstruction of the cranial base. Clin Plast Surg 1995; 22:551–61.
[75] Jones NF, Schramm VL, Sekhar LN. Reconstruction of the cranial base following tumour resection. Br J Plast Surg 1987;40:155–62.
[76] Janecka IP, Sekhar LN. Surgical management of cranial base tumours: a report on 91 patients. Oncology 1989;3:69–74.

[77] Disa J, Rodriquez VM, Cordeiro PG. Reconstruction of lateral skull base oncological defects: the role of free tissue transfer. Ann Plast Surg 1998;41:633–63.
[78] Thompson JG, Restifo RJ. Microsurgery for cranial base tumors. Clin Plast Surg 1995;22: 563–72.
[79] Fisher J, Jackson IT. Microvascular surgery as an adjunct to craniomaxillofacial reconstruction. Br J Plast Surg 1989;42:146–54.
[80] Gassner HG, Ponikau JU, Sherris DA, et al. CSF rhinorrhea: 95 consecutive surgical cases with long term follow up at the Mayo Clinic. Am J Rhinol 1999;13:439–47.
[81] Jones DT, McGill TJ, Healy GB. Cerebrospinal fistulas in children. Laryngoscope 1992; 102:443–6.
[82] Delfini R, Missori P, Iannetti G, et al. Mucoceles of the paranasal sinuses with intracranial and intraorbital extension: report of 28 cases. Neurosurgery 1993;32:901–6.
[83] Spetzler RF, Herman JM, Beals S, et al. Preservation of olfaction in anterior craniofacial approaches. J Neurosurg 1993;79:48–52.
[84] Shiley SG, Limonadi F, Delashaw JB, et al. Incidence, etiology, and management of cerebrospinal fluid leaks following trans-sphenoidal surgery. Laryngoscope 2003;113: 1283–8.
[85] Cappabianca P, Cavallo LM, Esposito F, et al. Sellar repair in endoscopic endonasal transsphenoidal surgery: results of 170 cases. Neurosurgery 2002;51:1365–71.
[86] Dessi P, Castro F, Triglia JM, et al. Major complications of sinus surgery: a review of 1192 procedures. J Laryngol Otol 1994;108:212–5.

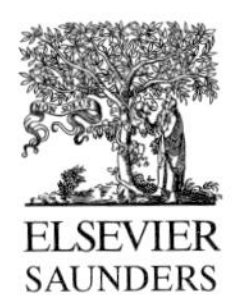

ELSEVIER
SAUNDERS

Otolaryngol Clin N Am
38 (2005) 613–629

OTOLARYNGOLOGIC
CLINICS
OF NORTH AMERICA

Innovations in Neuroimaging of Skull Base Pathology

Lucy W. Glenn, MD

Department of Radiology, Virginia Mason Medical Center, 1100 Ninth Avenue, Seattle, WA 98101, USA

The anatomy of the skull base is complex, and before recent innovations in imaging, often the only way to stage patients with skull base tumors accurately and to determine the extent of disease was through surgical exploration. This approach carried the inherent risks of cranial nerve and vascular injury, cerebrospinal fluid fistula, and infection resulting in significant morbidity and potential mortality. Advances in CT and magnetic resonance technology, in addition to the collaboration of a multispecialty surgical team, have allowed a more aggressive approach to skull base pathology by providing a precise preoperative assessment of tumor extent. Lesions previously considered unresectable are now being treated by skull base surgeons, with a resultant improvement in patient outcomes [1].

Current state

CT scanning and MRI have long been the main imaging modalities to evaluate skull base lesions. Preoperative imaging can (1) define the extent of tumor, (2) suggest the best surgical approach, (3) assess the involvement of adjacent critical structures, and (4) help identify pathologic entities that have a characteristic imaging profile. Arteriography has proven to be a helpful adjunct in the diagnosis of vascular lesions such as paragangliomas or angiofibromas. These diagnostic tools are widely available in community hospitals and have become standard of care in everyday practice of head and neck surgery [1].

E-mail address: radlwg@vmmc.org

doi:10.1016/j.otc.2005.03.007 **oto.theclinics.com**

Innovations

This article focuses on innovations in imaging of the skull base, including state-of-the-art CT imaging techniques, advances in MRI technology (including MR angiography), positron emission tomography (PET), and CT/PET techniques. Recent technological advances in CT and MRI allow high-resolution imaging of structures at the skull base that serves as a road map for the surgeon as well as for the radiation oncologist for planning treatment after surgery. PET and CT/PET are valuable aids in initial staging and for improved follow-up of head and neck cancer patients.

CT

Technology

CT has long been the mainstay for diagnosis of bony abnormalities involving the skull base. Original CT technology involved aiming an x-ray beam through the area of interest and passing in a full circle around the patient. After one revolution of the x-ray beam and detector, the patient was moved slightly to the next slice location, and another full revolution of the x-ray beam and detector occurred. The data were reconstructed using an algorithm that placed various pixels in two dimensions to create the CT image.

The next phase in CT development was the spiral scanner, which allowed movement of the patient while the x-ray beam gantry was rotating, thus creating a spiral of data. This development allowed faster scan times and greater anatomic coverage for similar scan times. The greatly reduced scan times allowed the acquisition of much thinner slices and therefore greatly increased spatial resolution. Most current CT scanners use spiral technology.

The next evolutionary step in CT technology was the development of multiple detectors (MDCT). With one revolution of the gantry, more than one slice could be obtained, and in the time previously required to obtain one slice of data, 4, 8, 16, 32, or 64 slices of data could be obtained. MDCT allows the acquisition of much thinner slices with much greater spatial resolution. In addition, the fast scan speeds allow imaging without degradation of image quality by patient motion. The use of multiple detectors makes possible imaging of the coronary arteries and similar structures that previously moved faster than the speed of the scanner. MDCT now creates true isometric voxels of information (ie, cubes of data that have the same dimension in all planes). This technology allows reconstruction of the data set in any sagittal, coronal, or oblique plane while maintaining the spatial resolution of the original axial data set. The reconstructions are therefore as accurate as the original plane of acquisition.

The current generation of MDCT scanners allows a slice thickness of 0.625 mm compared with the previous of thickness of 1.25 mm. In addition, the fast scan times allow an entire temporal bone scan to be completed in 4 seconds (Fig. 1). Now in development are volumetric CT scanners that use 64 detectors or more and provide 40 mm of coverage per rotation while providing 0.35-mm microvoxel resolution. These scanners will allow even higher resolution and 73% more coverage of anatomic structures than the current scanners in the same amount of time [2].

Image viewing

The proliferation of slices per study has led to a new paradigm in image interpretation. It is no longer feasible to print all images in a study, which now routinely number between 500 and 1000 images. Therefore, the images must be viewed on a workstation using a picture archival and communication system. Rather than viewing two-dimensional axial images, the new software allows volumetric displays of information in any plane. Such displays are particularly useful in the skull base, where both coronal and

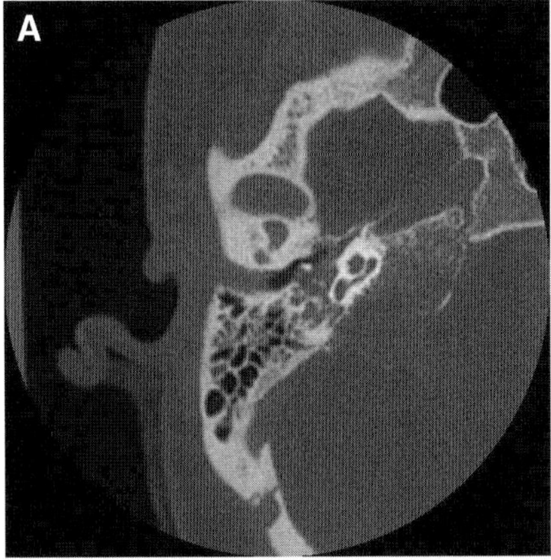

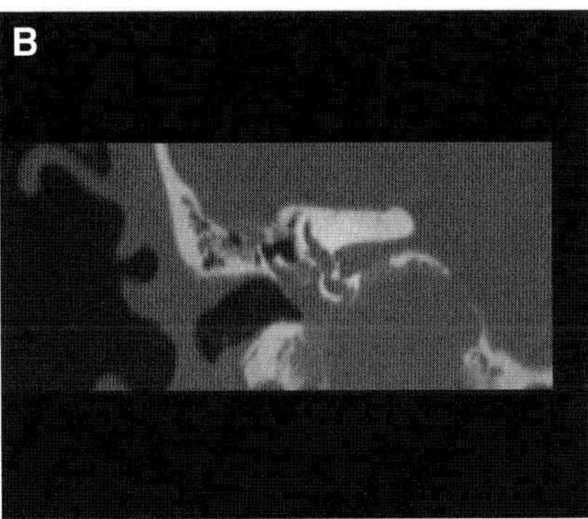

Fig. 1. CT temporal bone showing bone erosion from a glomus jugulare tumor. (*A*) Initial axial scans. (*B*) Coronal reconstructed image.

sagittal imaging are needed to evaluate accurately the intracranial extent of disease.

Three-dimensional reconstruction

Several different methods of three-dimensional (3-D) reconstruction are in common use. These methods include multiplanar reconstructions, maximum intensity projections, shaded surface display, and 3-D volume rendering. Multiplanar reconstructions are two-dimensional images that are obtained in a different plane from the original data set (Figs. 2 and 3). Shaded surface displays are 3-D reconstructions of the surface of objects, such as reconstructions of the entire mandible or skull (Fig. 4). Maximum intensity projections use the voxels of data with maximum density, such as contrast-enhanced vessels, to create an angiogram-like picture (Fig. 5).

Unlike shaded surface display and maximum intensity projections, volume rendering makes use of the full set of volumetric data to produce 3-D views. One can view all the structures, including bone, muscle, and vascular structures, simultaneously. Studies have shown that volume rendering is superior to other techniques for visualizing the size and extent of tumor, identifying and determining the size of lymph nodes, and the visualizing relationship between vessels, bone, muscles, and tumor. Thus, volume rendering preserves the full information contained within the data set (Fig. 6) [3].

Evaluation of bony anatomy

For optimal evaluation of bony structures of the skull base, 0.625-, 1.0-, or 1.25-mm scans should be obtained without intravenous contrast. If spiral CT scanning is performed, direct coronal scans must be obtained in addition to the axial scans. The non-isometric voxels obtained with a spiral scanner

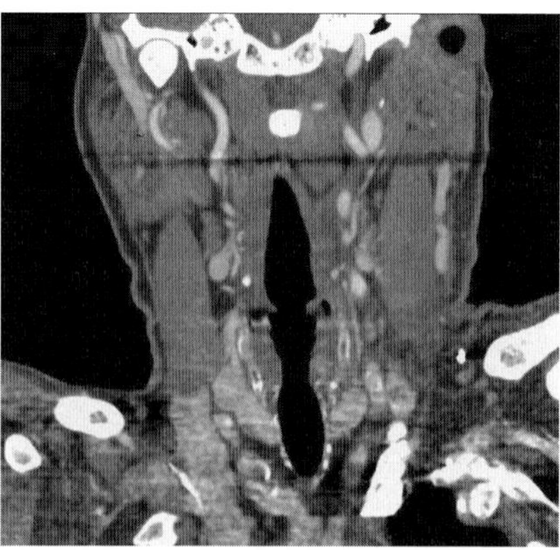

Fig. 2. Coronal two-dimensional reconstructed CT image.

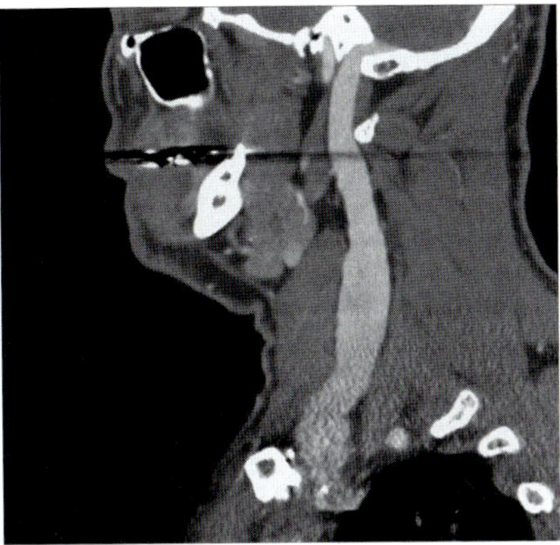

Fig. 3. Sagittal reconstructed CT image.

result in poorer resolution when reconstructions are performed in the coronal plane. With the use of MDCT, only axial scans need be obtained, because the reconstructed images have the same high resolution as the original data set. Sagittal and coronal reconstructions should be performed at 1-, 2-, or 3-mm intervals. Images are best viewed at a wide window width of 3500 Hounsfield units (HU) and a level of 200 HU. With MDCT scanners, the soft tissues and bone can be evaluated simultaneously. Scanning should be performed at 2.5-mm thickness during bolus infusion of intravenous (IV) contrast. Sagittal and coronal reformatted images should be performed at 2- or 3-mm intervals. Evaluation of soft tissue structures requires viewing the image at a window width of 400 HU and a window level of 50 HU.

CT angiography

CT angiography is also possible with MDCT scanners, allowing noninvasive vascular assessment of skull base lesions and carotid anatomy.

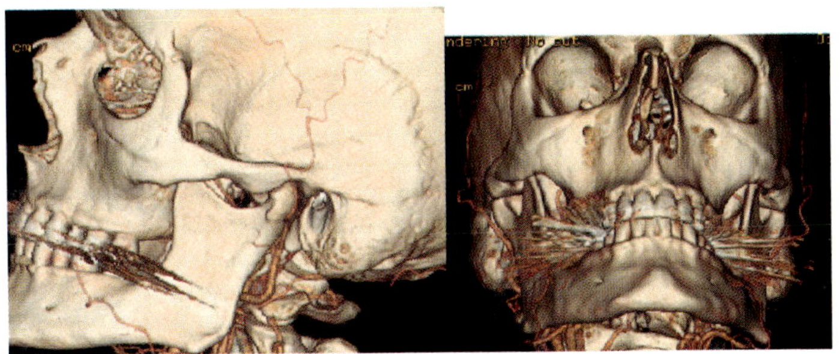

Fig. 4. 3-D CT reconstructions using shaded surface display.

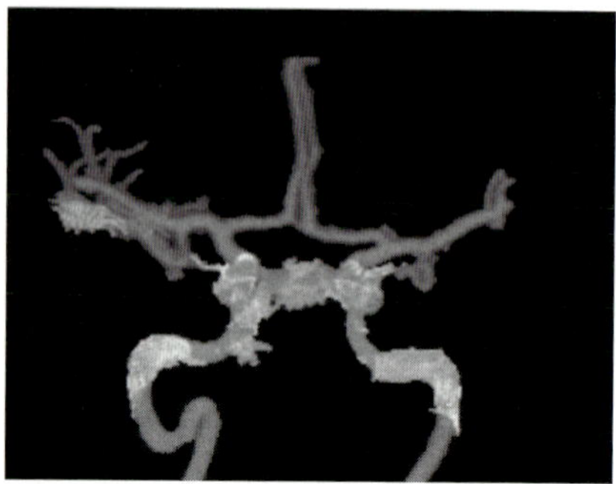

Fig. 5. 3-D reconstruction of the circle of Willis using maximum intensity projection. The bone of the skull base has been incompletely removed from this rendering.

High-resolution (0.625- or 1.25-mm) axial scans are obtained during the arterial phase of an IV bolus injection of contrast, and 3-D reconstructions are then performed. A limitation of this technique specifically at the skull base is that bone has a density similar to that of contrast-enhanced vessels, making it difficult to remove bone from the reconstructions selectively. Newer software has made it easier to delete bony structures from images, allowing unobstructed visualization of the vessels, although this process can still be time intensive. CT angiography may be helpful in evaluating paragangliomas, in detecting an aberrant course of the carotid artery, or in evaluating vascular malformations (Fig. 7).

CT perfusion studies

MDCT also allows CT perfusion studies to be performed. Early studies analyzing the usefulness of CT perfusion studies of head and neck lesions

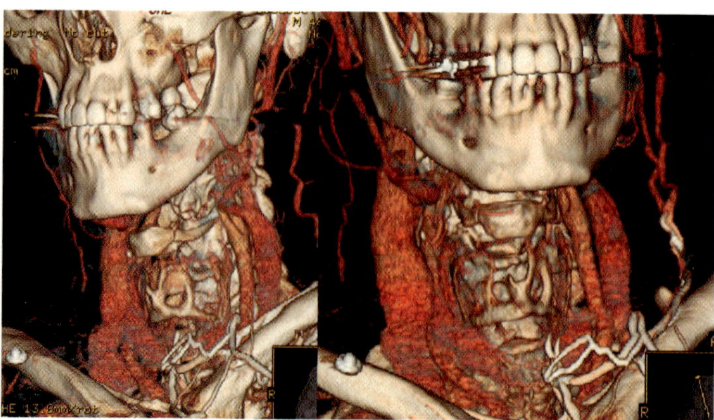

Fig. 6. Volume-rendered CT scans showing arterial and venous anatomy as well as bone detail.

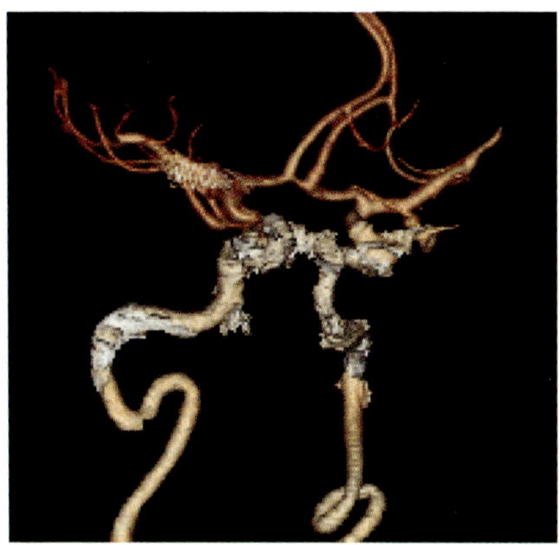

Fig. 7. 3-D CT angiogram using volume rendering.

show promise in distinguishing benign from malignant lesions by determining the tissue perfusion characteristics [4]. Scans of the lesion are obtained without contrast and then at 1-second intervals after a bolus IV injection of 40 to 50 cm^3 of contrast agent, for a total of 50 seconds. Using postprocessing software, images are analyzed for blood volume, blood flow, and mean transit time. Mean transit time provides the most reliable differentiation between malignant and nonmalignant lesions. Malignant lesions have much faster mean transit times than benign lesions. There may also be a role for CT perfusion studies in assessing the response of tumors to treatment with chemotherapy or radiation therapy [5].

MRI

MRI has been a critical factor in the improved diagnostic evaluation of skull base lesions. Because of the sharp contrast differentiation of different soft tissues, MRI superbly demonstrates dura, brain, cerebrospinal fluid, skeletal muscle, and tumor. The ability to image in any plane also allows better evaluation of masses that cross the skull base, either by direct extension or through perineural spread of tumor [6].

Existing standards in MRI

MR scanning is best performed with a high field strength (1.5- or 3.0-T) magnet using a head coil or head and neck coil. Imaging of the skull base should be performed using a smaller field of view (16–18 cm) and 3-mm-thick sections to optimize spatial resolution. The authors typically obtain T1 and T2 fat-saturated sequences in an axial and coronal plane. The T1-weighted images are useful to assess spatial anatomy and bone marrow invasion. The T2-weighted images with fat saturation allow tumors that are typically bright on T2 images, because of higher free water content, to stand out against the darker tissues [7]. IV contrast (gadolinium) is then administered, and axial and coronal T1-weighted images with fat saturation are obtained. The suppression of the fat signal makes the contrast enhancement of tumors much more conspicuous (Fig. 8). In addition, postgadolinium MR imaging can differentiate retained secretions from tumor in the paranasal sinuses or mastoid air cells. Occasionally, sagittal sequences are also obtained. Sagittal imaging is particularly useful in evaluation of anterior cranial fossa and sellar lesions.

Innovations in MRI

Advances in MR sequences have allowed high-resolution imaging of labyrinthine structures, cranial nerves, perineural spread of tumor, cavernous sinus invasion, and vascular abnormalities using MR angiography and MR venography.

Constructive interference steady-state sequences

Evaluation of the seventh and eighth cranial nerves in the cerebellopontine angle and the membranous labyrinthine structures can be evaluated using a bilateral temporomandibular joint coil and constructive interference steady-state (CISS) sequences. CISS sequences provide volumetric acquisition with thin-section collimation and strongly T2-weighted images. Unlike other gradient echo sequences, such as gradient recalled acquisition in the steady state or fast imaging with steady-state precession, CISS has inherent flow compensation that greatly reduces the artifact caused by cerebrospinal fluid pulsation [8]. Images can then be reconstructed in coronal and oblique sagittal planes, allowing assessment of the facial, cochlear, and superior and inferior vestibular nerves within the internal auditory canal (Figs. 9 and 10).

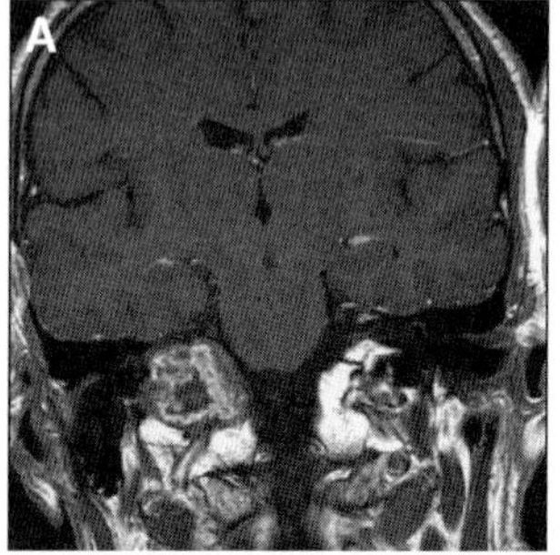

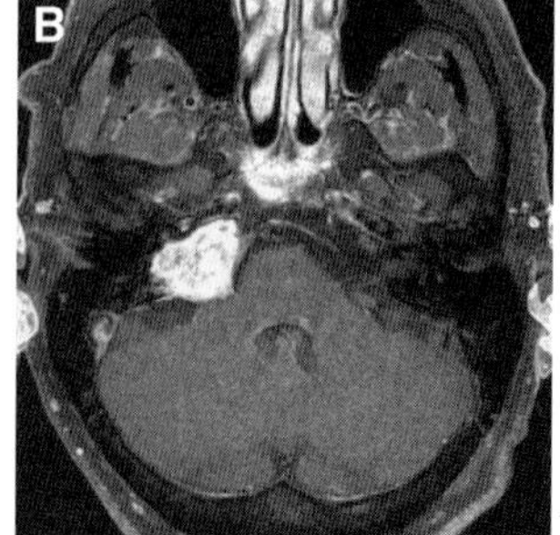

Fig. 8. Paraganglioma of the jugular foramen. (*A*) Coronal T1-weighted image after gadolinium enhancement with fat saturation. (*B*) Axial T1-weighted image after gadolinium enhancement with fat saturation.

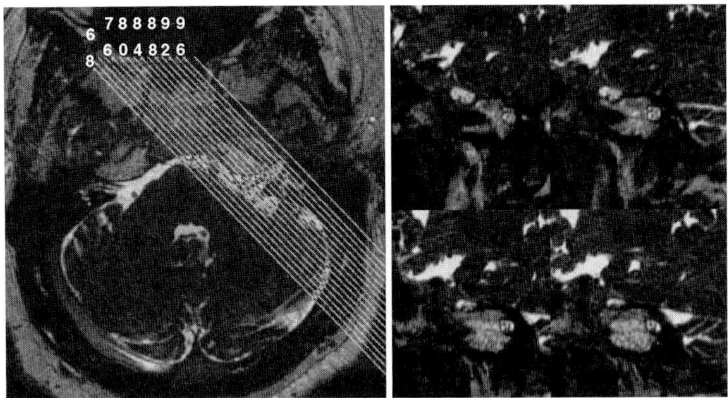

Fig. 9. (*Left*) Axial constructive interference steady-state image of the internal auditory canal construction plane for the oblique sagittal images. (*Right*) Sagittal images of the internal auditory canal show the normal four nerves.

CISS sequences also allow evaluation of the membranous labyrinth [9]. This ability is particularly useful in assessment before cochlear implantation. These sequences can detect cochlear nerve aplasia as well as obstruction of the membranous labyrinth (Figs. 11 and 12).

Magnetization-prepared rapid gradient echo sequences

A recently developed, small flip angle, gradient recalled echo sequence called magnetization-prepared rapid gradient echo (MP-RAGE) demonstrates excellent T1-weighted contrast enhancement with very thin section images of the brain. This technique allows acquisition of 3-D volume data at a 1- to 1.5-mm slice thickness and consequently high spatial resolution. There is also inherent signal suppression of fat tissue. Coronal and sagittal reformations can also be performed from the axial volume data set. This

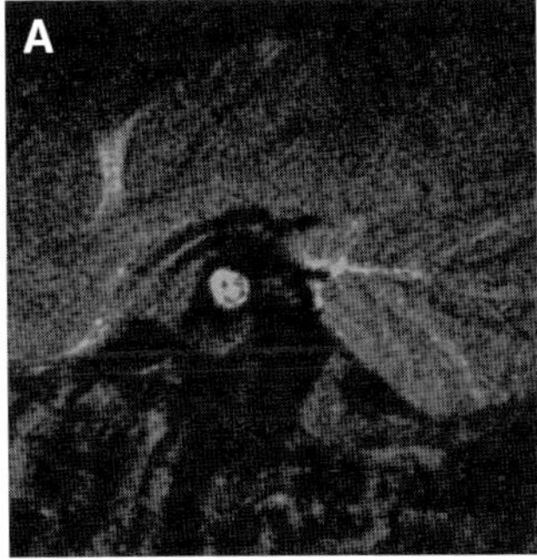

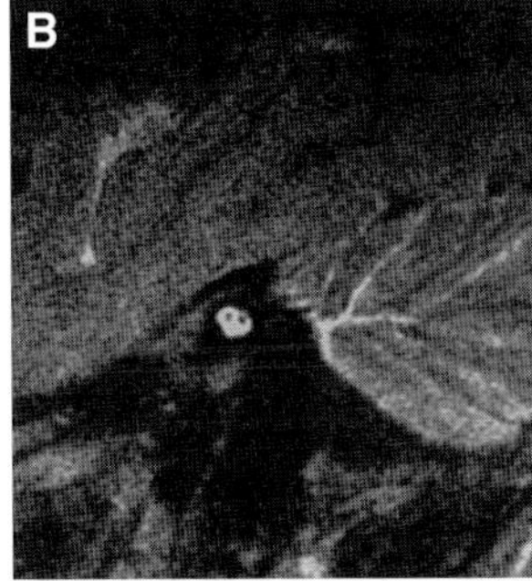

Fig. 10. (*A*) Normal oblique sagittal image of the internal auditory canal showing four nerves. (*B*) Abnormal side showing only facial and vestibular nerves.

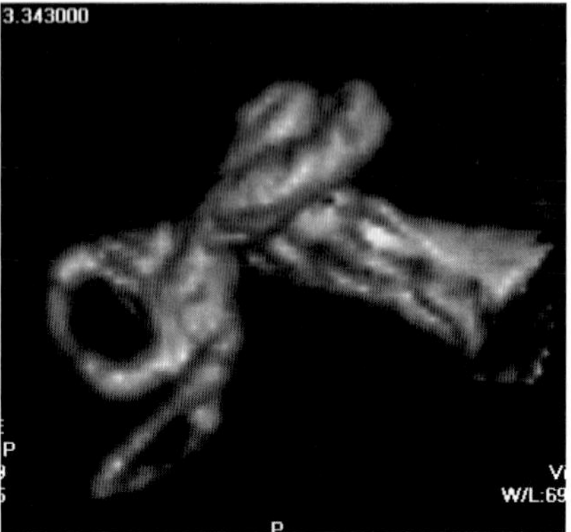

Fig. 11. Normal 3-D MRI using shaded surface display of the membranous labyrinthine structures.

ability makes it ideal for evaluating the extent of tumor at the skull base [10] and for detecting perineural spread (Fig. 13).

Findings that suggest perineural spread of tumor at the skull base include widening of the foramina and enhancing tissue extending through the foramina. A common site for perineural spread of tumor is through the foramen ovale along the V3 branch of the trigeminal nerve. One may also see enlargement and enhancement of the cavernous sinus (Fig. 14). Other common sites for perineural spread include the facial nerve through the stylomastoid foramen and the V2 branch of the trigeminal nerve in the pterygopalatine fossa or infraorbital canal, extending through foramen rotundum (Fig. 15) [11,12].

Dural invasion by tumor can also be assessed on postgadolinium T1-weighted images with fat saturation or MP-RAGE images. The dura

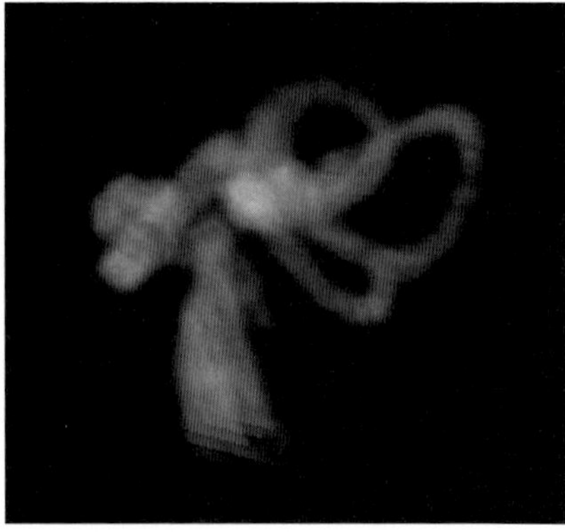

Fig. 12. Normal 3-D MRI using maximum intensity projection of the membranous labyrinth.

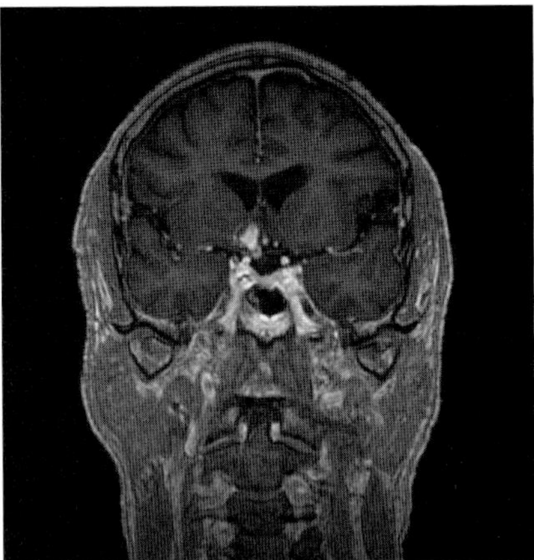

Fig. 13. Coronal magnetization-prepared rapid gradient echo image after gadolinium enhancement showing a partially thrombosed aneurysm of the right anterior communicating artery.

appears thickened and enhances intensely (Fig. 16). Leptomeningeal invasion and extension to the brain parenchyma can also be detected on these sequences (Fig. 17) [13].

MR angiography

Vascular lesions that cause vestibulocochlear symptoms include normal variants such as aberrant internal carotid artery and high jugular bulb with

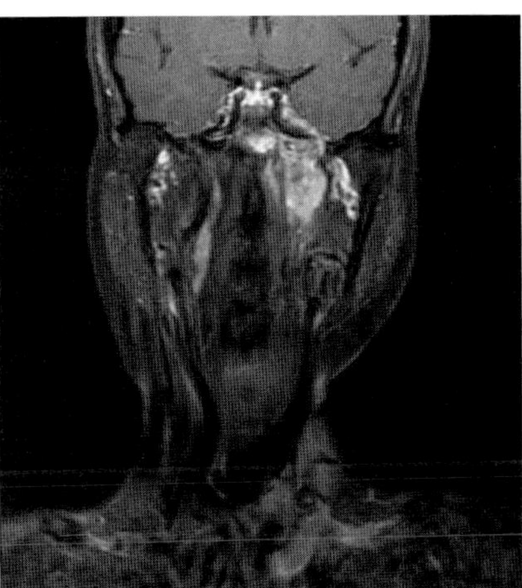

Fig. 14. Coronal T1-weighted image after gadolinium enhancement with fat saturation showing perineural extension of nasopharyngeal carcinoma along V3, through the foramen ovale on the left side.

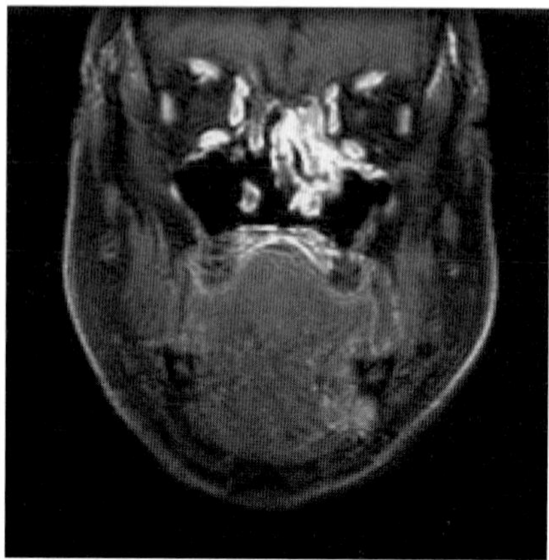

Fig. 15. Perineural spread of tumor along V2 in the left infraorbital canal.

dehiscence of the dome of the jugular fossa. Vascular abnormalities that occur at the skull base include dural fistulas, vertebral venous fistulas, aneurysms, stenosis, or carotid cavernous fistulas. Paragangliomas are often very hypervascular. MR angiography and venography may be helpful in diagnosis of these lesions [14].

MR angiography of neck vessels is performed with IV gadolinium and a coronal volumetric acquisition. Subtraction images and 3-D reconstruction software are used to obtain MR angiograms of the carotid and vertebral arteries. MR angiography can provide diagnostic images of aberrant vessels, aneurysms, and critical stenosis (Fig. 18).

MR venography is obtained without IV contrast by using a time-of-flight technique that shows flowing blood as bright. The arterial signal is

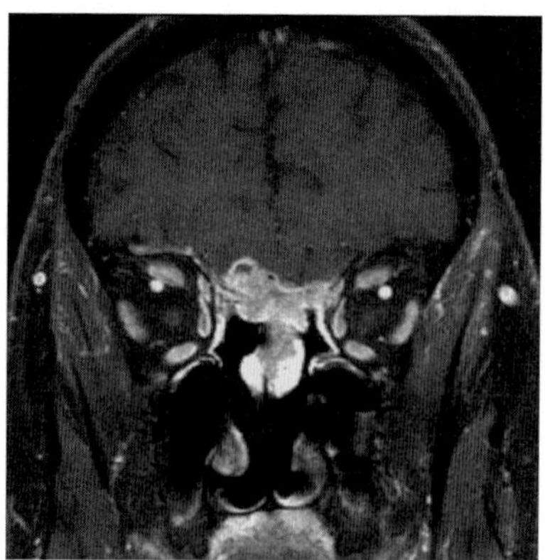

Fig. 16. Coronal T1-weighted image after gadolinium enhancement with fat saturation showing intracranial extension and dural invasion of sinonasal carcinoma.

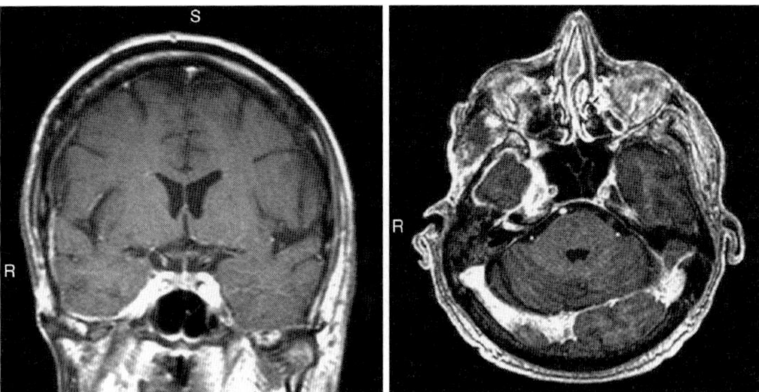

Fig. 17. (*Left*) Coronal T1-weighted image after gadolinium enhancement showing dural invasion by tumor. (*Right*) Axial magnetization-prepared rapid gradient echo image after gadolinium enhancement showing dural invasion surrounding the right temporal lobe.

suppressed by applying a saturation pulse inferior to the skull base. Thus, only flowing blood in the cerebral veins is displayed and reconstructed. MR venography often shows dural atrioventricular fistulas and secondary signs of transverse sinus occlusion. Angiography, however, is still the criterion standard for diagnosis and endovascular treatment in suspected cases of dural atrioventricular fistulas (Fig. 19).

Positron emission tomography

PET is currently performed using [^{18}F18] fluorodeoxyglucose (FDG). FDG uptake in tumors is proportional to the metabolic rate of viable tumor

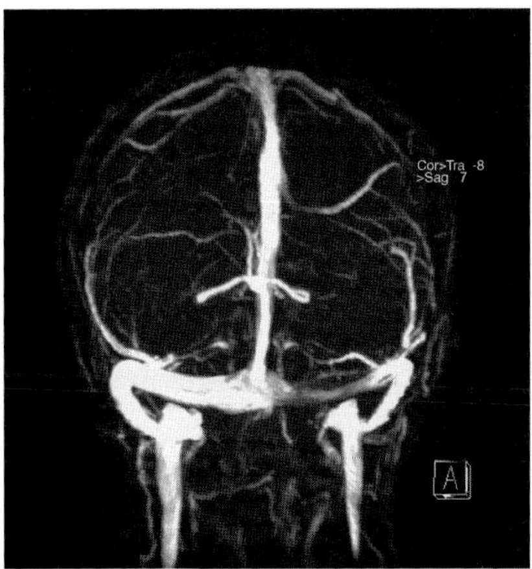

Fig. 18. 3-D maximum intensity projection MR venogram of the sagittal, transverse, and sigmoid sinuses.

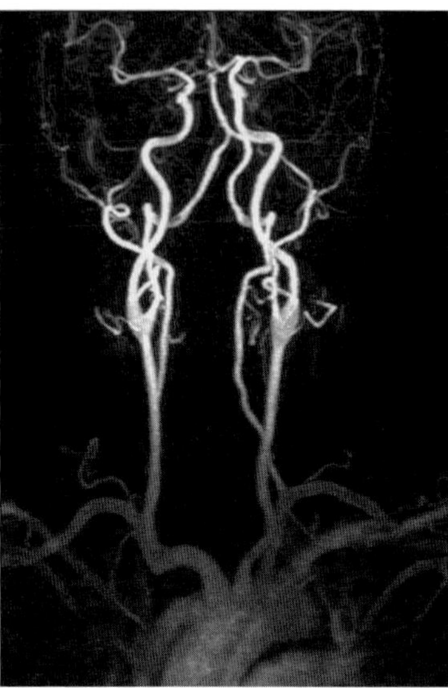

Fig. 19. 3-D MR angiogram of the carotids and vertebrobasilar arteries using maximum intensity projection.

cells, which have an increased demand for glucose. The increased glycolytic activity in tumor cells allows the differentiation of benign and malignant processes. There is some overlap between these two processes. The high sensitivity and high negative predictive value of FDG PET, as well as the ability to image the entire body in a single session, have made it a valuable tool in the initial diagnosis, staging, and restaging of tumors [15].

Normal distribution of fluorodeoxyglucose

There is normal uptake of FDG in the brain, liver, kidneys, intestine, and urinary bladder. There is also minimal uptake in the breasts, mediastinum, bone marrow, and myocardium. The biodistribution of FDG can be affected by blood glucose levels through competitive displacement of FDG by the circulating glucose. All patients should fast for at least 4 to 6 hours before the study, and patients with diabetes will need to have the blood glucose level checked before the study. Stress-related muscle uptake can be seen in the cervical, paraspinal, and trapezius muscles, as well as the vocal cords. Uptake in tonsils, parotid glands, and muscles of mastication may be seen as a normal variant.

Quantitative evaluation of fluorodeoxyglucose positron emission tomography

FDG PET provides quantitative data in the form of the standardized uptake value (SUV). The SUV is a measurement of the amount of glucose uptake by a particular tissue. Measurement of the SUV requires attenuation correction to take into account the variability of FDG uptake caused by varying tumor depth within the body. The SUV also normalizes the tumor FDG uptake with the dose injected and the body weight. SUVs of 2.5 or greater have been used as a cutoff value indicative of malignancy.

Initial staging of head and neck cancer

Medicare has approved payment of FDG PET for the diagnosis, initial staging, and restaging of head and neck cancer. Both CT and MRI have high sensitivity but lack specificity in evaluation of lymph nodes; FDG PET is more accurate for lymph node staging and assessing for unsuspected distant metastases. In detecting lymph node metastases, FDG PET has a sensitivity of 90% and a specificity of 94%, which compare favorably with the 82% sensitivity and 85% specificity for CT and 88% sensitivity and 79% specificity for MRI [15].

PET scanning can also be helpful in when there are neck nodal metastases but the primary cancer cannot be detected by traditional imaging. FDG PET can demonstrate up to 30% of previously undetected primary tumors [15].

Response to therapy and tumor recurrence

FDG PET can be used to assess a tumor's response to chemotherapy or radiation therapy. The decline of the SUV within a lesion may be the first sign of tumor, before actual shrinkage is detected by CT or MRI [16]. Chemotherapeutic regimens may be altered earlier, or salvage surgery may be performed earlier in nonresponders.

In addition, PET can be used in follow-up to detect tumor recurrence. The postsurgical and postradiation changes may make detection of tumor recurrence more difficult on CT and MRI scans. The sensitivity of FDG PET is comparable to that of CT and MRI for detecting tumor recurrence; however, PET has far greater specificity (75%–100%, versus 50%–57% for CT and MRI) [16]. A waiting period of 6 weeks after surgery is recommended to avoid false-positive findings seen with inflammatory hypermetabolism in the surgical bed. In addition, a waiting period of 4 months after completion of radiation therapy is recommended.

Positron emission tomography/CT imaging

The limited spatial resolution and lack of anatomic landmarks in PET images make accurate tumor localization difficult. Separately acquired CT and PET scans can be fused retrospectively using postprocessing software; however, patient movement and imprecise localization of points between CT and PET limit this approach. Computer algorithms to coregister the CT and PET scans are less useful in the head and neck region than in anatomically fixed organs (ie, the brain), because orientation can change between scans.

Combined PET/CT scanners acquire the CT scan and the PET scan in one sitting without moving the patient between the two studies. This technique allows precise functional data from the PET scan to be superimposed on the precise anatomical data from the CT scan.

PET/CT has great applicability in the early detection of recurrent head and neck cancer. The distortion of tissues after surgery and radiation therapy makes it difficult to detect small tumor recurrence. Differentiating scar tissue from recurrent tumor is quite difficult on CT and MRI scans without serial studies to assess for interval growth. In one study, PET identified recurrence in posttreatment necks with an accuracy of 100%, compared with 53% for CT [16].

Summary

Recent advances in CT and MR technology have allowed detailed imaging of the skull base with greater diagnostic accuracy. Innovations such as multidetector volumetric CT scanners with 3-D reconstructions provide soft tissue and bony detail with very high resolution for small structures such as the neural foramina. CT angiography can assess vascular structures noninvasively, and CT perfusion can help differentiate between malignant and benign tumors. MR technology has provided high-resolution, rapid volumetric sequences that are useful in skull base imaging. MR angiography and MR venography can also assess vascular structures noninvasively. PET scanning and CT/PET scanning will increasingly become a mainstay of head and neck tumor imaging for initial staging, monitoring response to therapy, and detecting recurrent disease or metastases. Many more diagnostic imaging options are available to the head and neck surgeon today than ever before.

References

[1] Durden D, Williams D. Radiology of skull base neoplasms. Otolaryngol Clin North Am 2001;34(6):1043–64.

[2] GE volume CT. GE Healthcare. Waukesha (WI): GE Healthcare; 2004.

[3] Franca C, Levin-Plotnik D, Sehgal V, et al. Use of three dimensional spiral computed tomography imaging for staging and surgical planning of head and neck cancer. J Digit Imaging 2000;13(2 Suppl 1):24–32.

[4] Rumboldt Z, Al-Okaili R, Roberts D, et al. CT perfusion in head and neck cancer: a pilot study. In: Programs and abstracts of the American Society of Neuroradiology. 2004. p. 54.

[5] Gandhi D, Chepeha DB, Sacco A, et al. Correlation between initial and early follow-up CT perfusion parameters with endoscopic tumor response in patients with advanced squamous cell carcinomas of the oral cavity/oropharynx treated with organ preservation therapy. In: Programs and abstracts of the American Society of Neuroradiology. 2004. p. 25.

[6] Weber AL. Imaging of the skull base. Eur J Radiol 1996;22(1):68–81.

[7] Fischbein NJ, Kaplan MJ. Magnetic resonance imaging of the central skull base. Top Magn Reson Imaging 1999;10(5):325–46.

[8] Laine FJ, Underhill T. Imaging of the lower cranial nerves. Magn Reson Imaging Clin N Am 2002;10(3):433–49.
[9] Davidson HC. Imaging of the temporal bone. Magn Reson Imaging Clin N Am 2002;10(4): 573–613.
[10] Yoshizumi K, Korogi Y, Sugahara T, et al. Skull base tumors: evaluation with MP-RAGE sequence. Comput Med Imaging Graph 2001;25(1):23–31.
[11] Ginsberg LE. MR imaging of perineural tumor spread. Magn Reson Imaging Clin N Am 2002;10(3):511–25.
[12] Wallace R, Dean B, Beals S, et al. Posttreatment imaging of the skull base. Semin Ultrasound CT MR 2003;24(3):164–81.
[13] Ishida H, Mohri M, Amatsu M. Invasion of the skull base by carcinomas: histopathologically evidenced findings with CT and MRI. Eur Arch Otorhinolaryngol 2002;259(10):535–9.
[14] Thornton J, Bashir Q, Aletich VA, et al. Role of magnetic resonance imaging and diagnostic interventional angiography in vascular and neoplastic diseases of the skull base associated with vestibulocochlear symptoms. Top Magn Reson Imaging 2000;11(2):123–37.
[15] Kostakoglu L, Agress H, Goldsmith S. Clinical role of FDG PET in evaluation of cancer patients. Radiographics 2003;23:315–40.
[16] Fukui M, Blodgett T, Meltzer C. PET/CT imaging in recurrent head and neck cancer. Semin Ultrasound CT MR 2003;24(3):157–63.

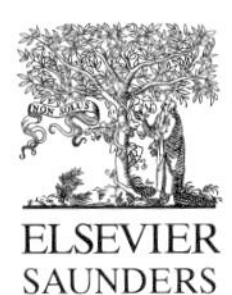
ELSEVIER
SAUNDERS

Otolaryngol Clin N Am
38 (2005) 631–642

OTOLARYNGOLOGIC
CLINICS
OF NORTH AMERICA

Intraoperative Neurophysiologic Monitoring: Indications and Techniques for Common Procedures in Otolaryngology–Head and Neck Surgery

Bruce M. Edwards, AuD*, Paul R. Kileny, PhD

Division of Audiology and Electrophysiology, Department of Otolaryngology–Head and Neck Surgery, University of Michigan Health System, 1500 East Medical Center Drive, TC 1904, Ann Arbor, Michigan 43109, USA

Indications

Intraoperative neurophysiologic monitoring (IOM) of cranial nerve activity is provided in the University of Michigan Health System and other centers for surgical procedures performed by head and neck surgeons, otologists, and neurotologists. These procedures include parotidectomy, posterior or middle fossa craniotomy for tumor, revision tympanoplasty/mastoidectomy, thyroidectomy, congenital aural atresia reconstruction, and cochlear implantation with selective use of facial nerve monitoring [1,2].

Surgical procedures that potentially involve peripheral nerves or sensory and motor divisions of cranial nerves can benefit from IOM that assesses the functional integrity of the patient's nervous system, aiding in the identification of neural structures in the surgical field to avoid their injury. Changes in baseline activity are sought, causative factors are identified, and appropriate measures are taken that may lead to a return to a recognized benchmark or standard. Successful realization of these steps leads to better postoperative outcomes in the short and long term.

This article reviews recent IOM literature and offers examples of the usefulness of IOM in selected, common procedures in otolaryngology-head and neck surgery. Examples of routinely encountered surgical events that directly affect IOM measures are discussed. It is hoped that readers will benefit by improved outcomes in their work.

* Corresponding author.
E-mail address: bedwards@umich.edu (B.M. Edwards).

doi:10.1016/j.otc.2005.03.002 **oto.theclinics.com**

Characterization of intraoperative neurophysiologic monitoring

Programmatic differences in the IOM model exist across institutions. The continuous model calls for an individual other than the surgeon to observe baseline cranial nerve activity closely and report to the surgical team a change from the established baseline, particularly when associated with a surgical event such as tumor dissection. That nonsurgeon must be familiar with the operative procedure and certain events that may be related to undesirable results. The authors find it helpful to be able to observe a surgeon's actions to correlate them with neurophysiologic events. Continuous IOM necessitates the observation of amplitude, duration, and frequency patterns of mechanically activated electromyogram (EMG) activity that can be associated with postoperative facial paralysis or paresis. Criteria exist that quantitatively assess the electrically triggered compound muscle action potential as a predictor of postoperative functional status [3–5]. A prospective study recently demonstrated that quantitative data acquired during continuous facial nerve monitoring (FNM) are good predictors of postoperative facial function [6]. Romstock and colleagues [6] determined FNM to be superior to electrically triggered EMG or so-called "remote" monitoring.

Arguably, the most commonly practiced form of monitoring, the remote model, uses black-box technology that requires a surgeon to attend to and discriminate between acoustic alarms that signal (1) baseline changes in free-running EMG associated with surgical events, (2) spurious noise emanating from contact between noninsulated instruments converging in the operative field, or (3) amplified noise originating from electrocautery devices that escapes muting circuitry. In this paradigm, the monitoring onus transfers to the surgeon. The recognition of a potentially adverse situation is based on the perception of a change in acoustic output from the monitoring loudspeaker, reinforced with visual confirmation of EMG activity displayed on the monitor screen. A disadvantage of this method is the potential for a gradual loss of vigilance, or willingness to avoid certain actions, if the surgeon considers that preceding acoustic warning signals represented false alarms.

When information about sensory function is needed, an individual other than the surgeon observes averaged activity that reflects sensory function, as in monitoring eighth cranial nerve responses during vestibular nerve sections or for planned hearing preservation surgery for vestibular schwannoma. The continuous or attended model previously described is the default scheme in such cases.

Neither continuous monitoring nor remote IOM protects the nonvisualized cranial nerve. A nonvisualized nerve remains at risk of iatrogenic injury if no EMG event signals its presence in or near the operative field, particularly if the nerve remains unseen, as may occur in revision surgery. Accordingly, during their residency training, otolaryngology surgeons are instructed that intraoperative monitoring is not an acceptable substitute for anatomic understanding or surgical experience and skill [7,8].

Standard of care, cost effectiveness, and clinical outcomes

IOM has found a place in neurotologic [3–6,9–16], selected otologic [17–19], skull base [20–22], and head and neck procedures involving the parotid [23–31] or thyroid glands/recurrent laryngeal nerve [32–40] and in neck dissections [41,42]. The National Institutes of Health published a consensus statement based on expert testimony summarizing then-current management options, including FNM, during surgical treatment for vestibular schwannoma [43,44]. The recently expired consensus statement suggested that similar methods have potential value for avoiding iatrogenic injury to structures served by other cranial motor nerves. Concurring with the consensus, the American Academy of Otolaryngology-Head & Neck Surgery (AAOHNS) acknowledges that competently performed IOM of the facial nerve is efficacious and may minimize the risk of iatrogenic injury [45].

Nonetheless, monitoring of cranial motor nerves is considered to exceed the standard of care for many procedures performed by otolaryngology-head and neck surgeons [7,29–30]. Although recognized by frequent users as having great value in the identification and potential safeguarding of the facial nerve [46], IOM seems to be used infrequently in chronic ear surgery [47,48]. Greenberg et al [47] randomly sampled 500 active AAOHNS members; most of the 223 respondents were private practitioners. Within that group, 82% of self-reported "otologists" used facial nerve monitoring as compared with 50% of self-reported general or "other" otolaryngologists. Seventy-six percent of all respondents reportedly had access to a facial nerve monitor when desired. Certain trends were described. Frequent users of FNM were employed in academia, were more recently trained, or were experienced otologic surgeons. Notably, most did not advocate mandatory monitoring for chronic ear surgery. Saravanappa et al [48] reported that of 234 respondents to their survey of 545 full members of the British Association of Otolaryngologists/Head and Neck Surgeons, 33% of those who regularly performed mastoidectomy used FNM, and 38% never used it. The greatest use of FNM occurred during combined approach tympanoplasty, with 49% of respondents reporting routine use.

Presumed considerable cost may be a barrier to the acceptance of IOM for both primary and revision ear surgery [17]. Wilson and colleagues [17] examined the cost effectiveness of FNM in middle ear and mastoid surgery, selecting as the primary outcome measure the incremental cost per incremental quality-adjusted life-year (QALY) saved. With a decision-tree matrix, they analyzed the cost effectiveness of FNM for three cohorts: patients who received FNM for all middle ear and mastoid surgery, patients who had selective FNM, and patients who received no monitoring. QALYs were obtained by multiplying life expectancy by estimated utility of patients living with facial paralysis. Calculations were made using the Short Form-36 questionnaire from the Facial Clinimetric Evaluation (FaCE) scale, a self-evaluation tool for patients with facial paralysis [49]. Results strongly favored FNM for all patients undergoing middle ear and mastoid surgery. A cost range of approximately $223.00 to 528.00 was reported. Rank ordering of QALYs supported a strategy to monitor primary and revision surgery (45.68), versus either revision-only or no-monitoring scenarios (45.67 and 45.65, respectively). Associated costs of facial paralysis increased with decreasing use of monitoring (ie, the highest costs were associated with no provision for monitoring).

Recent investigations of patient outcomes following continuous FNM demonstrate overall improvement in facial nerve morbidity after neurotologic surgical treatment for vestibular schwannoma [4] and a reduction in the incidence of short-term facial paresis in primary parotid gland surgery [25]. Isaacson et al [4] reported that IOM has led to significant improvements in facial nerve function in vestibular schwannoma surgery. Despite these and other surgical advances, some patients still have poor facial nerve outcomes. Monitoring may be able to predict poor long-term facial nerve outcomes and aid in rehabilitation planning. Following resection of eighth nerve lesions, Isaacson et al [4] reported that immediate postoperative facial function predicted outcome with 98.5% sensitivity, 59% specificity, and 94% positive predictive value. These investigators reported that after dissection a combination of stimulus thresholds and the calculation of proximal-to-distal amplitude ratios held promise in predicting postoperative facial outcomes. Terrell and colleagues [25] discovered that there was a 24% lower chance of transient paresis following primary parotidectomy using continuous monitoring. They reported that mean setup time for monitoring a simple parotidectomy was 11 minutes; the total of fixed and incremental costs associated with provision of IOM was $379.00 per case.

Utility of intraoperative neurophysiologic monitoring

Several recent reports underscore the utility of electrophysiologic measures in assorted surgeries that place cranial nerves at risk [50–53]. Harper [50] thoroughly discusses the growing body of evidence that supports the value of cranial nerve monitoring in a variety of surgical environments, pointing out that neural dysfunction follows from the effects of the underlying pathologic state of the patient or the surgical treatment of the diseased state. Thus, auditory brainstem responses (ABRs) are not easily predicted in patients with mass lesions that impinge on cranial nerve eight; preoperative testing clarifies them and avoids unintended surprises in the operating room. Similarly, facial EMG obtained intraoperatively from a patient with a parotid mass may discretely affect branches of the extracranial facial nerve during dissection (Fig. 1).

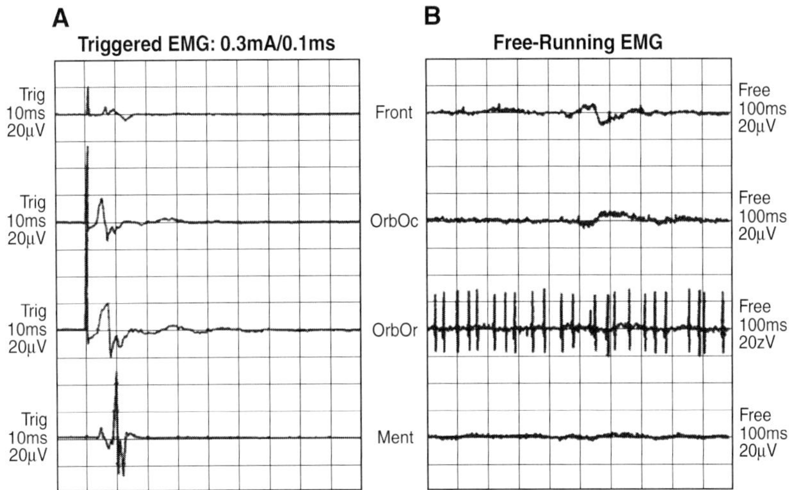

Fig. 1. (*A*) Triggered EMG. An electrical stimulus of 0.3 mA delivered to the main trunk of the facial nerve produces compound muscle action potentials that confirm seventh nerve function and integrity during parotidectomy. (*B*) Free-running EMG. Motor unit potentials are present in the orbicularis oris muscle innervated by the buccal branch of the facial nerve following mechanical activation.

Sala et al [51] systematically discuss IOM in the setting of pediatric neurosurgery, considering "why, when, and how" questions of monitoring. For instance, in answer to the question "Why is monitoring provided?" they reason that dynamic IOM enables a surgeon to alter a surgical plan, avoiding unsatisfactory postoperative functional outcomes. Well-conducted IOM can allow the surgeon to take more aggressive measures leading to complete extirpation.

Avoiding hazards of Intraoperative neurophysiologic monitoring

Edwards and Kileny [53] outline the components in a standardized cranial nerve monitoring program. Consideration of these issues in advance of surgery is the primary mechanism for avoiding many hazards and pitfalls of IOM that lead to losses of confidence in monitoring as well as unsatisfactory surgical outcomes [53]. Table 1 contains a simple checklist with suggestions for cranial nerve monitoring for selected otolaryngology-head and neck surgery. Several "pearls" follow that help in the delivery of neurophysiologic monitoring of cranial nerves in selected otolaryngology-head and neck surgery.

Notes on electromyography

Certain pitfalls can be anticipated in otolaryngology-head and neck surgical procedures. Mastery of them will lead to fewer technical

Table 1
Intraoperative cranial nerve monitoring schemes for selected surgical procedures that involve otolaryngology-head and neck surgeons

	Cranial Nerve									
Procedure	III	IV	V	VI	VII	VIII	IX	X	XI	XII
Otology										
Revision ear					•					
Aural atresia					•					
CI					•					
VNS					•	•				
Head & neck										
Parotid					•					
Thyroid								•		
Radical neck					•				•	
Neurotology										
VS			•		•	•				
ABI					•	•	•	•	•	
Skull base/other										
Petroclival	•	•		•						
Jugular foramen							•	•	•	
Sphenoid wing	•			•	•					
Parapharyngeal space								•	•	•
MVD		•[a]	•		•	•	•			

Abbreviations: ABI, auditory brainstem implant; CI, cochlear implant; CN, cranial nerve; MVD, microvascular decompression; VNS, vestibular nerve section; VS, vestibular schwannoma.

[a] Common injury during MVD for trigeminal neuralgia; monitoring may be useful [55].

interruptions and potentially better patient outcomes. (1) Long-lasting neuromuscular blockade by anesthesiology is contraindicated when monitoring free running and triggered EMG from cranial motor nerves. Suprathreshold repetitive stimulation [54] and threshold estimation are more difficult in the presence of partial blockade. (2) The use of warmer fluids can reduce the number of times that irrigation-induced motor units occur. Identification of EMG changes is enhanced when a quieter EMG noise floor is maintained; nursing can be valuable in providing warm irrigation fluids as needed. An alternative, anecdotal view holds that an irrigation-induced muscle spasm grossly confirms function of the monitored cranial nerve. (3) To verify that a functional circuit comprised of both the recording and stimulating components of the monitoring system exists, perform a positive control assessment before an expected negative test result is obtained [54]. For example, before stimulating the exposed capsule of a vestibular schwannoma, one must know that current delivered to the facial nerve will result in a compound muscle action potential. Once the return electrode and handheld probe are ready, stimulation of the greater superficial petrosal nerve at the geniculate ganglion results in retrograde stimulation of cranial nerve VII, confirming stimulability of the nerve and viability of the monitoring setup. (4) Before delivering current through the surgical stimulator, meticulously maintain the surgical field by removing cerebrospinal or irrigation fluids or blood. This precaution avoids shunting of the electrical stimulus. The result will be improved precision in obtaining positive responses and delineating stimulus thresholds. (5) Criteria have been published that correlate postoperative function with intraoperative events as represented by EMG changes; these criteria can serve as general guides when observing alterations in either free-running or triggered EMG [2–5,18,38,56].

Notes on auditory evoked potentials

Difficulties are routinely experienced when monitoring the eighth cranial nerve because of the compressive effects of vestibular schwannomas on neural and vascular structures. Some technical problems can be overcome or minimized by obtaining preoperative audiologic studies including pure tone and speech audiometry and ABR. Optimizing evoked potentials during preoperative testing is beneficial for monitoring [57]. Consider two strategic points. First, obtaining evoked potentials just before surgery minimizes the chance that significant decrements will occur in the interim. Second, once an intracranial mass lesion is discovered and plans are made for its extirpation, evoked potentials acquired just before surgery take on a different purpose. No longer is a tightly controlled neurodiagnostic test setting necessary. Test parameters should be adjusted with the goal of producing the best evoked responses possible. The results, and the modification of stimulus characteristics such as polarity, rate, and intensity and the recording parameters (eg, electrode montage, filtering) that led to acquiring them, should be reported to facilitate quality auditory nerve monitoring. Obtaining a first-rate baseline evoked response is essential for reporting any change relative to that metric. As an aside, evoked otoacoustic emissions may play a role in estimation of cochlear health generally [58–59], gauging cochlear vascular supply [60–61], and for differentiating cochlear versus sensory components of hearing loss for patients with vestibular schwannomas [62]. The predictive value of various otoacoustic emissions for postoperative auditory outcomes has been investigated [57–59,63–64].

Eighth nerve monitoring can be specified for certain neurotologic procedures using one or more methods appropriate to the case [11,65–68]. These techniques have inherent strengths and weaknesses and may be affected by pharmacologic agents or physiologic events during surgery. Table 2 lists some changes that can be anticipated in the course of neurophysiologic monitoring for otolaryngology-head and neck surgery cases. Legatt [65] offers a comprehensive discussion of intraoperative mechanisms that lead to changes in auditory potentials. For example, a commonly encountered problem involves the temporary deterioration of the ABR resulting from masking produced by temporal bone drilling and suction irrigation. Although disconcerting, it is predictable and resolves

Table 2
Effects of pharmacologic agents and physiologic events on intraoperative neurophysiologic monitoring

Pharmacologic agent	Effect
Modality: electrocochleography	Resistant to effects of anesthesia
Modality: auditory brainstem response	
Inhalation anesthetics (enflurane, halothane, isoflurane)	Delay of 0.5–1.0 ms prolongation of wave V; I–V interpeak latency prolonged when end-tidal concentration exceeds 1.5%
Thiopental	≥20 mg/kg dose, wave V prolonged, amplitude reductions noted with larger doses
Pentobarbital	>9 mg/kg, latencies prolonged, amplitudes reduced
Modality: facial electromyography	
Local anesthetics (lidocaine, bupivacaine, cocaine, tetracaine)	Latency and amplitude of CMAP following impaired propagation of potentials
Neuromuscular blockade (succinylcholine; atracurium, mivacurium, vecuronium; pancuronium, doxacurium, pipecuronium)	Spontaneous and triggered EMG abolished until worn off or reversed (can be lengthy time period)
Physiologic event	
Local or systemic hypothermia	ABR absolute, interpeak latencies prolonged, wave amplitudes diminish; neurotonic stimulation of EMG activity
Tissue compression, retraction	Averaged auditory responses degraded, abolished
Inadequate ventilation, hemodilution, systemic hypotension, regional ischemia	Reduced oxygen affects endocochlear potentials, decreases cochlear output

Abbreviations: ABR, auditory brainstem response; CMAP, compound muscle action potential; EMG, electromyogram.

From Edwards BM, Kileny PR. Intraoperative monitoring of cranial nerves. In: Canalis RF, Lambert PR, editors. The ear: comprehensive otology. Philadelphia: Lippincott Williams & Wilkins; 2000. p. 284; with permission.

quickly with cessation of drilling. Nevertheless, to create a setting in which the chance for iatrogenic injury is minimized, no assumptions should be made. High-quality two-way communication is key to avoiding unintended, permanent changes in evoked potentials and concomitant loss of hearing. Two recognized actions that correlate with hearing outcomes include tumor dissection at the fundus of the internal auditory canal (IAC) and drilling the posterior wall of the IAC [65].

The ABR represents afferent activity from the distal auditory nerve (wave I) to the brainstem's lateral lemniscus (wave V) and is the most commonly employed method for monitoring cranial nerve eight. Useful in planned hearing preservation, vestibular nerve section, and microvascular decompression for trigeminal neuralgia or hemifacial spasm, waveform morphology of the ABR is highly dependent on hearing sensitivity. For patients with larger vestibular schwannomas and elevated hearing sensitivity, an adequate ABR often takes 30 to 60 seconds of averaging. Simultaneous recording of electrocochleography (ECoG) can furnish information about the involved ear more quickly because the recording electrode is placed closer to the response generator [53,66–68]. A shortcoming of the ECoG, a representation of very early evoked potentials from cochlear hair cells and the distal eighth cranial nerve, is that it provides little information regarding the proximal nerve and surgical effects on it. To record the ECoG and the ABR simultaneously, preoperative plans should be made for placing a reference electrode deep in the external ear canal (or through the tympanic membrane onto the promontory) along with other monitoring leads, before the patient is prepped for surgery. Critically, the computer used for multimodality recording must support multiple channels with independent time bases and recording montages to record simultaneously evoked responses that occur at different points along the time continuum (Fig. 1) [53].

Surgical effects on the proximal auditory nerve can be quickly established by direct eighth nerve recordings comprised of a pair of positive peaks generated by the eighth nerve and the cochlear nucleus, respectively. Fewer stimuli are needed to generate this large-amplitude, virtually instantaneous response because of the proximity of the recording electrode to anatomic generators and an enhanced signal-to-noise ratio. Although efficacious, direct recordings cannot be realized until the cochlear nerve is visualized [69]. A variation of the procedure places an extradural electrode adjacent to the eighth nerve between the floor of the IAC and the dura. Once reflected anteriorly, the incised dura covers and stabilizes the reference electrode [70]. Using this method, cochlear nerve action potentials can be obtained in seconds with amplitudes many times larger than ABR.

References

[1] Edwards BM, Kileny PR, McCue J, et al. Intraoperative neurophysiologic monitoring: a contemporary brief. The ASHA Leader 2004;9(6):4–6, 16.

[2] Leonetti JP, Matz GJ, Smith PG, et al. Facial nerve monitoring in otologic surgery: clinical indications and intraoperative technique. Ann Otol Rhinol Laryngol 1990;99(11): 911–8.

[3] Nakao Y, Piccirillo E, Falcioni M, et al. Electromyographic evaluation of facial nerve damage in acoustic neuroma surgery. Otol Neurotol 2001;22(4):554–7.

[4] Isaacson B, Kileny PR, El-Kashlan H. Intraoperative monitoring and facial nerve outcomes after vestibular schwannoma resection. Otol Neurotol 2003;24(5):812–7.

[5] Goldbrunner RH, Schlake HP, Milewski C, et al. Quantitative parameters of intraoperative electromyography predict facial nerve outcomes for vestibular schwannoma surgery. Neurosurgery 2000;46(5):1140–8.

[6] Romstock J, Strauss C, Fahlbusch R. Continuous electromyography monitoring of motor cranial nerves during cerebellopontine angle surgery. J Neurosurg 2000;93:586–93.

[7] Roland PS, Meyerhoff WL. Intraoperative facial nerve monitoring: what is its appropriate role? Am J Oto 1993;14(2):1.
[8] Harner SG, Leonetti JP. Iatrogenic facial paralysis prevention. Ear Nose Throat J 1996; 75(11):1996.
[9] Schmerber S, Lavieille JP, Dumas G, et al. Intraoperative auditory monitoring in vestibular schwannoma surgery: new trends. Acta Otolaryngol 2004;124:53–61.
[10] Batra PS, Dutra JC, Wiet RJ. Auditory and facial nerve function following surgery for cerebellopontine angle meningiomas. Arch Otolaryngol Head Neck Surg 2002;128:369–74.
[11] Battista RA, Wiet RJ, Paauwe L. Evaluation of three intraoperative auditory monitoring techniques in acoustic neuroma surgery. Am J Otol 2000;21(2):244–8.
[12] Morikawa M, Tamaki N, Nagashima T, et al. Long-term results of facial nerve function after acoustic neuroma surgery, clinical benefit of intraoperative facial nerve monitoring. Kobe J Med Sci 2000;46:113–24.
[13] Frohne C, Matthies C, Lesinski-Schiedat A, et al. Extensive monitoring during auditory brainstem implant surgery. J Laryngol Otol 2000;114(S27):11–4.
[14] Matthies C, Samii M. Direct brainstem recording of auditory evoked potentials during vestibular schwannoma resection: nuclear BAEP recording. J Neurosurg 1997;86:1057–62.
[15] Axon PR, Ramsden RT. Assessment of real-time clinical facial function during vestibular schwannoma resection. Laryngoscope 2000;110:1911–5.
[16] Wedekind C, Klug N. Facial f wave recording: a novel and effective technique for extra- and intraoperative diagnosis of facial nerve function in acoustic tumor disease. Otolaryngol Head Neck Surg 2003;129:114–20.
[17] Wilson L, Lin E, Lalwani A. Cost-effectiveness of intraoperative facial nerve monitoring in middle ear or mastoid surgery. Laryngoscope 2003;113:1736–45.
[18] Noss RS, Lalwani AK, Yingling CD. Facial nerve monitoring in middle ear and mastoid surgery. Laryngoscope 2001;111:831–6.
[19] Graham JM, Phelps PD, Michaels L. Congenital malformations of the ear and cochlear implantation in children: review and temporal bone report of common cavity. J Laryngol Otol 2000;114(S25):1–14.
[20] Kawaguchi M, Ohnishi H, Sakamoto T, et al. Intraoperative electrophysiologic monitoring of cranial motor nerves in skull base surgery. Surg Neurol 1995;43:177–81.
[21] Schlake HP, Goldbrunner RH, Milewski C, et al. Intra-operative electromyographic monitoring of the lower cranial motor nerves (lcn IX–XII) in skull base surgery. Clin Neurol Neurosurg 2001;103:72–82.
[22] Schlake HP, Goldbrunner RH, Siebert M, et al. Intra-operative electromyographic monitoring of extra-ocular motor nerves (nn III, VI) in skull base surgery. Acta Neurochir (Wien) 2001;143:251–61.
[23] Doikov IY, Konsulov SS, Dimov RS, et al. Stimulation electromyography as a method of intraoperative localization and identification of the facial nerve during parotidectomy: review of 15 consecutive parotid surgeries. Folia Med 2001;4:23–6.
[24] Aimoni C, Lombardi L, Gastaldo E, et al. Preoperative and postoperative electroneurographic facial nerve monitoring in patients with parotid tumors. Arch Otolaryngol Head Neck Surg 2003;129:940–3.
[25] Terrell JE, Kileny PR, Yian C, et al. Clinical outcome of continuous facial nerve monitoring during primary parotidectomy. Arch Otolaryngol Head Neck Surg 1997;123(10):1081–7.
[26] Dulguerov P, Marchal F, Lehmann W. Postparotidectomy facial nerve paralysis: possible etiologic factors and results with routine facial nerve monitoring. Laryngoscope 1999;109(5): 754–62.
[27] Roland PS. Facial nerve monitoring for non-neurotologic procedures. Otol Neurotol 2002; 23(S1):S12–3.
[28] Rosenblum BN, Benecke JA. Combined transcervical transmastoid approach to giant parotid pleomorphic adenoma: a case report. Mod Med 2001;98(7):267–9.

[29] Brennan J, Moore EJ, Shuler KJ. Prospective analysis of the efficacy of continuous intraoperative nerve monitoring during thyroidectomy, parathyroidectomy, and parotidectomy. Otolaryngol Head Neck Surg 2001;124:537–43.
[30] Witt RL. Facial nerve monitoring in parotid surgery: the standard of care? Otolaryngol Head Neck Surg 1998;119:468–70.
[31] Suchy BH, Wolf SR. Bilateral mucosa-associated lymphoid tissue lymphoma of the parotid gland. Arch Otolaryngol Head Neck Surg 2000;126:224–6.
[32] Odegard KC, Kirse DJ, del Nido PJ, et al. Intraoperative recurrent laryngeal nerve monitoring during video-assisted thoracoscopic surgery for patent ductus arteriosus. J Cardiothorac Vasc Anesthes 2000;14(5):562–4.
[33] Affleck BD, Swartz K, Brennan J. Surgical considerations and controversies in thyroid and parathyroid surgery. Otolaryngol Clin North Am 2003;36:151–87.
[34] Stechison MT. Vagus nerve monitoring: percutaneous versus vocal fold electrode recording. Am J Otol 1995;16(5):703–6.
[35] Eisele DW. Intraoperative electrophysiologic monitoring of the recurrent laryngeal nerve. Laryngoscope 1996;106:443–9.
[36] Jonas J, Bahr R. Neuromonitoring of the external branch of the superior laryngeal nerve during thyroid surgery. Am J Surg 2000;179:234–6.
[37] Thomusch O, Sekulla C, Walls G, et al. Intraoperative neuromonitoring of surgery for benign goiter. Am J Surg 2002;183:673–8.
[38] Marcus B, Edwards BM, Yoo S, et al. Recurrent laryngeal nerve monitoring in thyroid and parathyroid surgery: the University of Michigan experience. Laryngoscope 2003;113: 356–61.
[39] Otto RA, Cochran CS. Sensitivity and specificity of intraoperative recurrent laryngeal nerve stimulation in predicting postoperative nerve paralysis. Ann Otol Rhinol Laryngol 2002; 11(11):1005–7.
[40] Fewins J, Simpson CB, Miller FR. Complications of thyroid and parathyroid surgery. Otolaryngol Clin North Am 2003;36:189–206.
[41] Midwinter K, Willatt D. Accessory nerve monitoring and stimulation during neck surgery. J Laryngol Otol 2002;116:272–4.
[42] Kierner AC, Burian M, Bentzien S, et al. Intraoperative electromyography for identification of the trapezius muscle innervation: clinical proof of a new anatomical concept. Laryngoscope 2002;112:1853–6.
[43] National Institutes of Health (NIH). Acoustic neuroma. NIH consensus statement, 1991;9(4):1–24. Available at: http://consensus.nih.gov/087/087_statement.htm. Accessed May 25, 2004.
[44] Eldridge R, Parry D. Summary: Vestibular Schwannoma (acoustic neuroma) Consensus Development Conference. Neurosurgery 1992;30(6):962–4.
[45] American Academy of Otolaryngology-Head & Neck Surgery, Inc. Policy statement: facial nerve monitoring. 1998. Available at: www.entlink.net/practice/rules/facial_nerve_monitoring.cfm. Accessed May 25, 2004.
[46] Lundy L. Intraoperative facial nerve monitoring for chronic ear surgery. Abstracts of the 9th International Facial Nerve Symposium. Otol Neurotol 2004;23(S1):14.
[47] Greenberg JS, Manolidis S, Stewart MG, et al. Facial nerve monitoring in chronic ear surgery: US practice patterns. Otolaryngol Head Neck Surg 2002;126(2):108–14.
[48] Saravanappa N, Balfour A, Bowdler DA. Use of laser, otoendoscopy and facial nerve monitoring in otological surgery: United Kingdom survey. J Laryngol Otol 2003;117:751–5.
[49] Kahn JB, Gliklich RE, Boyev KP, et al. Validation of a patient-graded instrument for facial nerve paralysis: the FaCE scale. Laryngoscope 2001;111(3):387–98.
[50] Harper CM. Intraoperative cranial nerve monitoring. Muscle Nerve 2004;29:339–51.
[51] Sala F, Krzan MJ, Deletis V. Intraoperative neurophysiological monitoring in pediatric neurosurgery: why, when, how? Childs Nerv Syst 2002;18:264–87.

[52] Noss RS, Lalwani AK, Yingling CD, et al. Facial nerve monitoring in middle ear and mastoid surgery. Laryngoscope 2001;111:831–6.
[53] Edwards BM, Kileny PR. Intraoperative monitoring of cranial nerves. In: Canalis RF, Lambert PR, editors. The ear: comprehensive otology. Philadelphia: Lippincott Williams & Wilkins; 2000. p. 279–94.
[54] Holland NR. Intraoperative electromyography. J Clin Neurophysiol 2002;19(5):444–53.
[55] Barker FG, Jannetta PJ, Bissonette DJ, et al. The long-term outcome of microvascular decompression for trigeminal neuralgia. N Engl J Med 1996;334(17):1077–83.
[56] Mandpe AH, Mikulec A, Jackler RK, et al. Comparison of response amplitude versus stimulation threshold in predicting early postoperative facial nerve function after acoustic neuroma resection. Am J Otol 1998;19(1):112–7.
[57] Schwartz DM, Morris MD. Strategies for optimizing the detection of neuropathology from the auditory brainstem response. In: Jacobson JT, Northern JL, editors. Diagnostic audiology. Austin (TX): Pro-ed; 1991. p. 141–60.
[58] Lanzino G, diPierro CG, Ruth RA, et al. Recovery of useful hearing after posterior fossa surgery: the role of otoacoustic emissions: case report. Neurosurgery 1997;41(2):469–73.
[59] Schaffer LA, Withnell RH, Dhar S, et al. Sources and mechanisms of DPOAE generation: implications for the prediction of auditory sensitivity. Ear Hear 2003;24:367–9.
[60] Widick MP, Telischi FF, Lonsbury-Martin BL, et al. Early effects of cerebellopontine angle compression on rabbit distortion-product otoacoustic emissions: a model for monitoring cochlear function during acoustic neuroma surgery. Otolaryngol Head Neck Surg 1994; 111(4):407–16.
[61] Kileny PR, Edwards BM, Disher MJ, et al. Hearing improvement after resection of cerebellopontine angle meningioma: case study of the preoperative role of transient evoked otoacoustic emissions. J Am Acad Audiol 1998;9(4):251–6.
[62] Telishi FF, Roth J, Stagner BB, et al. Patterns of otoacoustic emissions associated with acoustic neuromas. Laryngoscope 1995;105:675–83.
[63] Robinette MS, Bauch CD, Olsen WO, et al. Nonsurgical factors predictive of postoperative hearing for patients with vestibular schwannoma. Am J Otol 1997;18:738–45.
[64] Robinette MS. Clinical observations with evoked otoacoustic emissions. J Am Acad Audiol 2003;14:213–24.
[65] Legatt AD. Mechanisms of intraoperative brainstem auditory evoked potential changes. J Clin Neurophysiol 2002;19(5):396–408.
[66] Kileny PR, Edwards BM. Intraoperative cranial nerve monitoring. Semin Anesth 1997; 16(1):36–45.
[67] Martin WH, Mishler ET. Intraoperative monitoring of auditory evoked potentials and facial nerve electromyography. In: Katz J, editor. Handbook of clinical audiology. 5th edition. Philadelphia: Lippincott Williams & Wilkins; 2002. p. 323–48.
[68] Zappia JJ, Wiet RJ, O'Connor CA, et al. Intraoperative auditory monitoring in acoustic neuroma surgery. Otolaryngol Head Neck Surg 1996;115(1):98–106.
[69] Schmerber S, Lavielle JP, Dumas G, et al. Intraoperative auditory monitoring vestibular schwannoma surgery: new trends. Acta Otolaryngol 2004;124:53–61.
[70] Jackson LE, Roberson JB. Acoustic neuroma surgery: use of cochlear nerve action potential monitoring for hearing preservation. Am J Otol 2000;21:249–59.

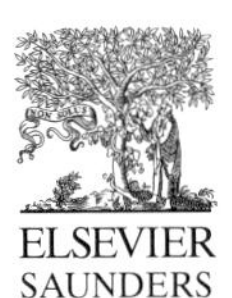
ELSEVIER
SAUNDERS

Otolaryngol Clin N Am
38 (2005) 643–652

OTOLARYNGOLOGIC
CLINICS
OF NORTH AMERICA

Counseling Patients on Surgical Options for Treating Acoustic Neuroma

Wayne J. Harsha, MD[a],
Douglas D. Backous, MD, FACS[b,c,*]

[a]*Otolaryngology–Head & Neck Surgery Service, Madigan Army Medical Center, Tacoma, WA, USA*
[b]*Department of Otology, Neurotology and Skull Base Surgery, Virginia Mason Medical Center, 1100 Ninth Avenue, Seattle, WA 98111, USA*
[c]*The Listen For Life Center at Virginia Mason, Virginia Mason Medical Center, 1100 Ninth Avenue, Seattle, WA 98111, USA*

Vestibular schwannomas, known more commonly as acoustic neuromas (AN), are benign tumors of Schwann cell origin that emanate from the superior or inferior vestibular nerves. AN have an average growth rate of 1 mm^3 per year, so observation with interval MRI scanning every 6 to 12 months is an option for a select subset of patients. Since Cushing's first report of successful removal of an AN through a suboccipital approach, however, surgical techniques have evolved to provide safe removal of acoustic tumors with preservation of cranial nerve function. In the last 3 decades, radiotherapy, using single-dose or fractionated regimens, has gained popularity as a definitive treatment option for these patients. Unfortunately, few studies comparing long-term results of surgery and radiotherapy with standard dosing protocols exist to assist in advising patients as to choice of therapy. Wackym addresses the topic of radiotherapy versus surgery elsewhere in this issue.

For patients who choose to have the tumor removed surgically, there are three principle approaches: the translabyrinthine (TLA), the retrosigmoid (RSA), and the middle cranial fossa (MCF). Two of these approaches, the MCF approach and the RSA, have the potential for hearing preservation, whereas the TLA usually sacrifices residual preoperative hearing.

* Corresponding author. Department of Otolaryngology-Head and Neck Surgery, 1100 Ninth Avenue, X10-0N, Seattle, WA 98111.
E-mail address: otoddb@vmmc.org (D.D. Backous).

doi:10.1016/j.otc.2005.01.006 **oto.theclinics.com**

The MCF approach is most suitable for the removal of predominantly intracanalicular tumors with minimal ($\leq$0.5 cm) extension into the cerebellopontine angle (CPA) in patients who have serviceable preoperative hearing. Recent articles report on the extended MCF approach for the removal of AN with medial extension of >1.0 cm. The MCF approach provides excellent exposure of the internal auditory canal (IAC) with the exception of the far lateral aspect, below the transverse crest, where small amounts of tumor can be left because of poor visualization in this area. The superior-directed entry into the IAC afforded by the MCF approach often necessitates more manipulation of the facial nerve during tumor removal than necessary with other approaches. The risk of new-onset temporal lobe seizures following prolonged retraction during removal of acoustic tumors using the MCF approach has been reported; diligent surveillance of the duration of retractor use is required to prevent this complication. The MCF approach is relatively contraindicated in patients over 65 years of age because of the thinning of the dura and the subsequent increased risk of cerebrospinal fluid (CSF) leakage.

The RSA is indicated primarily in patients who have serviceable hearing but whose tumor extends more than 0.5 cm into the CPA (ie, beyond the limits of tumor resection using the MCF approach). Because of the clear visibility and access to the brainstem and critical vasculature, this combined neurotologic/neurosurgical approach is also useful for removal of large tumors extending into the inferior CPA regardless of hearing status. As in the MCF approach, there is limited access to the far lateral IAC.

Since its introduction in 1960 by William F. House, the TLA remains a popular approach to the internal auditory canal for neurotologists. The TLA is indicated for tumors of any size in patients without serviceable hearing. It is particularly useful for the removal of tumors with lateral IAC extension in patients with poor hearing. Absolute contraindications include the desire for an attempt at hearing preservation or the removal of an acoustic tumor in an only-hearing ear. The exception is in cases of neurofibromatosis type II, when the TLA can be combined with placement of an auditory brainstem implant. Access to the CPA is remarkable, and tumors as large as 6 cm have been removed through a combined translabyrinthine/transotic approach. The TLA offers the best access to the lateral IAC and labyrinthine segment of the facial nerve.

Three principle factors determine the choice of surgical approach: surgical outcomes, complication rates, and the training and comfort level of the skull base team. The three main outcome measures used for comparing the approaches are long-term facial nerve function, rate of hearing preservation, and postoperative balance function. Because no standard exists for the reporting of postoperative vestibular impairment, the literature on this subject is scarce, and this issue is not discussed in this article. The three most frequent complications are CSF leakage, meningitis, and postoperative headache. The familiarity with specific approaches and skill of the skull base team (consisting of a neurotologist, neurosurgeon, neuroanesthesiologist, and neuro-monitoring team) are extremely important factors in choosing an approach.

This article reviews selected articles in the recent English-language literature on reported surgical outcomes and complications to provide the general otolaryngologist with a logical outline for counseling patients about surgical options for AN removal before referral to a skull base team. The article is not intended as a meta-analysis or a comprehensive review of the literature on AN surgery.

Methods

The authors performed a broad search of Medline for all articles pertaining to AN surgery, complications, and therapy published between 1994 and 2004. They found 1132 articles. They then restricted the search to include only English-language articles published on human data. Any articles pertaining to radiotherapy or observation were then eliminated, reducing the number of articles to 517. They reviewed these references and eliminated any review articles, articles on classification systems, on specific operative techniques, and on outcome predictive factors. The remaining abstracts were evaluated, and articles were chosen based on the following criteria:

1. Facial nerve outcomes were reported using the American Academy of Otolaryngology–Head & Neck Surgery (AAO-HNS)/House-Brackmann grading scale at the 6- to 12-month postoperative visit.
2. Postoperative hearing was reported using either the AAO-HNS scale or the Gardner-Robertson scale.
3. Complication rates were reported based on the approach used. Articles were excluded if outcomes and complications were not specifically referenced to the surgical approach used.

A total of 31 articles were chosen using these criteria, 14 of which compared one or more outcome measures or complication rates with different approaches within the same institution. The remainder reported outcomes or complications from a single surgical approach.

Outcomes

Hearing preservation

The authors define serviceable hearing as a four-frequency pure-tone average of better than 50 dB and a speech-discrimination score (SDS) of 50% or better (the "50/50 rule"). This definition corresponds to the AAO-HNS classification of class A or B hearing (Table 1), which is generally

Table 1
Classifications of hearing

	American Academy of Otolaryngology–Head & Neck Surgery Classification	
Class	Pure Tone Average (0.5, 1, 2, 3 kHz)	Speech Discrimination Score (%)
A	0–30 dB HL	70–100
B	31–50 dB HL	50–100
C	>50 dB HL	50–100
D	Any	<50
	Gardner-Robertson Classification	
Class	Pure Tone Average/Speech Reception Threshold	Speech Discrimination Score (%)
1	0–30 dB HL	70–100
2	31–50 dB HL	50–69
3	51–90 dB HL	5–49
4	>90	1–4

accepted as a good hearing outcome following AN surgery. An alternative reporting standard is the Gardner-Robertson hearing classification, in which class 1 patients have a speech reception threshold of 30 dB or less and a SDS of 70% to 100%, and class 2 patients have a speech reception threshold of 31 to 50 dB and a SDS of 50% to 69%. Thus, AAO-HNS class A/B hearing and Gardner-Robertson Class 1/2 hearing are comparable.

Sixteen articles reporting the rate of good hearing outcome (either AAO-HNS class A/B or Gardner-Robertson class 1/2) following AN removal were reviewed [1–16]. In all of these series, tumor removal and hearing preservation were a main goal of the operations. The overall rate of serviceable hearing preservation was 44% (662/1507 patients). The rate of hearing preservation was considerably higher in the group in which the MCF approach was used (53%, 479/896 patients) than in group in which the RSA approach was used (30%, 183/611 patients). Six of these articles compared the rate of hearing preservation for the MCF approach and the RSA within a given institution [1–6]. Ninety-six of 198 patients (48%) who underwent the MCF approach maintained serviceable hearing postoperatively, versus 62 of 202 patients (31%) operated on with the RSA. Eleven of these 16 articles reported the hearing results for each AAO-HNS hearing class (Table 2) [1–3,5–7,9–11,14,15]. Class A hearing was preserved in 210 of 830 patients (25%) in the MCF group and in 45 of 304 patients (15%) in the RSA group. Class B hearing was maintained by 220 of 830 patients (27%) in the MCF group and 50 of 304 patients (16%) in the RSA group. Five articles reported the outcomes of more than 100 patients operated on using a single approach [7,9,11,12,14]. Again, the rate of class A or B hearing preservation was considerably higher in the MCF group (56%, 342/611 patients) than in the RSA group (28%, 96/348 patients). These results are not controlled for preoperative hearing levels or tumor size, both of which have been linked with surgical outcome.

Table 2
Hearing outcomes (using AAO-HNS class A/B or Gardner-Robertson class 1/2) in the middle cranial fossa and retrosigmoid approaches to acoustic neuroma removal in papers reporting all classifications

	Postoperative Hearing Classification # Patients (%)			
Author [Reference #]	A/1	B/2	C/3	D/4
Middle cranial fossa approach				
Colletti [1]	3 (12)	10 (40)	3 (12)	9 (36)
Staecker [2]	5 (33)	3 (20)	2 (13)	5 (33)
Hecht [3]	4 (22)	3 (17)	1 (5)	10 (56)
Arriaga [4]	15 (44)	8 (24)	2 (6)	9 (26)
Sanna [6]	4 (7)	15 (26)	10 (17)	30 (50)
Slattery [7]	35 (25)	39 (27)	5 (4)	64 (45)
Brackmann [9]	109 (33)	87 (26)	16 (5)	121 (36)
Weber [10]	5 (10)	13 (27)	3 (6)	28 (57)
Satar [11]	30 (22)	42 (31)	18 (13)	64 (34)
Total	210 (25)	220 (27)	60 (7)	340 (41)
Retrosigmoid approach				
Colletti [1]	2 (8)	8 (32)	4 (16)	11 (44)
Staecker [2]	6 (40)	1 (7)	1 (7)	7 (46)
Hecht [3]	4 (10)	5 (12)	4 (10)	29 (68)
Arriaga [5]	8 (31)	6 (23)	1 (4)	11 (42)
Sanna [6]	8 (18)	7 (16)	4 (9)	29 (66)
Magnan [14]	17 (15)	18 (16)	23 (19)	61 (51)
Lassaletta [15]	0 (0)	5 (17)	1 (3)	23 (79)
Total	45 (15)	50 (16)	38 (13)	171 (56)
Overall total	255 (22)	270 (24)	98 (9)	511 (45)

Facial nerve preservation

The AAO-HNS (House-Brackmann) facial nerve grading scale is the standard for reporting facial nerve outcomes following AN surgery. Generally, good postoperative facial nerve function is defined as grade I/II at the 6- to 12-month postoperative visit; intermediate facial nerve function is considered grade III/IV motion; and poor facial nerve function is grade V or VI.

The authors reviewed 19 articles that reported facial nerve grading using the AAO-HNS scale at the 6- to 12-month postoperative visit [1,2,4,6,7,10, 11,13,14,16–25]. The overall rate of grade I/II facial nerve outcome was 82% (1723/2101 patients). Ninety-two percent of the RSA patients had good facial function, compared with 89% of the MCF patients and 73% of the TLA patients. Fourteen of the 19 papers reported facial nerve outcomes by each AAO-HNS grade (Table 3) [1,6,7,10,11,13,14,17–19,20,22,24,25]. Grade I (normal) function was seen in 432 of 571 patients (76%) in the MCF group, in 248 of 298 patients (83%) in the RSA group, and in 545 of 921 patients (59%) in the TLA group. In the only article that reported facial nerve outcomes from all three approaches within the same institution, the RSA had a higher rate of good outcomes (91%) than did the MCF (88%)

Table 3
Facial nerve outcomes (AAO-HNS/House-Brackmann grade) at 6 to 12 months with the middle cranial fossa, retrosigmoid, and translabyrinthine approaches to acoustic neuroma removal

	AAO-HNS facial nerve outcome # of patients (%)					
Author [Reference #]	I	II	III	IV	V	VI
Middle cranial fossa approach						
Colletti [1]	16 (64)	4 (16)	3 (12)	2 (8)	-	-
Holsinger [17]	31 (89)	4 (11)	-	-	-	-
Arriaga [18]	40 (69)	11 (19)	5 (9)	1 (2)	1 (2)	-
Sanna [6]	22 (39)	7 (13)	26 (47)	1 (2)	-	-
Slattery [7]	120 (82)	19 (13)	6 (4)	2 (1)	-	-
Weber [10]	37 (76)	9 (18)	2 (4)	1 (2)	-	-
Arriaga [19]	41 (85)	5 (10)	2 (4)	-	-	-
Satar [11]	125 (82)	14 (9)	12 (8)	1 (1)	-	1 (1)
Total	432 (76)	73 (13)	56 (10)	8 (1)	1 (0)	1 (0)
Retrosigmoid approach						
Colletti [1]	20 (80)	3 (12)	2 (8)	-	-	-
Holsinger [17]	11 (92)	1 (8)	-	-	-	-
Arriaga [18]	40 (87)	2 (4)	1 (2)	-	1 (2)	2 (4)
Sanna [6]	34 (83)	5 (12)	2 (5)	-	-	-
Ho [20]	24 (69)	3 (9)	5 (14)	2 (6)	-	1 (3)
Mamikoglu [13]	9 (53)	1 (6)	4 (24)	1 (6)	1 (6)	1 (6)
Magnan [14]	110 (92)	5 (4)	2 (2)	1 (1)	-	-
Total	248 (83)	20 (7)	16 (5)	4 (1)	2 (1)	4(1)
Translabyrinthine approach						
Arriaga [18]	125 (62)	31 (15)	25 (12)	8 (4)	3 (1)	11 (5)
Ho [20]	24 (69)	3 (9)	5 (14)	2 (6)	-	1 (3)
Mamikoglu [13]	43 (54)	11 (14)	9 (11)	3 (4)	2 (3)	11 (14)
Arriaga [19]	86 (74)	20 (17)	6 (5)	3 (3)	-	1 (1)
Lanman [22]	31 (33)	19 (20)	13 (14)	14 (15)	6 (6)	12 (13)
Andersson [24]	74 (55)	22 (16)	19 (14)	7 (5)	5 (4)	8 (6)
Mass [25]	162 (63)	34 (13)	30 (12)	16 (6)	7 (3)	9 (3)
Total	545 (59)	140 (15)	107 (12)	53 (6)	23 (2)	53 (6)
Overall total	1225 (69)	233 (13)	179 (10)	65 (4)	26 (1)	58 (3)

or the TLA (77%) [18]. When only the high-volume centers (>100 cases reported for each approach) were considered, the RSA patients continued to have the best outcome, with 97% (115/119) recovering grade I or grade II function, compared with 93% (278/300) MCF patients, and 78% (554/712) TLA patients [7,11,14,18,19,24,25]. Again, these results were irrespective of tumor size, which has been linked to outcome.

Complications

Cerebrospinal fluid leakage

CSF leakage is the most common complication following AN removal. This complication typically occurs within the first 2 to 3 days or later, at 10 to 14 days postoperatively, and may manifest as either wound leakage or CSF rhinorrhea. In pooling the data from 17 studies, the authors found 345 instances of CSF leakage in 4064 patients (8%) (Table 4) [2,7,10,13–15, 21–31]. The rate of CSF leakage was slightly lower in the MCF group (6%) than in the TLA group (9%) or the RSA group (11%). Three articles compared the rate of CSF leakage in all three approaches performed within the respective institutions [26–28]. The rate of CSF leakage at these three centers was 6% in the MCF group (37/588 patients), 8% in the TLA group (158/1925 patients), and 13% in the RSA group (20/158 patients). Slattery [28] reported data from the largest cohort (1697 patients) and found that 15% of the RSA group, 11% of the TLA group, and 6% of the MCF group

Table 4
Cerebrospinal fluid leak, meningitis, and postoperative headache in the different approaches to acoustic neuroma removal

Author [Reference #]	CSF Leak #/n (%)	Meningitis #/n (%)	Postoperative Headache #/n (%)
Middle cranial fossa approach			
Sanna [26]	2/54 (4)		
Becker [27]	10/100 (10)		
Slattery [28]	25/434 (6)		
Slattery [7]	9/151 (7)	3/151 (2)	
Staecker [2]	3/15 (20)		3/15 (20)
Weber [10]	3/49 (6)		2/49 (4)
Total	52/803 (6)	3/151 (2)	5/64 (8)
Retrosigmoid approach			
Sanna [26]	7/38 (18)	1/38 (3)	
Becker [27]	10/100 (10)		
Slattery [28]	3/20 (15)		
Mamikoglu [13]	0/17 (0)		
Brennan [29]	4/75 (5)		
Lassaletta [15]	10/65 (15)		
Yamakami [21]	2/50 (4)		
Staecker [2]	4/15 (27)		7/15 (47)
Magnan [14]			2/119 (2)
Schaller [30]			52/155 (33)
Total	40/380 (11)	1/38 (3)	61/289 (21)
Translabyrinthine approach			
Sanna [26]	11/600 (2)		
Becker [27]	13/100 (13)		
Slattery [28]	135/1225 (11)		
Brennan [29]	20/228 (9)		
Celikkanat [31]	8/129 (6)		
Mamikoglu [13]	7/81 (9)		
Mamikoglu [23]	12/70 (17)	3/70 (4)	
Lanman [22]	27/190 (14)	7/190 (4)	
Mass [25]	20/258 (8)	4/258 (2)	3/258 (1)
Andersson [24]			8/135 (6)
Total	253/2881 (9)	14/518 (3)	11/393 (3)
Overall total	345/4064 (8)	18/707 (3)	77/746 (10)

had postoperative CSF leakage. In a recent meta-analysis, however, Selesnick [32] found that the rate of CSF leakage was equal (10.6%) in the RSA and the MCF groups and lowest in the TLA group (9.5%).

Meningitis

The incidence of bacterial meningitis has decreased dramatically with the use of prophylactic perioperative intravenous antibiotics and antibiotic irrigation. Aseptic meningitis is more common and is believed to be caused by blood or bone dust in the subarachnoid space. Five recent papers reported the rate of meningitis following AN removal (Table 4) [7,22,23,25,26]. The rate of meningitis was 2% following the MCF approach, 3% following the RSA, and 3% following the TLA. The highest rate reported in these articles was 4% [22,23]. The authors did not find a single report comparing the incidence of meningitis in the three approaches.

Headache

Headaches are common in the immediate postoperative period and represent a form of postoperative pain. Prolonged postoperative headaches are defined as those persisting at least 3 months after surgery. Unfortunately, there is no uniform system for reporting the severity and frequency of postoperative headache; therefore, the literature varies widely in the reported incidence of this troublesome complication.

The authors found six articles reporting an overall 10% incidence of persistent headache (in 77/746 patients) following AN surgery (Table 4) [2,10,14,24,25,30]. The rate of postoperative headache following the RSA (21%) was more than double that for the MCF approach (8%) and seven times higher than that of the TLA (3%). In the only article comparing the rate of postoperative headache following the MCF approach and the RSA, Staecker [2] found that 20% of patients experienced troublesome headaches following the MCF versus 47% following the RSA.

Summary

The selection of surgical approach for the removal of AN is a complex one, depending on factors related to specific tumor anatomy, patient characteristics, and the familiarity and skill level of the skull base team. Overall, the literature supports that surgical outcomes are acceptable in regard to tumor removal, patient safety, and complication rates. The inconsistent reporting methods in the current literature make it difficult to assess logically the rates for hearing preservation, facial nerve outcome, and complications as controlled for tumor size and other preoperative patient characteristics. The best conclusions would be from prospective surgical trials controlling for patient factors, size of the tumor, and experience of the skull base team. In the absence of such studies, formal meta-analyses may help clarify specific differences among approaches.

References

[1] Colletti V, Fiorino F. Middle fossa versus retrosigmoid-transmeatal approach in vestibular schwannoma surgery: a prospective study. Otol Neurotol 2003;24:927–34.
[2] Staecker H, Nadol J, Ojeman R, et al. Hearing preservation in acoustic neuroma surgery: middle fossa versus retrosigmoid approach. Am J Otol 2000;21(3):399–404.
[3] Hecht C, Honrubia V, Wiet R, et al. Hearing preservation after acoustic neuroma resection with tumor size used as a clinical prognosticator. Laryngoscope 1997;107:1122–6.
[4] Irving R, Jackler R, Pitts L. Hearing preservation in patients undergoing vestibular schwannoma surgery: comparison of middle fossa and retrosigmoid approaches. J Neurosurg 1998;88:840–5.
[5] Arriaga M, Chen D. Facial function in hearing preservation acoustic neuroma surgery. Arch Otolaryngol Head Neck Surg 2001;127:543–6.
[6] Sanna M, Khrais T, Piccirillo E, et al. Hearing preservation surgery in vestibular schwannoma: the hidden truth. Ann Otol Rhinol Laryngol 2004;113:156–63.
[7] Slattery W, Brackmann D, Hitselberger W. Middle fossa approach for hearing preservation with acoustic neuromas. Am J Otol 1997;18:596–601.
[8] Friedman R, Kesser B, Brackmann D, et al. Long-term hearing preservation after middle fossa removal of vestibular schwannoma. Otolaryngol Head Neck Surg 2003;129(6):660–5.
[9] Brackmann D, Owens R, Friedman R, et al. Prognostic factors for hearing preservation in vestibular schwannoma surgery. Am J Otol 2000;21(3):417–24.
[10] Weber P, Gantz B. Results and complications from acoustic neuromas excision via middle cranial fossa approach. Am J Otol 1996;17:669–75.
[11] Satar B, Jackler R, Oghalai J, et al. Risk-benefit analysis of using the middle fossa approach for acoustic neuromas with >10 mm cerebellopontine angle component. Laryngoscope 2002;112:1500–6.
[12] Tonn J, Schlake H, Goldbrunner R, et al. Acoustic neuromas surgery as an interdisciplinary approach: a neurosurgical series of 508 patients. J Neurol Neurosurg Psychiatry 2000;69: 161–6.
[13] Mamikoglu B, Esquivel C, Wiet R. Comparison of facial nerve function results after translabyrinthine and retrosigmoid approach in medium-sized tumors. Arch Otolaryngol Head Neck Surg 2003;129:429–31.
[14] Magnan J, Barbieri M, Mora R, et al. Retrosigmoid approach for small and medium-sized acoustic neuromas. Otol Neurotol 2002;23:141–5.
[15] Lassaletta L, Fontes L, Melcon E, et al. Hearing preservation with the retrosigmoid approach for vestibular schwannoma: myth or reality? Otolaryngol Head Neck Surg 2003; 129(4):397–401.
[16] Mangham C. Retrosigmoid versus middle fossa surgery for small vestibular schwannoma. Laryngoscope 2004;114:1455–61.
[17] Holsinger F, Coker C, Newton J, et al. Hearing preservation in conservation surgery for vestibular schwannoma. Am J Otol 2000;21(5):695–700.
[18] Arriaga M, Chen D, Fukushima T. Individualized hearing preservation in acoustic neuroma surgery. Laryngoscope 1997;107:1043–7.
[19] Arriaga M, Luxford W, Berliner K. Facial nerve function following middle fossa and translabyrinthine acoustic tumor surgery: a comparison. Am J Otol 1994;15(5):620–4.
[20] Ho S, Hudgens S, Wiet R. Comparison of postoperative facial nerve outcomes between translabyrinthine and retrosigmoid approaches in matched-pair patients. Laryngoscope 2003;113(11):2014–20.

[21] Yamakami I, Uchino Y, Kobayashi E, et al. Removal of large acoustic neurinomas (vestibular schwannomas) by the retrosigmoid approach with no mortality and minimal morbidity. J Neurol Neurosurg Psychiatry 2004;75:453–8.
[22] Lanman T, Brackmann D, Hitselberger W, et al. Report of 190 consecutive cases of large acoustic tumors (vestibular schwannoma) removed via the translabyrinthine approach. J Neurosurg 1999;90:617–23.
[23] Mamikoglu B, Wiet R, Esquivel C. Translabyrinthine approach for the management of large and giant vestibular schwannoma. Otol Neurotol 2002;23(2):224–7.
[24] Andersson G, Ekvall L, Kinnefors A, et al. Evaluation of quality of life and symptoms after translabyrinthine acoustic neuroma surgery. Am J Otol 1997;18(4):421–6.
[25] Mass S, Wiet R, Dinces E. Complications of the translabyrinthine approach for the removal of acoustic neuromas. Arch Otolaryngol Head Neck Surg 1999;125:801–4.
[26] Sanna M, Taibah A, Russo A, et al. Perioperative complications in acoustic neuroma (vestibular schwannoma) surgery. Otol Neurotol 2004;25(3):379–86.
[27] Becker S, Jackler R, Pitts L. Cerebrospinal fluid leak after acoustic neuroma surgery: a comparison of the translabyrinthine, middle fossa, and retrosigmoid approaches. Otol Neurotol 2003;24(1):107–12.
[28] Slattery W, Sabina F, House K. Perioperative morbidity of acoustic neuroma surgery. Otol Neurotol 2001;22(6):895–902.
[29] Brennan J, Rowed D, Nedzelski J, et al. Cerebrospinal fluid leak after acoustic neuroma surgery: influence of tumor size and surgical approach on incidence and response to treatment. J Neurosurg 2001;94:217–23.
[30] Schaller B, Baumann A. Headache after removal of vestibular schwannoma via the retrosigmoid approach: a long-term follow-up-study. Otolaryngol Head Neck Surg 2003; 128(3):387–95.
[31] Cellikkanat S, Saleh E, Khashaba A, et al. Cerebrospinal fluid leak after translabyrinthine acoustic neuroma surgery. Otolaryngol Head Neck Surg 1995;112(6):654–8.
[32] Selesnick S, Liu J, Jen A, et al. The incidence of cerebrospinal fluid leak after vestibular schwannoma surgery. Otol Neurotol 2004;25:387–93.

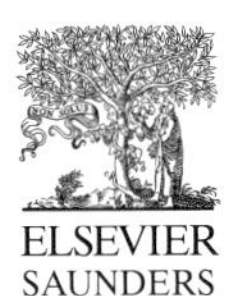

ELSEVIER
SAUNDERS

Otolaryngol Clin N Am
38 (2005) 653–670

OTOLARYNGOLOGIC
CLINICS
OF NORTH AMERICA

Stereotactic Radiosurgery, Microsurgery, and Expectant Management of Acoustic Neuroma: Basis for Informed Consent

P. Ashley Wackym, MD, FACS, FAAP

Department of Otolaryngology and Communication Sciences, Medical College of Wisconsin Milwaukee, 9200 West Wisconsin Avenue, Milwaukee WI 53226, USA

There are three primary treatment options available to patients with acoustic neuroma: expectant management, stereotactic radiation, and microsurgical resection. With the exception of patients with extremely large tumors producing hydrocephalus, patients always have time to decide which option they wish to select. The selection is a personal decision that must be made after thorough discussion of all available options. Each patient must first understand and then weigh the advantages and disadvantages of each management option. A dogmatic approach to patient counseling is inappropriate and dangerous, particularly if this approach is used by a surgeon who does not have direct experience in all categories of treatment.

Informed consent issues

Optimal outcome in managing patients with acoustic neuroma is facilitated by experienced multidisciplinary teams. A balanced discussion of all three options is essential, and direct experience with all options is ideal. Too often surgeons are biased toward one modality and allow these biases to taint their presentation to patients and their families. Worldwide, for historical reasons, centers of excellence have evolved that are primarily focused on either microsurgery or radiosurgery. There is typically polarization within each center. In some centers, the surgeons most experienced in radiosurgery of acoustic neuromas do not perform microsurgical resection of acoustic neuromas, whereas in other centers a tremendous experience in microsurgery

E-mail address: wackym@mcw.edu

doi:10.1016/j.otc.2005.03.018 **oto.theclinics.com**

coexists with lack of experience with radiosurgery. Although it could be argued that strength in one area is adequate; an increasing number of medicolegal judgments have been based on inadequate informed consent, particularly related to an uneven presentation of options.

In the author's experience, a typical detailed informed consent discussion requires approximately 60 minutes. In addition, the author sends patients home with three documents that summarize the discussion and usually raise additional questions that are important for patients to consider when making the decision. It is important to document this discussion and the written or web-based resources provided to each patient in the medical record. The three documents that the author provides are two chapters from the Jackler and Brackmann textbook *Neurotology*—the Jackler and Pfister [1] chapter on acoustic neuroma and the Wackym and Runge-Samuelson [2] chapter on radiosurgery of skull base tumors [2]—and the Acoustic Neuroma Association's brochure on acoustic neuroma [3]. In addition, the author points out the URL of the Acoustic Neuroma Association website (www.anausa.org), which can be found on the back cover of the brochure. The content of these materials represents the general areas of discussion and allows reinforcement of these issues once the patient leaves the office and refocuses consideration of which path to follow. Covering all of the relevant issues in detail is beyond the scope of this article. Instead, this article focuses on radiosurgery in the context of surgical or expectant management considerations.

General considerations

Decision-making for patients with acoustic neuromas is complex and must be individualized. Patients, except for those with very large acoustic neuromas, can select any of the three available options depending on their assessment of the relative advantages or disadvantages of each option, including the potential complications associated each clinical pathway. In addition to outcomes data and expectations, a large number of variables that affect outcome must be taken into account: tumor size, tumor position, patient age, neurofibromatosis type 2 (NF2), cystic tumor, only hearing ear, growth rate, degree of hearing loss, auditory brainstem response (ABR) wave morphology, and degree of vestibular loss. These key variables are important because they may affect the likelihood of an undesirable complication in a given patient. For example, with tumors larger than 1.5 cm in maximum axial dimension within the cerebellopontine angle (CPA), the risk of facial nerve injury is greater with microsurgical removal than with some forms of stereotactic radiosurgery. If the tumor is cystic, however, the facial nerve is at higher risk with microsurgery than with solid tumors. Likewise, a patient with a tumor confined to the internal auditory canal (IAC) and extending laterally into the fundus has a lower chance of hearing preservation than a patient with a medially based tumor, especially if poor wave morphology is seen on preoperative ABR.

In general terms, patients who select expectant management or radiosurgery must be comfortable living with the tumor. For several years, these patients undergo gadolinium-enhanced MRIs at 6-month intervals to determine tumor size over time. Based on new early outcomes data reported by this author [4], patients selecting Gamma Knife (Elekta AB, Stockholm, Sweden) radiosurgery must also understand that hearing and balance outcomes over time are generally reduced but variable (and some patients experience improvement), that there is a very low rate of facial nerve dysfunction and an excellent rate of tumor control, and that the surgery is an outpatient procedure with minimal disruption of the patient's personal life. Patients undergoing radiosurgery must also recognize that facial nerve outcome will be compromised in the unlikely event that microsurgical intervention is necessary in future years and that the largest tumor that can be treated is 3 cm in maximum axial diameter within the CPA. The principle advantage of microsurgery is that complete tumor resection may be achieved; however, this advantage comes at a cost of longer postoperative recovery, risk of headache, cerebrospinal fluid (CSF) leakage, and other surgical risks that are discussed later. With expectant management, the patient must understand the natural history of acoustic neuromas, including the fact that hearing will deteriorate over time or may drop suddenly.

Expectant management

Expectant management may be an excellent option, particularly for older patients and patients with a small acoustic neuroma. Assessment of growth rate over time may suggest that the tumor will never reach a size that places a patient into a higher risk category if they later select radiosurgery or microsurgery. Of course, this advantage must be tempered by the increased medical risks associated with delaying treatment into advanced age. The other major advantage is that expectant management allows ample time for the patient to work through the decision-making process.

Microsurgical resection

Optimal results in microsurgical resection of acoustic neuromas are obtained by experienced surgical teams in centers that maintain an institutional commitment to providing comprehensive care to this special patient population. The results of the surgeon who occasionally sees an acoustic neuroma cannot be compared with the outcomes of experienced surgical teams. Because there are so many issues to consider with microsurgical resection of acoustic neuromas, this article focuses on major complications unique to microsurgery. Complete and detailed discussions of these potential complications are beyond the scope of this article, as are discussions regarding rehabilitation options [1]. The fundamental advantage of microsurgical resection is that the tumor, if it is completely removed, will not recur.

The five most common major complications are hearing loss, CSF leakage, facial nerve injury, headache, and meningitis. Aside from meningitis, the surgical approach affects the likelihood of each of these complications. In addition, the size of the tumor is a major variable affecting outcome of the five most common major complications.

The three approaches used to resect acoustic neuromas are the middle fossa approach, the retrosigmoid (suboccipital) approach, and the translabyrinthine approach. The approach chosen depends on level of preoperative hearing, size of the tumor, position of the tumor, and experience of the team with each approach. The patient must understand that all these variables affect potential outcomes. For example, the "50:50 rule" (50 dB speech reception threshold and 50% speech discrimination score) is a standard guideline used to recommend that an approach with a goal of hearing preservation not be used. Values equal to or worse than this guideline lead to a recommendation that a patient to consider a translabyrinthine approach and resection of the tumor, resulting in an expected complete loss of hearing. Patients with useful hearing and a tumor wedged in the fundus of the internal auditory canal, however, may opt for a translabyrinthine approach and sacrifice hearing in exchange for lower risk of recidivistic tumor and lower risk to facial nerve function. One indication for using the middle fossa approach is the presence of such a tumor in a patient with useful hearing. The falciform crest, however, obscures the inferior half of the fundus [6,7], creating a pocket that cannot be visualized, which on average was found to be 1.82 × 2.33 mm. Thus, a patient with distal extension of the tumor, particularly if it is an inferior vestibular nerve tumor, may decide against the middle fossa approach because of concern for recidivism. The same patient may elect to undergo a retrosigmoid approach because the risk of facial nerve injury is lower than with the middle fossa approach or choose a translabyrinthine approach and sacrifice hearing in exchange for lower likelihood of recidivism and facial nerve injury. The retrosigmoid approach has the same disadvantage as the middle fossa approach, in that the distal internal auditory canal cannot be completely exposed, and an average unexposed length of 3 mm (32% of the internal auditory canal length) has been reported by Blevins and Jackler [8]. In a series of 108 patients undergoing acoustic neuroma resection by the retrosigmoid approach with adjunctive use of endoscopy, the author and colleagues [9] found that 19 patients (18%) had residual tumor at the fundus that was not seen with the operating microscope. These findings are similar to those reported in an earlier series [10]. In all of these patients, the residual tumor was removed endoscopically.

The goal of hearing preservation is confounded by a complicated set of issues. Tumor size is an important predictive factor in hearing preservation, but so are the position of the tumor within the IAC and preoperative hearing levels. Preoperative ABR is helpful in determining the ability to monitor auditory function during surgery. An additional technical challenge is that the observed delay or reduced amplitude of wave V temporally relative to the event that resulted in this change is a significant limitation of this intraoperative monitoring technique. Microvascular damage to the cochlear nerve or the cochlea is possible and can result in reduced or lost hearing during acoustic neuroma resection. Vasospasm, stretch injury of the cochlear nerve, shear injury of axons at the level of the habenula perforata, infiltration of the acoustic neuroma into the cochlear nerve, postoperative cochlear nerve edema, and thrombosis of the labyrinthine artery are all potential mechanisms of hearing loss during acoustic neuroma resection. Typically, guidelines for counseling a patient with "useful hearing" to consider a hearing preservation approach would be better than a 30-dB speech reception threshold and a 70% speech discrimination score. A normal ABR is also a good prognostic sign for attempting hearing preservation, whereas an abnormal and distorted ABR in the face of good hearing is a poor prognostic sign. The quality of preoperative hearing varies among centers and depends on the size of tumor, the point (early or late) in the natural history of the tumor that diagnosis is made, and the sense of urgency that the patient feels in evaluating unilateral hearing loss or tinnitus. With these factors in mind, approximately 10% to 15% of all acoustic neuroma patients in the author's practice who seriously consider microsurgical removal of the tumor are potential candidates for attempting hearing preservation. In the patient with the best prognostic factors—small tumor, medial position within the IAC, excellent hearing, normal ABR, and normal medical history—the chance of preserving hearing is approximately 50% whether the tumor is resected by the middle cranial fossa or the retrosigmoid approach. Patients should be counseled that the highest likelihood for outcome following microsurgical resection of their tumor is hearing loss. Discussion of contralateral routing of signal (CROS), binaural contralateral routing of signal (BiCROS), and bone-anchored hearing aids should also be included in preoperative discussions.

In most series of microsurgical resection of acoustic neuromas, CSF leakage is a common complication. CSF leakage may manifest through the incision, through the tympanic membrane as otorrhea when a perforation or tympanostomy tube exists, or through the eustachian tube and nasopharynx as rhinorrhea. The retrosigmoid, translabyrinthine, and middle cranial fossa approaches may expose pneumatized spaces of the temporal bone, allowing CSF to leak if not adequately sealed. More than 20 years ago, Harner and Laws [11] provided a detailed description of the possible communications within temporal bones in cases of CSF rhinorrhea after posterior fossa surgery. Communications may occur through the lateral end of the IAC, vestibule, and oval window into the middle ear; through the posterosuperior or posteromedial tracts; through air cells exposed during the retrosigmoid craniectomy; through the petrous apex and anterior air cell tract; and through the tubal openings of the peritubal cells directly into the osseous eustachian tube. Identification and sealing of open air cells are central to avoiding CSF leakage. The author and colleagues have applied endoscopy to identify these open air cells; in their series of 128 endoscope-assisted acoustic neuroma cases, 52 (40.6%) had air cells that were identified with the endoscope that were not seen with the microscope [9]. Only 1 (0.9%) of their 111 patients who underwent a retrosigmoid or middle cranial fossa approach for resection of acoustic neuroma experienced transient CSF rhinorrhea that resolved by lumbar drainage of CSF [9]. The author and colleagues believe that the improved visualization and sealing the identified open air cells is a critical factor in reducing the rate of postoperative CSF rhinorrhea to levels well below the reported rate of 5% to 20% [1].

Facial nerve injury is the greatest worry that most patients have when considering microsurgical removal of the tumor. Although multiple factors affect facial nerve outcome, the two most important are tumor size and the relationship between the tumor and the facial nerve. The tumor diameter within the CPA is a critical variable, because the facial nerve becomes stretched and splayed over the surface of the tumor as the diameter increases. The likelihood of anatomic and functional preservation during microsurgical resection is much greater with tumors smaller than 1.5 cm within the CPA plus the IAC component than with medium-sized, large, or giant acoustic neuromas. There are also multiple phenotypes of acoustic neuromas that range from vascular to relatively avascular, from soft to fibrous to cystic, and from slowly growing to rapidly growing. In all these phenotypes the tumor is most adherent to the facial nerve just outside the porus acusticus. Although the degree of adherence varies among tumors, cystic tumors tend to be more adherent. Facial nerve monitoring (electromyography) has radically improved facial nerve outcome, and stimulus dissection instruments further enhance the safe separation of the tumor from the facial nerve.

Headache and neck pain are common postoperative experiences; however, significant headaches persisting beyond the first month postoperatively occur in a minority of patients. Headaches rarely persist longer than 1 year postoperatively. The incidence of headaches is greater after a retrosigmoid approach than after a translabyrinthine approach. Parving et al [12] identified postoperative headache risk factors including a retrosigmoid approach, postoperative gait disturbance, preoperative headaches, and small tumors. Four basic mechanisms are thought to play a role in the development of headache after acoustic neuroma surgery: bone debris in the posterior fossa and subsequent aseptic meningitis, entrapment of the occipital nerve in the nuchal muscle scar tissue, scarring of nuchal musculature to the dura, and migraine. The presence of retained bone debris in the posterior fossa certainly explains the higher incidence of headache after the retrosigmoid approach than after the translabyrinthine approach, because in the latter approach the bone work is completed before the dura is opened. The use of absorbable gelatin sponge (eg, Gelfoam, Pharmacia & Upjohn Co., Kalamazoo, MI) to trap the bone debris created during intracranial opening of the IAC and subsequent removal of tumor has been reported to reduce the amount of retained bone debris and postoperative headaches [13]. The role of aseptic meningitis is further supported by steroid responsiveness in some patients with postoperative headaches. Scarring of the nuchal musculature to the dura is another important cause of headache after the retrosigmoid approach and resection of acoustic neuromas, and this mechanism explains the induction of headache that can occur with straining, neck turning, and exertion. The abnormal coupling of the dura to the nuchal musculature results when the cranial defect is not repaired. Thus the primary way to avoid this complication is to perform a cranioplasty at the conclusion of the retrosigmoid resection of the acoustic neuroma [14].

Bacterial meningitis is infrequent after acoustic neuroma resection, but, because it is a potentially serious complication, it warrants discussion with every patient. Most cases of bacterial meningitis occur in association with CSF leakage. The peak incidence is 3 to 5 days postoperatively. In a prospective trial of almost 3000 patients by Korinek [15], meningitis or deep abscess was seen in 2.5% of the craniotomy patients, with symptoms developing by postoperative day 10 (range, 2–18 days; mean, 10 days; median 7 days). *Staphylococcus aureus* was the most common cause [15]. The author and colleagues reported a case of Enterobacter meningitis resulting in paraplegia after percutaneous gastrostomy tube placement 15 days after acoustic neuroma resection [16]. The most likely clinical scenario is that the Enterobacter, which is normally found in the gastrointestinal tract, was introduced to the blood stream either through direct inoculation during the percutaneous endoscopic gastrostomy tube placement, through aspiration of refluxed gastric contents, or through a nosocomial infection. From there, the bacteria could have spread to the CSF and to the hydroxyapatite cement graft. Once the mesh and graft were inoculated, the bacteria could have showered the CSF, causing persistently positive CSF cultures until the graft material was removed. The lack of radiologic evidence supporting an infiltrative process in the lungs decreases the likelihood of aspiration being the source of the infection. Rapid identification and targeted antibiotic treatment is critical to minimize sequelae. Aseptic meningitis is common, occurring in up to 20% of patients [17,18]. The onset is usually later than that of bacterial meningitis, and the inflammation is induced by blood products, bone dust, or aseptic necrosis of free-fat grafts in the posterior fossa. Steroids, followed by nonsteroidal anti-inflammatory agents over a prolonged course, typically resolve the inflammation.

Stereotactic radiosurgery

Although stereotactic radiosurgery can be applied to a wide range of skull base diseases, it is used most frequently in the treatment of acoustic neuromas. Like microsurgery, stereotactic radiosurgery has advantages and disadvantages that must be thoroughly discussed with the patient. Although there are several forms of stereotactic radiosurgery, the largest experience to date is with Gamma Knife radiosurgery. Consequently the discussion that follows focuses on this treatment modality. For the patient, an outpatient procedure is more attractive than the much longer period of care required with microsurgical management. For example, for a typical acoustic neuroma managed by microsurgery, surgery takes place on the day of admission, and an overnight stay in the ICU followed by 5 to 7 days of hospitalization and a postdischarge recovery of 2 to 4 weeks is typical. Gamma Knife radiosurgery is performed on an outpatient basis. Tumor control has been clearly demonstrated, and with current methods cranial nerve morbidity is low. Unfortunately, advertised claims are sometimes misleading to patients. Fig. 1 demonstrates this problem: although the tumor appears smaller at 6 months after radiation, 1 year after radiation, and 3 years after radiation than before radiation, 6 months after radiation, and 1 year after radiation, the MRIs are photographed at different levels, artificially changing the apparent size of the tumor. This example illustrates the critical need for accurate measurement and reporting of tumor volume over time. Similar reporting using distorted images unfortunately has occurred with other systems, as well. In fact, the MRI images used to illustrate "tumor shrinkage" in the classic *New England Journal Medicine* article reporting outcomes of a cohort of patients treated with Gamma Knife radiosurgery suffer from this problem [19].

Gamma knife radiosurgery applications and outcomes

Like other forms of medical and surgical therapy, the outcomes of Gamma Knife radiosurgery for the treatment of acoustic neuromas and other skull base tumors has evolved and improved over time. This evolution, based on patient outcome, is described in the initial portion of this section. The article then addresses remaining questions that need to be answered and gives examples of good and poor hearing outcome after Gamma Knife radiosurgery. Finally, the use of the technology in inappropriate areas is discussed.

The first Gamma Knife unit model U was installed at the University of Pittsburgh in 1987, and this group has the longest and largest clinical experience in treating acoustic neuromas with Gamma Knife radiosurgery. There have been several reports of this series, and in 1998, Kondziolka and colleagues [19] summarized their experience with 162 acoustic neuromas treated between 1987 and 1992. The average dose at the tumor margin was

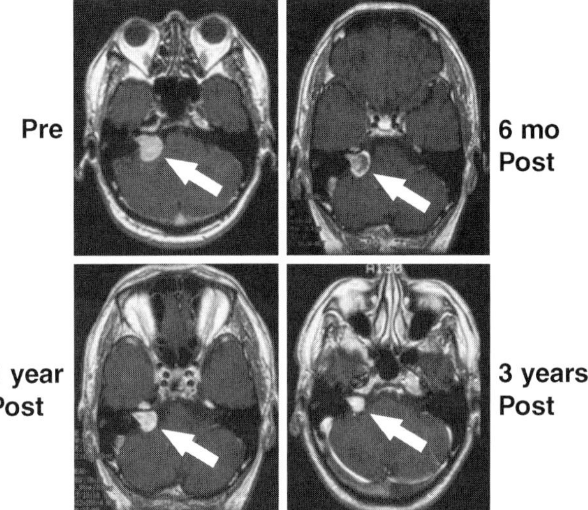

Fig. 1. CyberKnife (Accuray, Sunnyvale, CA) radiosurgery treatment of a right acoustic neuroma. As shown on the CyberKnife Society website, this patient was imaged before radiosurgery and 6 months, 1 year, and 3 years after radiosurgery. The gadolinium-enhanced axial MR images of the acoustic neuroma (*arrows*) at each post-radiosurgery time point seem to demonstrate progressive shrinking of the tumor. The level of the 6-month follow-up study shown is higher than that of the preradiosurgery image, however. The levels of the 1-year and 3-year post-radiosurgery images are progressively lower, and both are lower than the preradiosurgery MRI shown. This presentation of images at different levels falsely suggests that the tumor is decreasing in size. The website content does not make this claim; however, such imagery is misleading to patients relying on the internet to supplement information provided by their physician. (*Adapted from* CyberKnife Society [Accuray Incorporated, Sunnyvale, CA]. Available at (http://www.cksociety.org/PatientInfo/MedicalConditions/acousticneuroma.asp#treatment) with permission, copyright © 2004. Accessed May 15, 2005; with permission.)

16 Gy, and they reported a tumor control rate of 98%. They also reported normal facial nerve function in 79% of patients after 5 years of observation. They likewise reported normal trigeminal nerve function in 73% of these patients; stated conversely, this is an astounding rate of trigeminal nerve dysfunction of 27%. They reported "no change in hearing ability" in 51% of these patients; this means of reporting auditory performance points to the difficulty in interpreting the outcome of most of the studies that report hearing outcome in patients with acoustic neuroma who have been treated with Gamma Knife radiosurgery. Although tumor control is excellent (98%), the poor facial nerve and trigeminal nerve outcomes, combined with the poor hearing ability, led to reduction in the average dose delivered to the tumor margin.

In a series of an additional 190 acoustic neuroma patients, Flickinger et al [20] reviewed the University of Pittsburgh experience from 1992 to 1997. The average dose to the tumor margin was reduced to 13 Gy, and excellent tumor control (97.1%) was still achieved. There was a marked reduction in both facial nerve dysfunction (in 1.1 ± 0.8% of patients) and trigeminal nerve dysfunction (in 2.6 ± 1.2% of patients). In this study, issues highlighted earlier with reporting of hearing outcome are equally apparent. The authors reported "hearing-level preservation" in 71% ± 4.7% of patients. They also reported a "preservation of testable speech discrimination ability" in 91% ± 2.6% of subjects. Obviously, testable speech discrimination ability is far different from useful hearing, and it is unfortunate that these authors did not report the actual auditory thresholds or speech discrimination ability. Most importantly, these results were not reported as a function of time after Gamma Knife radiosurgery. An interesting finding was that facial paresis did not develop in any patient who received a marginal dose of less than 15 Gy (163 patients of 190 patients). In addition, the authors reported that "hearing levels improved" in 10 (7%) of 141 patients who exhibited decreased hearing defined as Gardner-Robertson [21] classes II to V before undergoing Gamma Knife radiosurgery.

The Medical College of Wisconsin Acoustic Neuroma and Skull Base Program has established a protocol for all patients undergoing Gamma Knife radiosurgery for primary or secondary treatment of tumors. After completion of stereotactic radiosurgery, each patient undergoes a gadolinium-enhanced MRI an audiometric test battery and caloric testing to assess peripheral vestibular function at 6-month interval. Before treatment patients undergo a complete electronystagmography test battery, a complete audiometric assessment, and facial nerve electromyography. The author and colleagues have recently analyzed and published these early outcomes data [4]. Figs. 2 through 4 summarize the hearing and vestibular outcomes over time. As shown, these data are presented for individual patients over time, reporting that is unique in the stereotactic radiosurgery literature. Gamma Knife radiosurgery, observation, and microsurgery remain options, and advantages and disadvantages are associated with each of these three treatment modalities. The systematic study of outcomes with each of these methods will ultimately determine which patient cohorts are best suited for each treatment.

Another issue to consider is the accuracy of stereotactic radiosurgery. The author and colleagues have recently found that there is a distortion in the MRI data set produced by the stereotactic headframe used in Gamma Knife radiosurgery [22]. In this study, they reviewed each axial, sagittal, and coronal slice in MR images containing Gamma Knife treatment plans. The length of the greatest displacement of the treatment plan, relative to the CT scan, was measured, and the volume of the treatment plan that fell outside of the IAC was calculated. Known clinical measurements of audiometric, vestibular, facial, and trigeminal nerve functions were then compared with current measurements of tumor size. Twenty-two of the 23 patients had measurable image shifts on the axial images. The range of the image shift was 0 to 5.8 mm, with a mean shift of 1.92 mm (SD ± 1.29 mm). Tumor

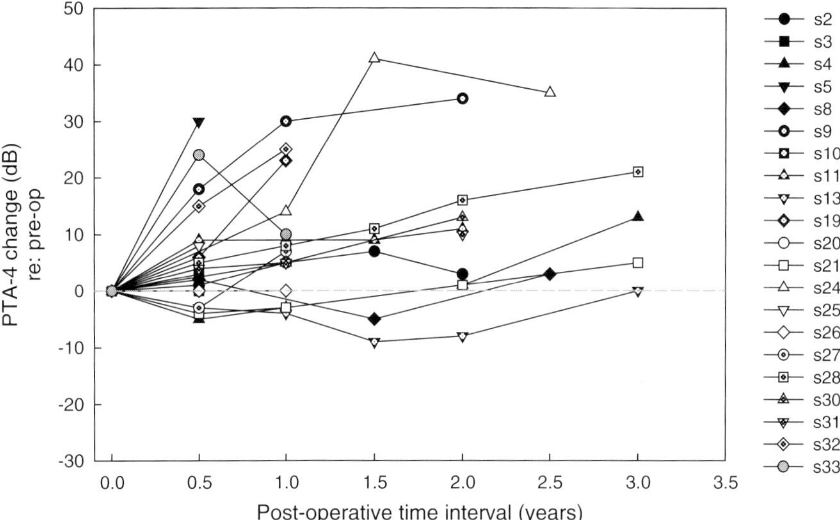

Fig. 2. Auditory function over time after Gamma Knife radiosurgery treatment of unilateral acoustic neuromas (Medical College of Wisconsin series). Four-frequency averages of pure-tone thresholds (PTA-4) in dB HL at 0.5, 1, 2, and 4 kHz were determined for all patients with measures at the preoperative interval and at least one postoperative interval. For each time interval, the PTA-4 difference was calculated relative to the preoperative PTA-4. The differences are plotted as a function of postoperative time interval, with zero representing the preoperative interval. A positive difference value indicates a higher (poorer) postoperative PTA-4. In general, over time, patients had PTA-4s that were poorer than or similar to preoperative PTA-4s, even though a few individuals showed some initial improvement. (Copyright © 2004, P.A. Wackym, MD; reproduced with permission.)

volumes of the treatment plan that fell outside of the IAC ranged from 0 to 414 mm^3 (mean, 90.5 mm^3). The mean percentage of that fell outside the IAC was 16.7% of total tumor volume (range, 2.4%–77.6%). The authors could not draw any consistent correlations between degree of image shift and tumor growth or objective examination findings. A software feature now allows blending of the MRI and CT images for use in treatment planning, and this shift may prove to affect the treatment outcomes of patients already treated with Gamma Knife radiosurgery. It should also be noted that several Gamma Knife Centers use MRI exclusively to build the three-dimensional work space and complete the treatment planning, raising questions about long-term treatment outcomes if regions of the tumor are undertreated and adjacent structures, such as the facial nerve, are overtreated.

One statistic that is particularly alarming to patients considering Gamma Knife radiosurgery for the treatment of acoustic neuroma and which is often quoted by those who are biased against Gamma Knife radiosurgery is that eight cases of malignancy within acoustic neuromas have been reported to date. These cases have been summarized by Bari et al [23] in 2002. Four of

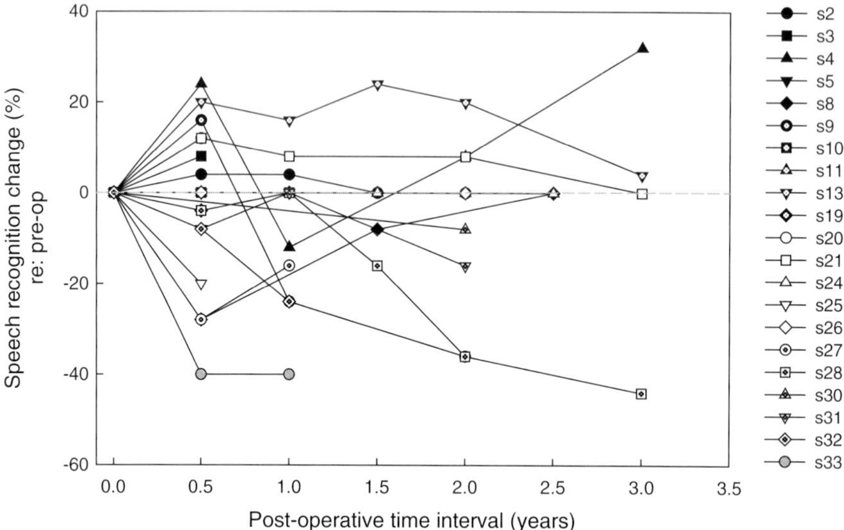

Fig. 3. Speech recognition testing was performed using the Northwestern University Auditory Test No. 6 (NU-6; Tillman and Carhart [5]) monosyllabic words (Medical College of Wisconsin series). The stimuli were presented at 40 dB sensation level (ie, above the speech-recognition threshold), or, if this was too loud, at the patient's most comfortable listening level. Speech recognition was scored in percent correct. As with PTA, the differences between pre- and postoperative speech recognition were calculated and plotted as a function of postoperative time interval. Positive values are consistent with an improvement in speech recognition. Approximately half of the patients showed improvement in speech recognition at 6 months after treatment; the other half showed a decrease in performance. Over time, patients generally demonstrate speech recognition similar to or poorer than pretreatment performance. (Copyright © 2004, P.A. Wackym, MD; reproduced with permission.)

these tumors had been treated previously with radiosurgery, and four other cases did not receive radiation. Although it is possible that these four cases developed after the radiation treatment, it is more likely that these malignant tumors were misdiagnosed at the outset of evaluation and treatment. The concept of delayed development of radiation-induced neoplasms was addressed by Pollock et al [24] in 1995. They reviewed the 26-year experience with radiosurgery in more than 20,000 patients worldwide and found no increased incidence in the development of new neoplasm. They defined neoplasm as a new growth of tissue serving no physiologic function, a definition that would include both benign and malignant disease. Despite the limitations of the studies just reviewed, it is important to counsel patients about this possibility. It is likewise appropriate to counsel them about the possible origins of these malignant schwannomas. To be diagnosed as a radiation-induced malignancy, four criteria must be satisfied:

1. The second neoplasm must arise in the irradiated field.
2. A latent period of at least several years must have elapsed between the radiation exposure and the development of the second neoplasm.

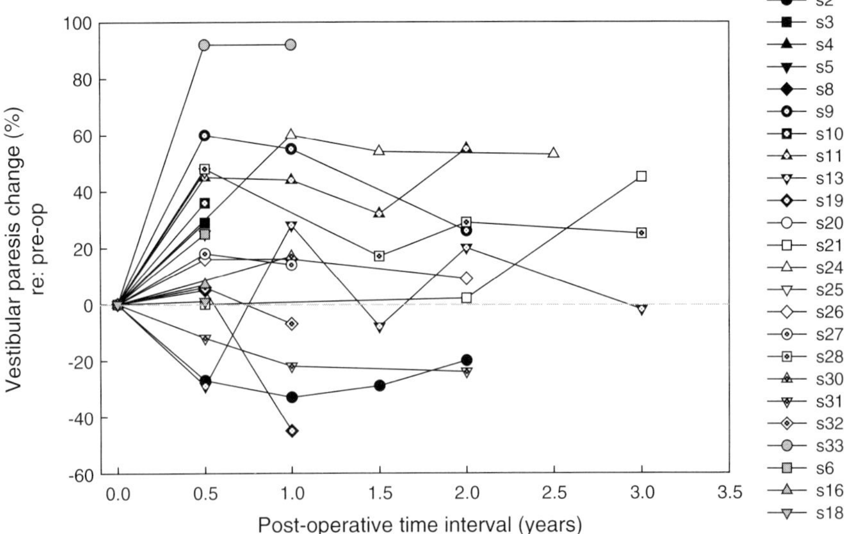

Fig. 4. Vestibular paresis was determined by bithermal caloric testing (Medical College of Wisconsin series). A positive difference value indicates greater vestibular paresis after Gamma Knife radiosurgery. Both degradation and improvement in vestibular paresis are observed across patients. For individual patients, the postoperative degree of vestibular paresis generally tends to remain stable over time. (Copyright © 2004, P.A. Wackym, MD; reproduced with permission.)

3. There must be histologic and radiographic evidence of the preexisting condition, in addition to microscopic proof of a tumor.
4. The second tumor must be of a different histologic type from that previously irradiated to eliminate the possibility of recurrence of the original tumor or a missed diagnosis of the original tumor.

With these criteria in mind, in 1997 Lustig et al [25] reported the development of a squamous cell carcinoma following radiation treatment of an acoustic neuroma. In addition, Hanabusa et al [26] reported the malignant transformation of an acoustic neuroma following Gamma Knife radiosurgery. There was histologic evidence of acoustic neuroma after a retrosigmoid resection of the tumor. Four years after this resection, recidivistic tumor was identified, and the patient was subsequently treated with Gamma Knife radiosurgery. Six months after treatment, the tumor had grown, and the patient underwent surgical resection through a combined retrosigmoid-translabyrinthine approach. Abnormal mitotic figures were observed on histologic sections, and the diagnosis of malignancy was assigned. The patient died 6.5 years after the initial treatment of the malignant disease.

A early trend in stereotactic radiosurgery that is cause for concern is the debulking subsequent radiation of the tumor for the purposes of "hearing preservation" and "facial nerve preservation." The single biggest variable during this process is how much tumor is resected before radiation. Without using intraoperative MRI to visualize the remaining tumor volume, it is difficult to be certain when or if the preoperative goal for debulking has been achieved. This approach is not used in high-volume acoustic neuroma programs nationally, and the traditional neuro-otologist/neurosurgeon team is not involved with the "innovative" surgical approach. Fig. 5 shows an example of a case where a neurosurgeon completed a debulking procedure, which, as shown in Fig. 5B, was essentially a biopsy. Aside from the unnecessary expense of completing both the craniotomy and Gamma Knife radiosurgery, the ethical and moral questions presented by this example are troubling. In light of the current outcomes in microsurgery or stereotactic radiosurgery [27,28], there is no justification for this type of management algorithm. In contrast, Iwai et al [29] applied this concept more appropriately. They reported a series of 14 patients managed over a 6-year interval with acoustic neuromas too large (range, 3.0–5.8 cm) to treat primarily with radiosurgery. Subtotal resection was achieved in 13 patients; because of hypervascularity, partial resection was performed in one patient. After recovery, the residual tumor was treated with radiosurgery.

One final issue is tumor growth after radiosurgery. Pretreatment include counseling should the information that tumor increases in size after radiosurgery. This posttreatment edema typically persists for 6 months but may remain for up to 1 year. Anecdotal cases have been discussed and occasionally reported describing increased tumor size early after radiosurgery. The challenge lies in making a decision about whether or when to operate on these tumors [24,30–33]. Pollock et al [24] emphasized the need to demonstrate sustained tumor growth by serial MRI and to review the case

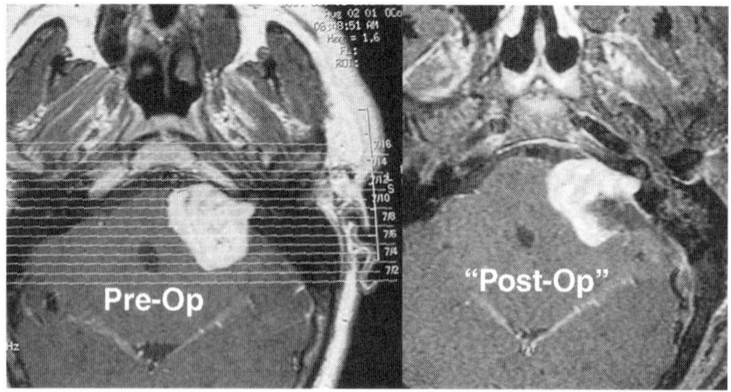

Fig. 5. Gamma Knife radiosurgery. An example of what has been described as an innovative combined microsurgical and radiosurgical approach to the management of acoustic neuromas. Advocates anecdotally assert that better hearing preservation and facial nerve outcome can be achieved of this method. This example, essentially a biopsy of the tumor with subtotal resection followed by Gamma Knife radiosurgery, raises ethical and cost-effectiveness issues. (Copyright © 2004, P.A. Wackym, MD; reproduced with permission.)

with the surgeon who performed the radiosurgery before making a surgical decision. The other related controversy is whether the facial nerve dissection and subsequent preservation is more difficult during microsurgical resection after radiosurgery. On one end of the spectrum [24], descriptions of no increased difficulty have been reported; on the other end of the spectrum [31–33], markedly increased difficulty in separating the tumor from the facial nerve and poorer facial nerve function outcome have been reported. The report of Watanabe et al [32] included a histopathologic analysis of the resected facial nerve. They found microvasculitis of the facial nerve, axonal degeneration/loss of axons, and proliferation of Schwann cells. Given the mechanism of delayed effects following radiosurgery, these findings are not surprising. Moreover, these findings emphasize the need for the neuro-otologist to be certain that the treatment plan avoids high radiation doses adjacent to the facial nerve. As discussed earlier, a dose of 12 Gy delivered to the 50% isodose line means that the maximum tumor dose is 24 Gy. If the treatment plan delivers this maximal dose to the area of the facial nerve, greater radiation effects should be expected. For this reason, if the neuro-otologist and the patient have made a decision to resect a tumor previously treated with radiosurgery, it is important to review the treatment plan to determine the amount of radiation delivered to the facial nerve and to counsel the patient appropriately preoperatively.

Fractionated stereotactic radiosurgery

The preceding section of this article, which focused on Gamma Knife radiosurgery, illustrates many principles of radiation biology and stereotactic surgery. Many of these principles hold true for fractionated stereotactic radiosurgery. Historically, the maximum radiation dose that could be given to a tumor site was restricted by the tolerance and sensitivity of the surrounding nearby healthy tissues. One-session Gamma Knife systems and other one-session linear accelerator (LINAC) technologies are available. In addition, several manufacturers currently offer conformal radiation treatment systems that can involve multiple fractionated treatments. The most widely known systems at this time are the Peacock (NOMOS Radiation Oncology Division of North American Scientific, Cranberry Township, PA), the SmartBeam IMRT (Varian Medical Systems Inc., Palo Alto, CA), The Precise (Elekta, Inc., Stockholm, Sweden), and the CyberKnife (Accuray, Sunnyvale, CA).

Conformal radiation differs from conventional radiation therapy in that radiation therapy targets a uniform shape to a total area to cover the tumor. Thus, with convention radiation therapy, some healthy tissue is always irradiated, and the target area receives a homogeneous or even dose of radiation across the entire target area. Conformal radiation treatments have the ability to deliver a higher dose within the tumor and thus can cause more damage to the tumor target and less damage to the surrounding healthy tissue than with conventional external beam radiation treatment. With the various methods of accomplishing fractionated stereotactic radiosurgery, the patient is fitted with some type of reusable localization device, which may be a mask or a body frame. This device assists reproducibility in targeting and consequently allows greater accuracy. Typically, with skull base tumors, including acoustic neuromas, the localization device is molded to fit the precise contours of the individual patient. This molded device is placed on the patient at each treatment. Conformal radiation usually requires multiple (1–28) treatments, but fewer treatments are required than with conventional radiation therapy. The treatment time for each session is typically longer than with conventional radiation therapy because of the complexity of the treatment. The outcomes after treatment of acoustic neuromas with fractionated stereotactic radiosurgery are being reported; however, fewer patients to date have been treated with these modalities than with Gamma Knife radiosurgery [34–36].

Summary

There is diversity in the techniques and instrumentation used to perform stereotactic radiosurgery. The field continues to evolve rapidly, and improvements are being made in accuracy, effective radiation dose, and parameters necessary to maximize patient outcome. Stereotactic radiosurgery, like any other treatment modality, has advantages and disadvantages that must be discussed with a patient who has an acoustic neuroma or other skull base tumor. An informed decision to pursue observation, microsurgery, stereotactic radiosurgery, or a combination of these methods must be made, and it remains the responsibility of the surgeon to provide a balanced view of the relative advantages and disadvantages of each method.

References

[1] Jackler RK, Pfister MHF. Acoustic neuroma (vestibular schwannoma). In: Jackler RK, Brackmann DE, editors. Neurotology. 2nd edition. St. Louis (M): Elsevier Mosby; 2005. p. 727–82.

[2] Wackym PA, Runge-Samuelson CL. Gamma Knife radiosurgery and other forms of radiosurgery for management of skull base tumors. In: Jackler RK, Brackmann DE, editors. Neurotology. 2nd edition. St. Louis (MO): Elsevier Mosby; 2005. p. 1164–86.

[3] Acoustic neuroma basic overview. Cumming (GA): Acoustic Neuroma Association; 2001. p. 1–11.

[4] Wackym PA, Runge-Samuelson CL, Poetker DM, et al. Gamma Knife radiosurgery for acoustic neuromas performed by a neurotologist: early experiences and outcomes. Otol Neurotol 2004;25(5):752–61.

[5] Tillman TW, Carhart R. An expanded test for speech recognition utilizing CNC monosyllabic words Northwestern University Auditory Test No. 6. Technical Documentary Report (No. SAM-Tr-66–55). Brooks Air Force Base (TX): USAF School of Aerospace Medicine Technical Report; 1966.

[6] Haberkamp TJ, Meyer GA, Fox M. Surgical exposure of the fundus of the internal auditory canal: anatomic limits of the middle fossa versus the retrosigmoid approach. Laryngoscope 1998;108:1190–4.
[7] Driscoll CL, Jackler RK, Pitts LH, et al. Is the entire fundus of the internal auditory canal visible during the middle fossa approach for acoustic neuroma? Am J Otol 2000;21(3): 382–8.
[8] Blevins NH, Jackler RK. Exposure of the lateral extremity of the internal auditory canal through the retrosigmoid approach: a radioanatomic study. Otolaryngol Head Neck Surg 1994;111:81–90.
[9] Wackym PA, King WA, Meyer GA, et al. Endoscopy and endoscopic stereotactic surgery during acoustic neuroma resection. In: Wackym PA, Rice DH, Schaefer SD, editors. Minimally invasive surgery of the head, neck, and cranial base. Philadelphia: Lippincott Williams & Wilkins; 2002. p. 83–100.
[10] Wackym PA, King WA, Poe DS, et al. Adjuctive use of endoscopy during acoustic neuroma surgery. Laryngoscope 1999;109:1193–201.
[11] Harner SG, Laws ER. Translabyrinthine repair for cerebrospinal fluid otorhinorrhea. J Neurosurg 1982;57:258–61.
[12] Parving A, Tos M, Thomsen J, et al. Some aspects of life quality after surgery for acoustic neuroma. Arch Otolaryngol Head Neck Surg 1992;118:1061–4.
[13] Catalano PJ, Jacobowitz O, Post KD. Prevention of headache after retrosigmoid removal of acoustic tumors. Am J Otol 1996;17(6):904–8.
[14] Poetker DM, Pytynia KB, Meyer GA, et al. Complications rate of transtemporal hydroxyapatite cement cranioplasties: a case series review of 76 cranioplasties. Otol Neurotol 2004;25(4):604–9.
[15] Korinek AM. Risk factors for neurosurgical site infections after craniotomy: a prospective multicenter study of 2944 patients. Neurosurgery 1997;41:1073–9.
[16] Poetker DM, Edmiston CE, Smith MM, et al. Meningitis due to *Enterobacter aerogenes* subsequent to resection of acoustic neuroma and percutaneous endoscopic gastrostomy tube placement: a rare nosocomial event. Infect Control Hosp Epidemiol 2003;24(10):780–2.
[17] Blomstedt GC. Post-operative aseptic meningitis. Acta Neurochir (Wien) 1987;89:112–6.
[18] Hwang P, Jackler RK. Lipoid meningitis due to aseptic necrosis of free fat graft placed during neurotologic surgery. Laryngoscope 1996;106:1482–6.
[19] Kondziolka D, Lunsford LD, McLaughlin MR, et al. Long-term outcomes after radiosurgery for acoustic neuroma. N Engl J Med 1998;339:1426–33.
[20] Flickinger JC, Kondziolka D, Niranjan A, et al. Results of acoustic neuroma radiosurgery: an analysis of 5 years' experience using current methods. J Neurosurg 2001;94(1):1–6.
[21] Gardner G, Robertson JH. Hearing preservation in unilateral acoustic neuroma surgery. Ann Otol Rhinol Laryngol 1998;97(1):55–66.
[22] Poetker DM, Jursinic PA, Runge-Samuelson CL, et al. Distortion of magnetic resonance images used in Gamma Knife radiosurgery treatment planning: Implications for acoustic neuroma outcomes. Otol Neurotol 2005, in press.
[23] Bari ME, Forster DM, Kemeny AA, et al. Malignancy in a vestibular schwannoma. Report of a case with central neurofibromatosis, treated by both stereotactic radiosurgery and surgical excision, with a review of the literature. Br J Neurosurg 2002;16(3):284–9.
[24] Pollock BE, Lunsford LD, Kondziolka D, et al. Vestibular schwannoma management. Part II. Failed radiosurgery and the role of delayed microsurgery. J Neurosurg 1998;89(6): 949–55.
[25] Lustig LR, Jackler RK, Lanser MJ. Radiation-induced tumors of the temporal bone. Am J Otol 1997;18(2):230–5.
[26] Hanabusa K, Morikawa A, Murata T, et al. Acoustic neuroma with malignant transformation. Case report. J Neurosurg 2001;95(3):518–21.
[27] Kaylie DM, McMenomey SO. Microsurgery vs gamma knife radiosurgery for the treatment of vestibular schwannomas. Arch Otolaryngol Head Neck Surg 2003;129(8):903–6.

[28] Yamakami I, Uchino Y, Kobayashi E, et al. Conservative management, gamma-knife radiosurgery, and microsurgery for acoustic neurinomas: a systematic review of outcome and risk of three therapeutic options. Neurol Res 2003;25(7):682–90.
[29] Iwai Y, Yamanaka K, Ishiguro T. Surgery combined with radiosurgery of large acoustic neuromas. Surg Neurol 2003;59(4):283–9.
[30] Pitts LA, Jackler RK. Treatment of acoustic neuromas. N Engl J Med 1998;339:1471–3.
[31] Ho SY, Kveton JF. Rapid growth of acoustic neuromas after stereotactic radiotherapy in type 2 neurofibromatosis. Ear Nose Throat J 2002;81(12):831–3.
[32] Watanabe T, Saito N, Hirato J, et al. Facial neuropathy due to axonal degeneration and microvasculitis following gamma knife surgery for vestibular schwannoma: a histological analysis. J Neurosurg 2003;99(5):916–20.
[33] Lee DJ, Westra WH, Staecker H, et al. Clinical and histopathologic features of recurrent vestibular schwannoma (acoustic neuroma) after stereotactic radiosurgery. Otol Neurol 2003;24(4):650–60.
[34] Andrews DW, Suarez O, Goldman HW, et al. Stereotactic radiosurgery and fractionated stereotactic radiotherapy for the treatment of acoustic schwannomas: comparative observations of 125 patients treated at one institution. Int J Radiat Oncol Biol Phys 2001; 50(5):1265–78.
[35] Williams JA. Fractionated stereotactic radiotherapy for acoustic neuromas. Int J Radiat Oncol Biol Phys 2002;54(2):500–4.
[36] Perks JR, St George EJ, Hamri K, et al. Stereotactic radiosurgery XVI: isodosimetric comparison of photon stereotactic radiosurgery techniques (gamma knife vs. multileaf collimator linear accelerator) for acoustic neuroma—and potential clinical importance. Int J Radiat Oncol Biol Phys 2003;57(5):1450–9.

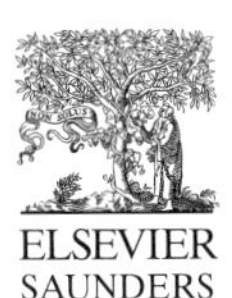
ELSEVIER
SAUNDERS

Otolaryngol Clin N Am
38 (2005) 671–684

OTOLARYNGOLOGIC
CLINICS
OF NORTH AMERICA

Current Concepts in the Evaluation and Treatment of Neurofibromatosis Type II

Brian A. Neff, MD[a], D. Bradley Welling, MD, PhD[b,*]

[a]*Department of Otolaryngology, Mayo Clinic, Rochester, MN, USA*
[b]*Department of Otolaryngology–Head and Neck Surgery, The Ohio State University College of Medicine, 456 West 10th Avenue, Columbus, OH 43210, USA*

Neurofibromatosis type II (NF2) is an autosomal dominant, highly penetrant disease whose hallmark is bilateral vestibular schwannomas [1]. The diagnostic prevalence of symptomatic NF2 has been estimated at 1 in 210,000 people [2]. Other disease features of NF2 include intracranial and spinal meningiomas, ependymomas, gliomas, presenile lens opacities, and peripheral, spinal, and cranial nerve schwannomas [3–6]. Skin tumors are predominantly schwannomas, however, Peripheral neurofibromas can also be seen in NF2, although they are more common in neurofibromatosis (NF1), von Recklinghausen's disease [7]. The skin can also be affected with café-au-lait spots (usually fewer than six in number), although to a much lesser degree than in NF1 [8–9]. The Manchester criteria, summarized in Table 1, are the most sensitive of the four different sets of diagnostic criteria for NF2 [10]. NF2 is now recognized as a distinctly different disease from NF1. NF1 is caused by a mutation in the *NF1* tumor-suppressor gene on chromosome 17, whereas NF2 is caused by a mutation in the *NF2* tumor-suppressor gene on chromosome 22 [11–12].

NF2 is currently divided into three clinical subgroups [2,13]. The Wishart type has a more severe clinical presentation. In addition to bilateral vestibular schwannomas, patients often suffer from multiple intracranial tumors and associated spinal tumors. The typical age at onset is in the late teens or early twenties [14]. The Gardner type has a later onset and a less severe presentation. Although patients present with bilateral schwannomas, associated intracranial tumors are less common [15]. A more recently recognized third category of NF2 has been termed segmental NF2.

* Corresponding author.
E-mail address: welling.1@osu.edu (D.B. Welling).

doi:10.1016/j.otc.2005.01.002 **oto.theclinics.com**

Table 1
Manchester criteria for the diagnosis of NF2 (Baser et al [10])

A. Bilateral vestibular schwannomas
B. First-degree relative with NF2 AND unilateral vestibular schwannoma OR any two of the following: meningioma, schwannoma, glioma, neurofibroma, juvenile posterior subcapsular lens opacity
C. Unilateral vestibular schwannoma AND any two of the following: Meningioma, schwannoma, glioma, neurofibroma, posterior subcapsular lenticular opacities
D. Multiple meningiomas (two or more) AND unilateral vestibular schwannoma OR any two of the following: schwannoma, glioma neurofibroma, cataract

Segmental NF2 may be caused by somatic mosaicism in which a mutation occurs during embryogenesis rather than in the germline DNA; therefore, only a portion of the patient's cells carry the mutation [16–17]. (Patients with traditional NF2 inherit the mutation from a parent and consequently carry the mutation in all their cells.) It recently has been estimated that mosaicism may account for 25% of NF2 cases of any subtype among patients whose parents did not have NF2 [17]. Patients with somatic mosaicism can display bilateral vestibular schwannomas if the postzygotic mutation occurred early in embryogenesis. Alternately, if the postzygotic mutation occurred late in development the patient may display an atypical presentation of segmental NF2 with a unilateral vestibular schwannoma and an ipsilateral, additional intracranial tumor, such as a meningioma [16]. Unlike the traditional forms of NF2, the risk of passing NF2 caused by mosaicism to future offspring is low [18].

Clinical presentation

Patients affected with NF2 are usually diagnosed between the second and fourth decade, but up to 18% of patients present under the age of 15 years [19]. Up to 41% of patients who eventually develop NF2 do not present with bilateral vestibular schwannomas; therefore, some adult patients can present with unilateral sensorineural hearing loss (SNHL) rather than symmetric or asymmetric bilateral SNHL [10]. The hearing loss is usually progressive, but sudden SNHL can occur. The patient can also present with tinnitus, disequilibrium, and headache. Cranial nerve symptoms, such as facial numbness or weakness, dysphagia, or hoarseness, can also be present if these cranial nerves develop separate schwannomas or become compressed by a large vestibular schwannoma [7]. Patients may present with skin or spinal tumors before the appearance of hearing loss associated with vestibular schwannomas [10]. This presentation is particularly common in children (<15 years), who present with symptoms unrelated to vestibular schwannomas in 70% to 85% of cases [19]. Spinal tumors have been reported to occur in up to 80% to 90% of NF2 patients, but they are usually asymptomatic [20–21]. Only 25% to 30% of spinal tumors develop symptoms such as compressive myelopathy [13,22].

Clinical and genetic screening for neurofibromatosis type II

The evaluation of a patient at risk for developing NF2 should begin with audiometric testing. A T1-weighted, gadolinium-enhanced MRI of the brain and internal auditory canals should be obtained if there is asymmetric hearing loss, or if the hearing is normal and there is a family history or other stigmata of NF2 disease. Some physicians advocate auditory brainstem response and acoustic reflex studies, which can be helpful but should not replace the MRI as a screening procedure because they have a lower sensitivity in detecting small tumors [23–24]. Additionally, an MRI of the entire spinal column has been suggested to screen for spinal tumors; however, nonsurgical management is usually recommended for asymptomatic tumors (Fig. 1) [22]. The authors suggest obtaining a baseline spinal MRI at the time of presentation but repeating the scan only if symptoms or findings on physical examination suggest a new or progressive spinal tumor.

A parent with a nonmosaic form of NF2 has a 50% chance of passing the affected *NF2* allele along to offspring. A child who inherits an abnormal

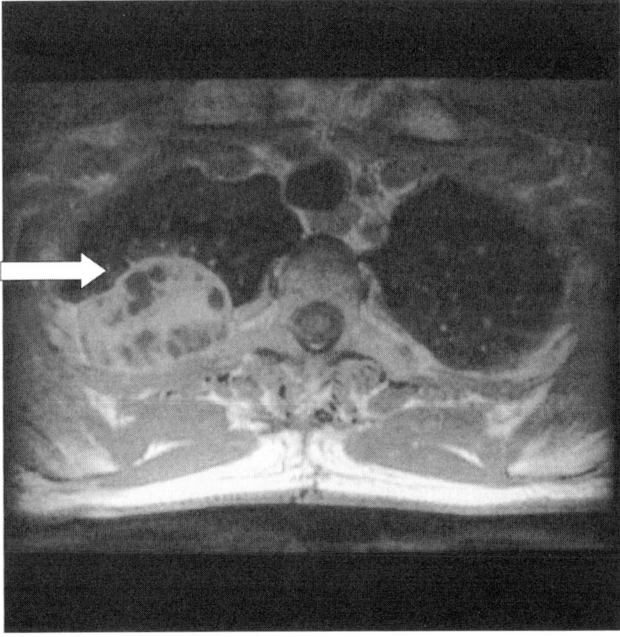

Fig. 1. Axial MRI of the thoracic spine with gadolinium contrast. The MRI demonstrates a 4.6-cm thoracic spinal nerve root schwannoma (*white arrow*) on the right side in a patient with NF2. Nonsurgical management was recommended because the tumor was asymptomatic.

copy of the *NF2* tumor-suppressor gene has a 95% chance of developing bilateral vestibular schwannomas. About one half of NF2 patients have no family history of NF2 disease; thus, they represent new germline or mosaic mutations that were not inherited [3–6]. Because of the autosomal dominant transmission and because early intervention is important in clinical outcome, clinical and genetic screening for at-risk patients has been advocated.

Routine clinical and radiologic examinations are required for patients with a first-degree relative with NF2, patients younger than 30 years old with a unilateral vestibular schwannoma, or any patient with multiple intracranial or spinal tumors or other stigmata associated with NF2. Any offspring of patients with NF2 should have annual ophthalmologic examinations starting soon after birth and annual neurology examinations starting at 7 years of age. Biannual audiograms and annual MRI evaluations should be performed beginning at age 7 years. Others have recommended starting a similar screening process at 10 years of age with an MRI every other year and annually if a vestibular schwannoma is found [9]. The important point is to begin some form of screening at an early age to pick up tumors while hearing-preservation surgery is still possible.

Mutation screening for the children of a NF2 parent is controversial. Several authors recommend routine genetic screening of first-degree relatives of NF2 patients [9,21]. This screening is reasonable if the patient also receives appropriate genetic counseling and has available resources to obtain the genetic screening. Currently, the authors do not recommend routine genetic screening in these cases unless there are special circumstances pertaining to family planning. The primary reason they do not routinely perform mutation screening is that screening detects mutations in only about 75% of patients; therefore, this test has a significant false-negative rate in predicting patients who will develop NF2 [25–29]. Therefore children who had a negative test would still need an annual MRI and biannual audiograms. Additionally, if a mutation were detected during DNA sequencing, the authors would still recommend annual MRIs and biannual audiometric testing to detect the development of vestibular schwannomas at the earliest possible stage. Current genetic screening for NF2 costs about $2000.

Screening first-degree relatives of persons in whom a *NF2* mutation has already been identified is considerably less costly (~$250 per screen). The sensitivity of genetic testing in this circumstance is extremely high (~100%) because the DNA being screened can be compared directly with the known mutation of the family member. In this case, knowing with near certainty that a child does not carry a *NF2* mutation can avoid the frequent MRI examinations that otherwise would be required. Therefore, if more than two members of a family have been diagnosed with NF2, it may be worthwhile to identify the mutation in at least one family member so that future family members can be screened. The authors will reevaluate their current position as the sensitivity of screening increases and the cost of detecting mutations decreases.

Hearing rehabilitation

Early in the course of NF2, conventional hearing aids may be useful for moderate hearing loss. There are two options for bilateral hearing restoration in severely to profoundly deafened individuals with NF2. Both cochlear implant (CI) and auditory brainstem implants (ABI) can be used in specific situations to provide hearing for the NF2 patient. A CI is used to stimulate auditory neurons in the cochlea and requires preservation of an intact cochlear nerve during tumor removal. Even though the blood supply of the cochlear nerve may be interrupted, and the postoperative hearing is lost, a CI may still be possible. Response to promontory stimulation may be absent early in the postoperative period but return 6 to 8 weeks after surgery.

Long-term hearing outcomes in six patients who have received a CI following vestibular schwannoma removal showed very good speech understanding. Central Institute for the Deaf sentence scores ranged from 90% to 100%, and hearing in noise testing results ranged from 83% to 96% with an average follow-up period of 5.5 years (range, 2–10 years). Five of six NF2 patients with a CI were able to use the telephone at most recent follow-up. This small collection of patients suggests the efficacy of CI in carefully selected NF2 patients [30–33].

It is also helpful to compare CI performance in NF2 patients with the performance of ABI users with NF2. Approximately 160 patients have received an ABI with surface electrodes stimulating the cochlear nucleus, but few obtain any open-set speech understanding, although lip reading cues and awareness of environmental sound is noteworthy [34]. ABI performance provides only 3% to 7% solely auditory, open-set speech understanding. Additionally, 85% to 96% of patients perceived auditory stimulation only, but with no speech understanding [35–36]. Currently, CI performance exceeds that of ABI for most NF2 patients. The authors believe that an ABI is an excellent rehabilitation option for NF2 patients whose cochlear nerves have been sectioned during tumor removal or for patients with intact cochlear nerves that do not respond with promontory stimulation. New multichannel ABIs that use electrodes that penetrate the cochlear nucleus rather than surface stimulation are under investigation and may hold promise for improved speech understanding [37].

Treatment

The initial treatment decisions are influenced by tumor size, location, patient age, and hearing status. Early surgical intervention with attempted hearing preservation in NF2 patients, as opposed to delaying tumor removal until after all useful hearing has been lost by tumor compression or invasion, is a greatly debated topic. The authors believe that early detection and treatment of NF2 tumors provides much greater opportunity for hearing preservation [7,38]. Additionally, they believe that the postresection use of

CI in select patients gives a second reason to intervene early with these tumors. Maintaining an intact cochlear nerve becomes increasingly difficult with increased tumor size. Consequently, early intervention with preservation of the anatomic integrity of the cochlear nerve seems to be warranted even if hearing preservation is not accomplished at the time of tumor removal.

The following discussion summarizes the authors' approach to patients with bilateral vestibular schwannomas.

Both tumors large; good hearing bilaterally

If the tumors are both larger than 2.0 cm and the speech discrimination score (SDS) is better than 50% bilaterally, the authors suggest initial observation of the tumor growth rate unless the tumor is causing brainstem compression. The rates of hearing and facial nerve preservation in NF2 patients traditionally have been worse than in patients with sporadic unilateral tumors [39–40], probably because NF2 tumors tend to splay and envelop the cranial nerves instead of displacing them [41–42]. Consequently, the authors suggest observation for patients with tumors larger than 2 cm to preserve natural hearing as long as possible. Once the SDS falls below 50% in either ear, removal of the tumor through the translabyrinthine approach is recommended. To rehabilitate hearing with a CI, the authors attempt to preserve an intact cochlear nerve during tumor resection; however, they are often unable to perform complete tumor resection in tumors larger 2.0 cm without sacrificing the cochlear nerve. Most of these patients will require an ABI for hearing rehabilitation.

The authors recognize that some physicians will attempt hearing preservation for patients with tumors as large as 2.5 to 3.0 cm [38–39], but they have not been successful in preserving useful hearing in patients with NF2-associated tumors of this size. The small chance of preserving hearing with tumors larger than 2.0 cm does not justify a hearing-preservation approach. Visualization of the facial nerve with tumors this size is better with the translabyrinthine approach than with the extended middle fossa and suboccipital approaches. This treatment approach may give better facial nerve outcomes, which is extremely important when treating bilateral tumors.

Another option during the observation period is to perform a middle fossa decompression at the first sign of fluctuation or decline in the hearing. This procedure involves bony removal over the internal auditory canals without opening the dura or debulking the tumor. Tumor decompression can result in stabilization and even improvement in hearing [38,44,45]. On the other hand, tumor debulking is thought to increase the risk of hearing loss dramatically without preventing the risk of future tumor growth [38,43,45]. Samii et al [39] would disagree, because 83% (8/11) of their debulking procedures did not experience postoperative hearing loss. They did not comment on tumor regrowth or hearing loss after long-term follow-up, however. The authors rarely use tumor debulking (eg, when a tumor compresses the brainstem in the only ear with hearing and for patients with brainstem decompression who are too medically unfit to undergo prolonged surgery for very large tumors).

Both tumors small; good hearing bilaterally

If both tumors are smaller than 2.0 cm, and the patient has a SDS of more than 50% bilaterally, the authors suggest removal of the smaller vestibular schwannoma because they believe this approach gives a better chance of hearing preservation [7,46]. Many propose an alternate approach, initially removing the larger tumor [43]. The authors would operate on a larger tumor in an ear with good hearing before a contralateral intracanalicular tumor in an ear with good hearing only if the larger tumor showed signs of significant brainstem compression. If there are small (<2.0 cm) tumors of equal size, and the patient possesses serviceable but asymmetric bilateral hearing, the authors first would perform hearing-preservation surgery on the ear with worse hearing (Fig. 2).

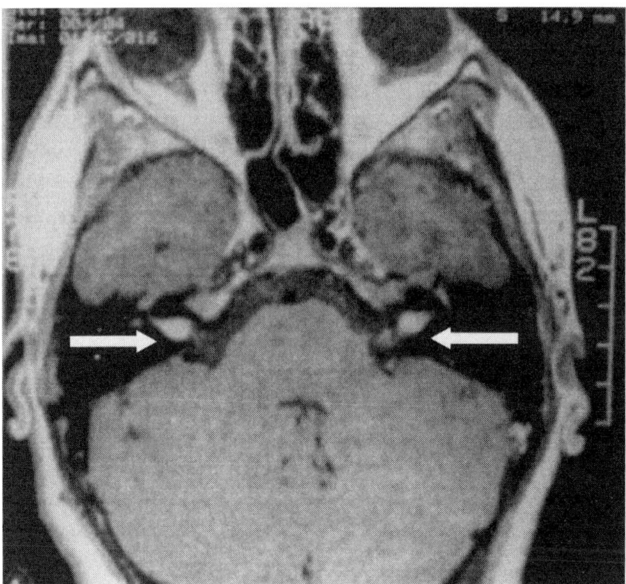

Fig. 2. Axial MRI of the brain and internal auditory canals with gadolinium contrast. The patient has a diagnosis of NF2 with small intracanalicular vestibular schwannomas (*white arrows*) and good hearing bilaterally. The tumors were of equal size, but the tumor on the left side was excised first through a middle fossa approach because the hearing in that ear was slightly worse (SDS 84%).

Based on the location of the tumor, a middle fossa, extended middle fossa, or suboccipital approach should be used in attempting to remove the smaller tumor in the ear with serviceable hearing. If the hearing in the first ear is preserved, the tumor in the other ear is removed using a hearing-preservation approach after the patient has recovered from surgery sufficiently and the postoperative hearing has stabilized. If tumor resection in the first ear results in profound hearing loss, but the cochlear nerve is anatomically preserved, a postoperative promontory stimulation test helps in making further management decisions. If there is a positive promontory stimulation test in the operated ear, the authors suggest tumor observation in the contralateral ear (the only ear with hearing) until the tumor begins to compress the brainstem or causes the SDS to drop below 50%. At that time, a translabyrinthine excision of the tumor in the second ear is indicated, in addition to a CI in the first ear with the intact cochlear nerve.

On the other hand, if the hearing is lost in the first ear, and the cochlear nerve has been transected, a CI in the first ear is not possible. Again, the authors suggest observing the tumor in the unoperated ear (the only ear with hearing) until the hearing declines to a SDS of less than 50% or there is radiographic evidence of brainstem compression. The patient needs to understand that during the period of observation, the tumor may grow to a size that makes maintaining a cochlear nerve in the second ear for a CI nearly impossible. As mentioned previously, during periods of tumor observation, decompression of the internal auditory canals and tumor can help preserve hearing if it begins to fluctuate or decline. Once surgery is indicated, the authors would remove the tumor using a translabyrinthine approach, making every effort to maintain the integrity of the cochlear nerve for a subsequent CI in the second ear. They would sacrifice the cochlear nerve if attempts to preserve it compromise complete tumor resection. Anecdotally, the authors have found it difficult to remove tumors larger than 2 cm reliably and preserve an intact cochlear nerve that is capable of stimulation postoperatively. If they are unable to save the hearing or the cochlear nerve on either side, they would implant an ABI at the time the second tumor is removed.

Small tumor with good hearing; large tumor with poor hearing

A patient may present with involves a larger tumor (>2 cm) in one ear with a SDS of less than 50% and a small (<2.0 cm) tumor in the contralateral ear with a SDS greater than 50%. In this case, the authors would immediately remove the larger tumor using the translabyrinthine approach. They would suggest an observation protocol similar to that described previously for the small tumor in the unoperated ear (the only ear with hearing). Once the tumor caused a significant hearing decline (SDS < 50%) or brainstem compression, the second tumor should be removed using the translabyrinthine approach. Again, if either cochlear nerve was preserved, and there was a positive promontory stimulation, the authors would offer a CI; otherwise, an ABI would be indicated.

Small tumor with poor hearing; large tumor with good hearing

If the patient presents with one ear containing a smaller tumor (<2.0 cm) and a SDS of less than 50%, and the other ear has a large tumor (>2.0 cm) and a SDS greater than 50%, the authors would remove the smaller tumor using the translabyrinthine approach and would attempt to preserve the cochlear nerve for a later CI. The larger tumor would then be located in the only ear with hearing, and the authors would observe the tumor and offer decompression of the internal auditory canals if indicated. They would wait to perform surgery until the hearing was lost if there were no signs of significant brainstem compression. Hearing rehabilitation with CI or ABI is similar to the protocol previously described.

Both tumors large or both tumors small; poor hearing

The last clinical scenarios involve both ears with a large tumor (>2.0 cm) and a SDS of less than 50% (Fig. 3) or both ears with a small tumor (<2.0 cm) with a SDS of less than 50% bilaterally. In both cases, the authors would first remove the larger tumor using a translabyrinthine approach, making every effort to preserve the continuity of the cochlear nerve. Because the patient has poor hearing bilaterally, an ABI may be considered during this first resection if the cochlear nerve is not preserved, and if the patient desires hearing restoration at that time. The authors would suggest, however, that the patient wait to see if a CI is possible on either side. They would remove the second tumor when the patient has sufficiently recovered and would perform an ABI at the time of the second tumor removal if neither cochlear nerve is preserved.

Surgical outcomes

Samii et al [39] reported complete tumor resection in 88% (105/120) of NF2 cases with no cases of tumor recurrence after short-term follow-up. Excluding patients with concomitant facial nerve schwannomas or pre-operative facial nerve weakness, they preserved House-Brackmann grade I facial nerve function in 77% (66/86) of patients. The overall rate of hearing preservation was 36% but improved to 57% in patients with tumors that were smaller than 3 cm. It is difficult to compare these rates to those reported for radiation treatment, because this series contained 51 tumors larger than 3 cm, and most radiation centers rarely treat tumors larger than 3 cm or tumors with brainstem compression. Brackmann et al [38] reviewed 40 middle fossa excisions of NF2-associated tumors with an average size of 1.1 cm. They were able to preserve normal facial function in 92% of patients, and postoperative hearing class was unchanged in 55%. Follow-up

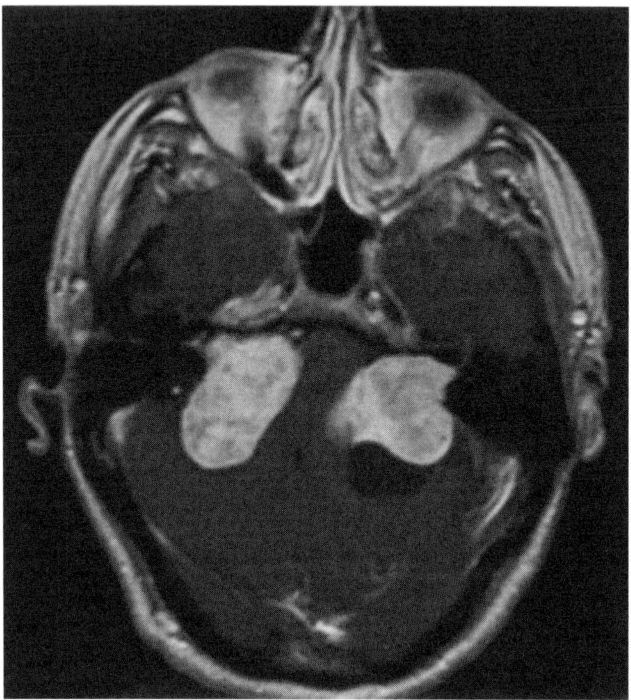

Fig. 3. Axial MRI of the brain and internal auditory canals with gadolinium contrast demonstrates bilateral, large (>3 cm) vestibular schwannomas in a NF2 patient with nonserviceable hearing bilaterally (SDS < 50%). Although the tumors were about the same size, the tumor on the left side was removed first using a translabyrinthine approach because it was causing a greater degree of midline shift and brainstem compression.

was too short to assess tumor control. Again, this report emphasizes that patient outcomes are much improved with early detection and removal of small tumors.

Stereotactic radiation

There are no randomized prospective trials comparing stereotactic radiation and microsurgical treatment of NF2-associated vestibular schwannomas. It has been reported that NF2 tumors do not respond as well as sporadic unilateral tumors to stereotactic radiation [21]. Rowe et al [47], however, showed a 79% control rate of 92 NF2 tumors at 8 years. These tumors received between 10 and 15 Gy using the gamma knife. This same series reported hearing preservation in 40% of patients and facial nerve preservation in 95%. The rate of facial nerve preservation did not factor in the 21% of patients with uncontrolled tumors who went on to surgical salvage. Most, but not all, physicians agree that these patients have a poor prognosis for facial nerve function because it is reportedly difficult to preserve facial nerve function after surgical salvage in an irradiated field [43,48–52].

Subach et al [53] showed a 98% tumor control rate in treating 45 NF2 tumors, but their follow-up was much shorter (average, 3 years), and additional failures, as seen in the series by Rowe et al [47], are likely to occur. Additionally, the radiation dose delivered to the tumor margin decreased over time from 18 to 20 Gy to 12 to 16 Gy to improve cranial nerve functional outcome. This modification was successful: they reported preservation of normal facial function in 84% and hearing preservation in 67% (six of nine tumors) of patients receiving 12 to 16 Gy of radiation. Data concerning long-term tumor control are not yet available for this group of NF2 patients receiving low-dose therapy, however, [53]. Moreover, the long-term incidence of second primary tumors in the radiated field is also not known and is a concern in younger NF2 patients.

Because of the short experience with the lower radiation dosages, the authors do not routinely encourage stereotactic radiotherapy as first-line therapy in this predominantly young population of patients with NF2. In NF2 patients whose tumors demonstrate growth, the authors currently recommend stereotactic radiation therapy for patients who refuse surgery or who are medically unfit to undergo surgery.

Potential future therapies

The *NF2* gene encodes a tumor-suppressor protein product, merlin [12]. It is hoped that understanding merlin's interactions with other proteins, signaling pathways, and regulation of the *NF2* gene will lead to the development of novel treatments for vestibular schwannomas. Ultimately, targeted molecular interventions and drug therapies will be designed to stop schwannoma progression or to eradicate preexisting tumors altogether. Such treatments will offer alternatives to the current options of untreated observation of tumor growth, stereotactic radiation, or surgical removal.

For example, several studies have suggested that merlin plays a role in the regulation of signaling of Rho geranylgeranyltransferases (GTPases) [54–56]. It has also been demonstrated that expression of RhoB GTPase is increased in vestibular schwannomas and may respond to target-specific therapy with farnesyl transferase inhibitors [57].

Another treatment approach may involve reducing the blood supply to vestibular schwannomas. Inhibition of angiogenic growth factor may reduce the rate of vestibular schwannoma growth [58]. In addition, the expression of osteonectin, a mediator of angiogenesis, was found to be increased significantly in several vestibular schwannomas and may offer a potential target for angiogenesis inhibitors [59–61].

With the use of viral vectors, introduction of the normal *NF2* genetic sequence (and hence the normal merlin protein product) into vestibular schwannoma cells may be possible. The complete molecular mechanism of schwannoma formation and the precise role of merlin must be defined more clearly before this goal is realized [9].

References

[1] Prevention and control of neurofibromatosis: memorandum from a joint WHO/NNFF meeting. Bull World Health Organ 1992;70:173–82.

[2] Evans DG, Huson SM, Donnai D, et al. A genetic study of type 2 neurofibromatosis in the United Kingdom: I. Prevalence, mutation rate, fitness, and confirmation of maternal transmission effect on severity. J Med Genet 1992;29:841–6.

[3] Fontaine B, Rouleau GA, Seizinger BR, et al. Molecular genetics of neurofibromatosis 2 and related tumors (acoustic neuroma and meningioma). Ann N Y Acad Sci 1991;615:338–43.

[4] Kaiser-Kupfer M, Freidlin V, Datiles MB, et al. The association of posterior capsular lens opacities with bilateral acoustic neuromas in patients with neurofibromatosis type 2. Arch Ophthalmol 1989;107(4):541–4.

[5] Kanter WR, Eldridge R, Fabricant R, et al. Central neurofibromatosis with bilateral acoustic neuroma: genetic, clinical and biochemical distinctions from peripheral neurofibromatosis. Neurology 1980;30:851–9.

[6] Martuza RL, Eldridge R. Neurofibromatosis 2 (bilateral acoustic neurofibromatosis). N Engl J Med 1988;318:684–8.

[7] Glasscock ME III, Woods CI, Jackson CG, et al. Management of bilateral acoustic tumors. Laryngoscope 1989;99:475–84.

[8] Mautner VF, Lindenau M, Baser ME, et al. Skin abnormalities in neurofibromatosis 2. Arch Dermatol 1997;133:1539–43.

[9] Evans DGR, Sainio M, Baser ME. Neurofibromatosis type 2. J Med Genet 2000;37:897–904.

[10] Baser ME, Friedman JM, Wallace AJ, et al. Evaluation of clinical diagnostic criteria for neurofibromatosis 2. Neurology 2002;59(11):1759–65.

[11] Marchuk DA, Saulino AM, Tavakkol R, et al. cDNA cloning of the type 1 neurofibromatosis gene: complete sequence of the NF1 gene product. Genomics 1991; 11(4):931–40.

[12] Trofatter JA, MacCollin MM, Rutter JL, et al. A novel Moesin-, Exrin-, Radixin-like gene is a candidate for the neurofibromatosis 2 tumor-suppressor. Cell 1993;72:791–800.

[13] Evans DGR, Huson SM, Donnai D, et al. A clinical study of type 2 neurofibromatosis. Q J Med 1992;84:603–18.

[14] Wishart JH. Case of tumors in the skull, dura mater, and brain. Edinburgh Med Surg J 1822; 18:393–7.

[15] Gardner WJ, Frazier CH. Bilateral acoustic neurofibromatosis: a clinical study and field survey of a family of five generations with bilateral deafness in thirty-eight members. Arch Neurol Psychiatry 1930;23:266–302.

[16] Ruggieri M, Huson SM. The clinical and diagnostic implications of mosaicism in neurofibromatosis. Neurology 2001;56(11):1433–43.

[17] Kluwe L, Mautner V, Heinrich B. Molecular study of frequency of mosaicism in neurofibromatosis 2 patients with bilateral vestibular schwannomas. J Med Genet 2003; 40(2):109–14.

[18] Moyhuddin A, Baser MG, Watson C. Somatic mosaicism in neurofibromatosis 2: prevalence and risk of disease transmission to offspring. J Med Genet 2003;40(6):459–63.

[19] Evans DGR, Birch JM, Ramsden R. Pediatric presentation of type 2 neurofibromatosis. Arch Dis Child 1999;81:496–9.

[20] Mautner VF, Lindenau M, Baser ME, et al. Spinal tumors in patients with neurofibromatosis type 2: MR imaging study of frequency, multiplicity, and variety. AJR Am J Roentgenol 1995;165:951–5.

[21] Moffat DA, Quaranta N, Baguley DM, et al. Management strategies in neurofibromatosis type 2. Eur Arch Otorhinolaryngol 2003;260:12–8.
[22] Mautner VF, Lindenau M, Baser ME, et al. The neuroimaging and clinical spectrum of neurofibromatosis 2. Neurosurgery 1996;38:880–5.
[23] Welling DB, Glasscock ME III, Woods CI, et al. Acoustic neuroma: a cost-effective approach. Otolaryngol Head Neck Surg 1990;103(3):364–70.
[24] Zealley IA, Cooper RC, Clifford KM, et al. MRI screening for acoustic neuroma: a comparison of fast spin echo and contrast enhanced imaging in 1233 patients. Br J Radiol 2000;73(867):242–7.
[25] Welling DB, Guida M, Goll F, et al. Mutational spectrums in the neurofibromatosis type 2 gene in sporadic and familial schwannomas. Hum Genet 1996;98:189–93.
[26] Merel P, Khe HX, Sanson M, et al. Screening for germ-line mutations in the NF2 gene. Genes Chromosomes Cancer 1995;12:117–27.
[27] MacCollin M, Ramesh V, Jacoby LB, et al. Mutational analysis of patients with neurofibromatosis 2. Am J Hum Genet 1994;55:314–20.
[28] Zucman-Rossi J, Legoix P, Der Sarkissian H, et al. NF2 gene in neurofibromatosis type 2 patients. Hum Mol Genet 1999;7:2095–101.
[29] Welling DB. Clinical manifestations of mutations in the neurofibromatosis type 2 gene in vestibular schwannomas (acoustic neuromas). Laryngoscope 1998;108:178–89.
[30] Welling DB, Neff BA, Wiet M, et al. Cochlear implantation in the profoundly deafened NF2 patient. Presented at the VIII International Cochlear Implant Conference, Indianapolis, IN, May 10–13, 2004.
[31] Hoffman RA, Kohan D, Cohen NL. Cochlear implants in the management of bilateral acoustic neuromas. Am J Otol 1992;13(6):525–8.
[32] Temple RH, Axon PR, Ramsden RT. Auditory rehabilitation in neurofibromatosis type 2: a case for cochlear implantation. J Laryngol Otol 1999;113(2):161–3.
[33] Hulka GF, Bernard EJ, Pillsbury HC. Cochlear implantation in a patient after removal of an acoustic neuroma. The implications of magnetic resonance imaging with gadolinium on patient management. Arch Otolaryngol Head Neck Surg 1995;121(4):465–8.
[34] Otto SR, Brackmann DE, Hitselberger WE, et al. Multichannel auditory brainstem implants: update on performance in 61 patients. J Neurosurg 2002;96(6):1063–71.
[35] Nevison B, Laszig R, Sollmann WP, et al. Results from a European clinical investigation of the nucleus multichannel auditory brainstem implant. Ear Hear 2002;23(3): 170–83.
[36] Ebinger K, Otto S, Arcaroli J, et al. Multichannel auditory brainstem implant: US clinical trial results. J Laryngol Otol Suppl 2000;27:50–3.
[37] Shannon RV, Otto S, Brackmann DE, et al. Psychophysical and speech results from the first patients with the penetrating auditory brainstem implant (PABI). Presented at the VIII International Cochlear Implant Conference, Indianapolis, IN, May 10–13, 2004.
[38] Brackmann DE, Fayad JN, Slattery WH, et al. Early proactive management of vestibular schwannomas in neurofibromatosis type 2. Neurosurgery 2001;49(2):274–83.
[39] Samii M, Matthies C, Tatagiba M. Management of vestibular schwannomas (acoustic neuromas): auditory and facial nerve function after resection of 120 vestibular schwannomas in patients with neurofibromatosis 2. Neurosurgery 1997;40(4):696–706.
[40] Hughes GB, Sismanis A, Glasscock ME III, et al. Management of bilateral acoustic neuromas. Laryngoscope 1982;92:1351–9.
[41] Linthicum FH. Unusual audiometric and histologic findings in bilateral acoustic neurinomas. Ann Otol 1972;81:433–7.
[42] Jääskeläinen J, Paetau A, Pyykkö I, et al. Interface between the facial nerve and large acoustic neurinomas. Immunohistochemical study of the cleavage plane in NF2 and non-NF2 cases. J Neurosurg 1994;80:541–7.
[43] Briggs RJS, Brackmann DE, Baser ME, et al. Comprehensive management of bilateral acoustic neuromas. Arch Otolaryngol Head Neck Surg 1994;120:1307–14.

[44] Gadre AK, Kwartler JA, Brackmann DE, et al. Middle fossa decompression of the internal auditory canal in acoustic neuroma surgery: a therapeutic alternative. Laryngoscope 1990; 100:948–52.
[45] Slattery WH, Brackmann DE, Hitselberger W. Hearing preservation in neurofibromatosis type 2. Am J Otol 1998;19(5):638–43.
[46] Glasscock ME III, Hart MJ, Vrabec JT. Management of bilateral acoustic neuromas. Otolaryngol Clin North Am 1992;25:449–69.
[47] Rowe JG, Radatz MWR, Walton L, et al. Clinical experience with gamma knife stereotactic radiosurgery in the management of vestibular schwannomas secondary to type 2 neurofibromatosis. J Neurol Neurosurg Psychiatry 2003;74:1288–93.
[48] Pollack BE, Lunsford LD, Kondziolka D, et al. Vestibular schwannoma management: II. Failed radiosurgery and the role of delayed microsurgery. J Neurosurg 1998;89:949–55.
[49] Battista RA, Wiet RJ. Stereotactic radiosurgery for acoustic neuromas: a survey of the American neurotology society. Am J Otol 2000;21:371–81.
[50] Schulder M, Gangadhar SS, Kwartler JA, et al. Microsurgical removal of a vestibular schwannoma after stereotactic radiosurgery: surgical and pathological findings. Am J Otol 1999;20:364–8.
[51] Slattery WH, Brackmann DE. Results of surgery following stereotactic irradiation for acoustic neuromas. Am J Otol 1995;16(3):315–21.
[52] Lee DJ, Westra WH, Staecker H, et al. Clinical and histopathologic features of recurrent vestibular schwannoma (acoustic neuroma) after stereotactic radiosurgery. Otol Neurotol 2003;24(4):650–60.
[53] Subach BR, Kondziolka D, Lunsford LD, et al. Stereotactic radiosurgery in the management of acoustic neuromas associated with neurofibromatosis type 2. J Neurosurg 1999;90:815–22.
[54] Shaw RJ, Paez JG, Curto M, et al. The Nf2 tumor suppressor, merlin, functions in Rac-dependent signaling. Dev Cell 2001;1:63–72.
[55] Kissil JL, Johnson KC, Eckman MS, et al. Merlin phosphorylation by p21-activated kinase 2 and effects of phosphorylation on merlin localization. J Biol Chem 2002;277:10394–9.
[56] Xiao GH, Beeser A, Chernoff J, et al. p21-activated kinase links Rac/Cdc42 signaling in merlin. J Biol Chem 2002;277:883–6.
[57] Allal C, Pradines A, Hamilton AD, et al. Farnestylated RhoB prevents cell cycle arrest and actin cytoskeleton disruption caused by the geranylgeranyltransferase I inhibitor GGTI-298. Cell Cycle 2002;1(6):430–7.
[58] Takamiya Y, Friedlander RM, Brem H, et al. Inhibition of angiogenesis and growth of human nerve-sheath tumors by AGM-1470. J Neurosurg 1993;78:470–6.
[59] Welling DB, Lasak JM, Akhmametyeva EM, et al. cDNA microarray analysis of vestibular schwannomas. Otol Neurotol 2002;23(5):736–48.
[60] Vajkoczy P, Menger MD, Vollmar B, et al. Inhibition of tumor growth, angiogenesis, and microcirculation by the novel Flk-1 inhibitor SU-5416 as assessed by intravital multi-fluorescence videomicroscopy. Neoplasia 1999;1:31–41.
[61] Vajkoczy P, Menger MD, Goldbrunner R, et al. Targeting angiogenesis inhibits tumor infiltration and expression of the pro-invasive protein SPARC. Int J Cancer 2000;87:261–8.

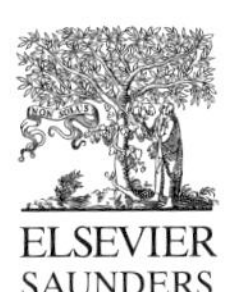
ELSEVIER
SAUNDERS

Otolaryngol Clin N Am
38 (2005) 685–710

OTOLARYNGOLOGIC
CLINICS
OF NORTH AMERICA

Facial Nerve Rerouting in Skull Base Surgery

Nooshin Parhizkar, MD, David H. Hiltzik, MD, Samuel H. Selesnick, MD*

Department of Otolaryngology, Weill Medical College of Cornell University, New York, 530 East 70th Street, New York, NY 10021, USA

Resection of skull base tumors is limited by the intratemporal course of the facial nerve. These tumors include glomus tumor jugulare, neuromas of cranial nerves IX–XI, infralabyrinthine cholesteatomas, mesenchymal tumors, and meningiomas. These tumors may extend into the posterior fossa, the middle fossa, and the infratemporal components of the skull base. Facial nerve rerouting techniques were developed to facilitate resection of extensive tumors occupying the skull base. Facial nerve rerouting, however, has its own limitations and risks, requiring microsurgical expertise, additional surgical time, and often some degree of facial nerve paresis. The first portion of this article presents different degrees of anterior and posterior facial nerve rerouting, techniques of facial nerve rerouting, and a comprehensive review of outcomes. The concluding portion reviews anatomic and functional preservation of the facial nerve in acoustic neuroma resection, technical aspects of facial nerve dissection, options for intracranial facial nerve repair, and outcomes for successful acoustic neuroma surgery.

Intratemporal anatomy of the facial nerve

The facial nerve courses intracranially from the brainstem to the porus acousticus and then intratemporally from the internal auditory canal (IAC) to the stylomastoid foramen before moving on to the muscles of facial expression. As the facial nerve travels through the petrous temporal bone in the bony fallopian canal, it can be divided into the intracanalicular, labyrinthine, tympanic, and mastoid segments.

* Corresponding author. Department of Otolaryngology, Weill Medical College of Cornell University, 520 East 70th Street, Room 541, New York, NY 10021.

E-mail address: shselesn@med.cornell.edu (S.H. Selesnick).

doi:10.1016/j.otc.2005.01.003 ***oto.theclinics.com***

The facial nerve arises from the facial nuclei and exits the brainstem at the level of the pontomedullary junction. It crosses the cerebellopontine angle to enter the IAC at the porus acousticus and exits the IAC superior to the transverse crest and anterior to the vertical bar (Bill's bar). After exiting the IAC, the nerve enters the labyrinthine segment. The labyrinthine segment originates at the meatal foramen, which is the narrowest point in the intratemporal bony canal, measuring on average 0.7 mm in diameter [1]. It is also the shortest segment in the fallopian canal, measuring approximately 3.5 mm to 4 mm in length [2]. At this level the nerve is 1 mm directly posterior to the cochlea. It is also 3 mm anterior to the superior semicircular canal and rests on the anterior part of the vestibule [2]. Because the labyrinthine segment is the narrowest part of the facial nerve, it is most susceptible to compression secondary to edema. Furthermore, it is the only segment that lacks anastomosing arterial cascades, thus making the area vulnerable to ischemia.

At the distal portion of the labyrinthine segment, the main trunk of the facial nerve changes direction at the geniculate ganglion. With the anterior exit of the greater superficial petrosal nerve at the geniculate ganglion, the main trunk of the nerve turns abruptly posteriorly, forming the tympanic segment that ends at the second genu [2]. The tympanic segment extends from the geniculate ganglion to the region of the horizontal semicircular canal. It measures approximately 8 to 11 mm in length. In its posterior course within the tympanic segment, the nerve is superior to the cochleariform process. The facial nerve forms the second genu between the oval window and the lateral semicircular canal and then turns inferiorly to begin the mastoid segment [3]. The mastoid segment is the vertical segment of the facial nerve and descends to the stylomastoid foramen, where it exits the fallopian canal through the stylomastoid foramen (SMF). This is the longest segment of the intratemporal course, approximately 10 to 14 mm long [3].

The facial nerve has both an intrinsic and an extrinsic vascular supply. The extrinsic blood supply is through the stylomastoid artery (a branch of the postauricular artery of the external carotid system), the greater petrosal artery (a branch of the middle meningeal artery, from the external carotid system), and the internal auditory artery (a branch of the anterior inferior cerebellar artery, a division of the vertebro-basilar system) [4]. In mobilization of the facial nerve, the blood supply to the facial nerve is at risk as it courses between the epineurium and the bony periosteum, especially when the nerve is mobilized at the first genu [4].

Anterior facial nerve rerouting

Historical perspective

Capps [5] first reported facial nerve rerouting in 1952. In 1949, he undertook an exploration of the middle ear and the jugular bulb for resection of a glomus jugulare tumor. He described a transmastoid approach with mobilization of the facial nerve, stating that the "facial nerve was exposed, freed, and drawn out of the way." He does not describe the extent of facial nerve mobilization, but he reports that postoperatively the patient had an incomplete resection, facial paralysis, and meningitis. The facial paralysis recovered after 2 years. In 1964, Shapiro and Neues [6] reported rerouting the vertical component of the facial nerve for access to the hypotympanum and jugular bulb in resection of glomus jugular tumors. Using an extensive transmastoid approach, they completely exenterated the mastoid cavity, widely exposed the sigmoid sinus, removed the mastoid tip, ligated the external carotid artery above the facial artery, and traced the facial nerve forward into the parotid gland from to the middle ear. Once the bony posterior and inferior canal walls were removed, the facial nerve was "carefully displaced from the canal and reflected forward and upward out of the way." The facial nerve was repositioned at the end of the surgery. Postoperatively, this patient had temporary facial nerve paralysis for 2 months with subsequent complete recovery [6]. In 1974, Glasscock [7] published a series of 21 patients with glomus tumors. He described two cases in which the facial nerve was mobilized and rerouted. In both cases the patient had large glomus jugulare tumors requiring an extended facial recess technique with skull base exposure similar to the one Shapiro and Neues [6] described in 1964. In describing his surgical technique, Glasscock [7] reported that to obtain better exposure, the bone over the facial nerve was thinned until "its sheath can be seen through the bone from its genu to the SMF." The facial nerve was then "taken out of the canal at the oval window and held along the posterior canal wall" to obtain access to the hypotympanum and jugular bulb. The external auditory canal (EAC) wall, the tympanic membrane, and the ossicles were preserved. Immediate facial nerve function was preserved. In his second facial nerve rerouting, "the 7th nerve was removed from its canal and temporarily laid across the middle ear." The posterior EAC wall was removed along with tympanic membrane and the ossicles. Although there was immediate facial nerve paralysis, the patient was reported to have complete facial nerve recovery in 2 months. Glasscock's original descriptions do not specify further extent or degree of anterior facial nerve transposition.

In 1977 Fisch [8] introduced the infratemporal fossa type A (ITFA) approach, which better defined the surgical exposure for resection of glomus jugulare tumors. In the ITFA approach, a radical mastoidectomy is followed by removal of the tympanic membrane, malleus, and incus and rerouting of the facial nerve from the SMF to the geniculate ganglion. In this technique, the facial nerve is dissected into the parotid gland, and permanent anterior transposition of the facial nerve is completed. At least temporary facial nerve paresis and conductive hearing loss are expected postoperative results.

Brackmann [9] descried modifications of the ITFA approach in 1987. The major difference between Brackmann's technique and Fisch's technique is the management of the facial nerve at the level of the SMF. Brackmann recommended that the soft tissue contents of the SMF be displaced en bloc with the facial nerve when it is anteriorly rerouted. This technique is believed to reduce unnecessary trauma to the nerve caused by dissection in the SMF region. He also recommended that the nerve be transposed only temporarily to reduce trauma that was believed to be more significant with the Fisch technique.

Degrees of facial nerve rerouting

Anterior rerouting of the facial nerve is a subtotal rerouting. The labyrinthine, intracanalicular, and intracranial portions of the facial nerve and their blood supply are left intact. In anterior facial nerve rerouting, rerouting begins at the stylomastoid foramen. Depending on the degree of exposure necessary, rerouting may extend proximally all the way to the geniculate ganglion to allow access to the jugular foramen and the ascending intrapetrous carotid artery as well as to the sigmoid sinus, the upper neck, the infratemporal region, and posterior fossa anterior to the sigmoid.

Kinney [10], Glasscock et al [11], and Jackson et al [12] describe a short and a long anterior rerouting depending on the extent of exposure indicated. In the short rerouting technique described by Glasscock [10] in 1984, the facial nerve is mobilized from the SMF to the second genu. This method is indicated when carotid involvement is limited. Because the facial nerve is fixed 10 mm anterior to the SMF, if the EAC wall remains intact, the vertical segment of the nerve can be rerouted anteriorly at an angle of $13.25^\circ \pm 2.52^\circ$ from the second genu with a maximum anterior displacement of 4.18 ± 0.83 mm from the fallopian canal at the level of the superior jugular bulb.

The facial nerve can be mobilized along its entire mastoid and tympanic course up to the geniculate ganglion. This method, the ITFA approach, was popularized by Fisch [8] for resection of glomus tumors (stages class C or D in the Fisch classification). The ITFA approach is the long rerouting technique in which the EAC, tympanic membrane, malleus, and incus are removed. Long rerouting allows a 10.8 ± 2.44–mm maximum anterior displacement of the second genu of the facial nerve, and a 14.5 ± 1.62–mm maximum anterior displacement of the nerve from the fallopian canal at the level of superior jugular bulb [13].

In both the short and long rerouting techniques, management of the nerve at the SMF is critical to postoperative facial nerve contents. The epineurium, vascular connective tissue, and periosteum of the fallopian canal are the components of the sheath of the facial nerve and a funnel-shaped structure [14,15]. As the nerve exits the SMF along with its sheath, the epineurium fuses with a thick layer of fascia from the digastric muscle and the periosteum of the skull base. The stylomastoid artery and veins are also enclosed within this sheath of dense connective tissue [1,17–20]. This fibrous tissue creates difficulty in identifying the nerve at the SMF [16]. En bloc transposition of the SMF with its contents is advocated to reduce mechanical trauma that can occur with dissection of the facial nerve at the level of SMF [9].

Anterior facial nerve rerouting: long technique

A postauricular skin incision is made extending into the neck, exposing the lower cranial nerves, carotid artery, and jugular vein. A mastoidectomy is performed exposing the sigmoid sinus, digastric ridge, vertical facial nerve, the middle cranial fossa tegmen, the mastoid antrum, incus, and the semicircular canals. Once the second genu of the facial nerve is identified, and the facial recess is opened widely, the malleus and incus, the tympanic membrane, and the skin of EAC are removed. The posterior external auditory canal bone is resected, and the chorda tympani is divided. The facial nerve is skeletonized from the SMF to the second genu and subsequently to the geniculate ganglion using diamond burrs. Any remaining bony fragments on the nerve are removed with a dissector. The epineurium is kept intact, and the nerve is gently dissected out of the fallopian canal [18]. Care is taken to identify and divide the branches of the stapedius and digastric muscles so that the nerve can be freely displaced anteriorly. The SMF, the posterior belly of the digastric muscles, and the undissected parotid gland are reflected anteriorly en bloc. The facial nerve should not be dissected out of the upper neck and the parotid gland, to avoid additional trauma and disruption of the nerve's blood supply. For the duration of the surgery, the facial nerve and its surrounding structures are temporarily mobilized and retracted over the angle of the mandible. At this point there is excellent access to the carotid artery anteriorly, the jugular bulb inferiorly, and the sigmoid sinus posteriorly [19]. Fig. 1A shows the facial nerve in its normal anatomic position within the right temporal bone. Fig. 1B demonstrates the facial nerve displaced forward up to the second genu, and Fig. 1C demonstrates full anterior mobilization of the facial nerve from the first genu to the stylomastoid foramen.

Posterior rerouting of the facial nerve

Historical background

In 1904 Panse first introduced a translabyrinthine approach with sacrifice of the facial nerve for resection of a cerebellopontine angle tumor [20]. Because of its high rate of complications, this approach was abandoned until the 1960s, when House [21,22] reintroduced the translabyrinthine approach preserving the facial nerve for access to the CPA. To obtain

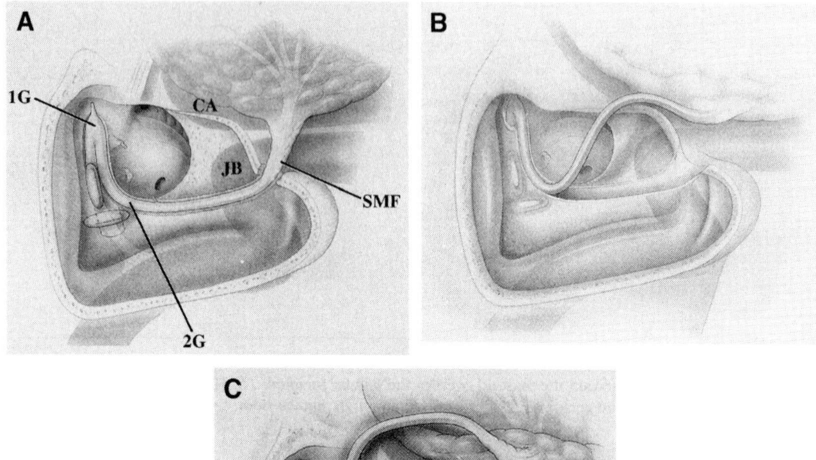

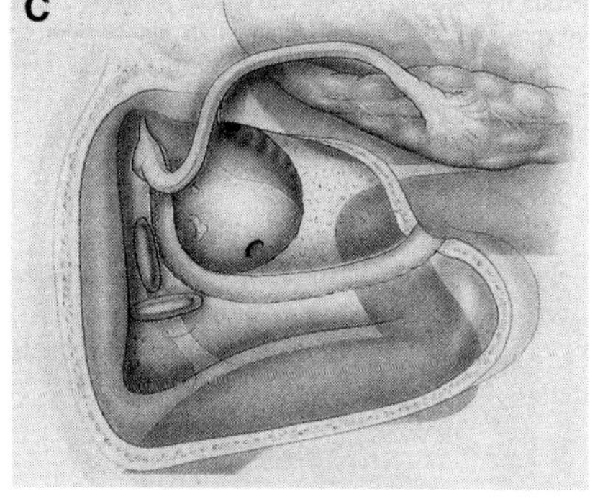

Fig. 1. (*A*) The facial nerve viewed in its normal anatomic position within the right temporal bone. (*B*) Anterior rerouting of the facial nerve after the ear canal is removed: the facial nerve is displaced forward up to the second genu. (*C*) Full anterior mobilization of the facial nerve from the second genu to the stylomastoid foramen. CA, carotid artery; 1G, first genu; 2G, second genu; JB, jugular bulb; SMF, stylomastoid foramen. (*From* Jackler RK. Atlas of neurotology and skull base surgery. St Louis (MO): Mosby-Year Book; 1996. p. 163 & 164; with permission.)

further exposure to the brainstem, petrous pyramid, and the clivus, House and Hitselberger [23] introduced the transcochlear approach in 1976. This additional exposure requires the posterior rerouting of the entire facial nerve, including the labyrinthine and the intracanicular segments. The petrous apex and part of the clivus can be removed to expose tumors such as petroclival meningiomas or other intradural or extradural tumors in the prepontine region and CPA. Pellet et al [24] subsequently described the transcochlear approach in combination with the ITFA approach to create a widened transcochlear method for resection of saddle-shaped tumors with both infratemporal and posterior fossa components.

Technique of posterior nerve rerouting

A postauricular skin incision is made, and an extended mastoidectomy is performed. The sigmoid sinus and the retrosigmoid area, the digastric ridge, and the vertical facial nerve along with the middle cranial fossa dura, the mastoid antrum, the fossa incudis, and the vestibular apparatus are identified. A complete labyrinthectomy is followed by the identification of the facial nerve from the SMF to the IAC. Once the IAC is identified, troughs are drilled superior and inferior to the canal to expose its contents further. The tympanic bone, the EAC skin, malleus, incus, and tympanic membrane are then resected [24,25]. The chorda tympani nerve is then divided. The horizontal portion of the facial nerve can be isolated after the tensor tympani and the stapedius tendons are divided and the ossicles have been removed. The bone of the middle cranial fossa floor is removed so the geniculate can be reached from a posterior superior approach. After removal of the gross bony covering of the fallopian canal with diamond burrs, the tympanic and mastoid segments can be dissected out of the bony canal (Fig. 2A, B). To mobilize the facial nerve from its fallopian canal, the greater superficial petrosal nerve is divided (Fig. 2C).

In the IAC, the facial nerve can be found in the anterior superior region. Once the facial nerve is rerouted, the cochlea can be removed completely and the intrapetrous genu of the internal carotid artery identified and traced both proximally and distally. The petrous apex bone can now be resected up to and including the clivus. At this point, the posterior fossa dura is exposed from the sigmoid sinus to the clivus, and dural incisions can be made and tumor dissection initiated (Fig. 2D).

Outcomes of rerouting

It is difficult to summarize the results of facial nerve rerouting objectively, because each series is different with regard to tumor histology, extent of tumor resections, preoperative facial nerve function, type of facial nerve manipulation, and descriptions of postoperative facial nerve function. Some authors assessed facial nerve function solely on subjective percentage of facial function as assessed by the patient using patient questionnaires, whereas others used the objective House-Brackmann (HB) scale. Postoperative follow-up often ranged from 6 months to 1 year.

In 1996 Selesnick and colleagues [26] published a comprehensive review of facial nerve rerouting from 1977 to 1996. These data are summarized in Tables 1 and 2. Analysis of the preceding studies showed that patients with short anterior rerouting had the least facial nerve dysfunction, with 47% having HB grade I and grade II function at short term follow-up and 93% having grade I and grade II function at long-term follow-up. Analysis of the series on long anterior rerouting showed that 41% of patients had grade I and grade II function at short-term follow-up and 73% had grade I and grade II function at long-term follow-up.

In a review of posterior facial nerve rerouting, only 26% recovered to HB grades I and grade II function in long-term follow-up. Grade III facial nerve dysfunction was the most common grade in patients with posterior

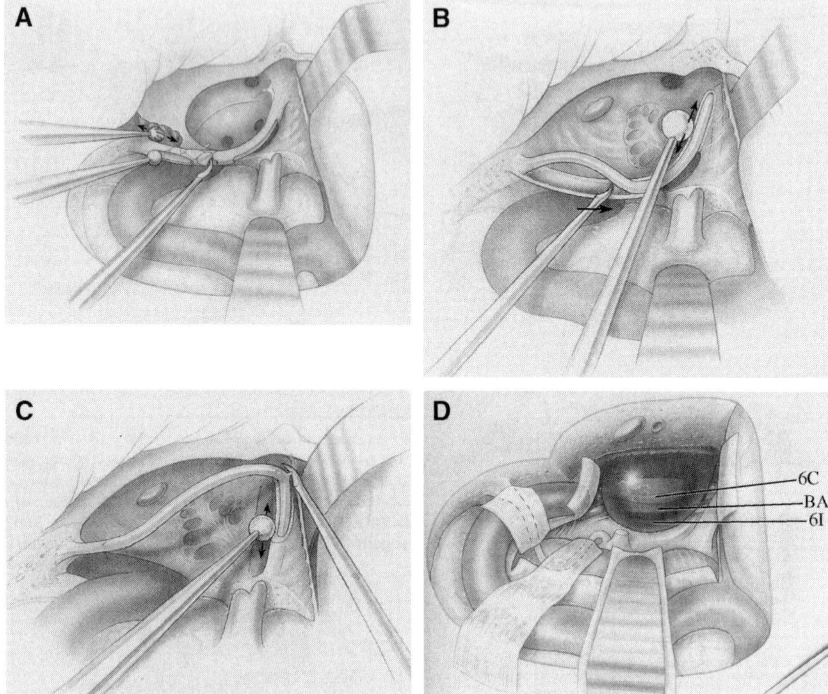

Fig. 2. The left ear with the EAC, tympanic membrane, and ossicles removed. Labyrinthectomy has been performed, and the IAC is delineated. (*A*) Dissection with various instruments is demonstrated. From left to right: dense bone is removed with the cutting burr, the bone over the facial nerve is exposed with the diamond burr, and residual bony fragments are dissected with fine instrumentation. (*B*) To minimize risk of nerve injury, dissection is performed parallel to the facial nerve using a diamond burr. (*C*) To mobilize the facial nerve fully, the greater superficial petrosal nerve is divided, and the facial nerve is reflected posteriorly. (*D*) Final exposure of the tumor after the facial nerve is rerouted (under cottonoids); the prepontine tumor is exposed. BA, basilar artery; 6C, contralateral abducens nerve; 6I, ipsilateral abducens nerve. (*From* Jackler RK. Atlas of neurotology and skull base surgery. St Louis: Mosby-Year Book; 1996. p. 52, 55, 56, & 59; with permission.)

rerouting, occurring in 53% of all patients. Only 7% of patients had grade VI facial paralysis.

These data are not surprising, because in long facial nerve rerouting interruption of the deep petrosal artery leads to perigeniculate ischemia and penetrates the vascular supply. There also is an increased chance of mechanical trauma with the mobilization of the facial nerve from the narrow labyrinthine segment and manipulation of the epineurium in the IAC [26]. Table 3 summarizes these cumulative data.

Since 1996, there have been a few large series analyzing facial nerve function after rerouting. In 1998 von Doersten et al [27] performed a retrospective review of 217 patients who underwent lateral skull base

Table 1
Facial nerve function after long* anterior rerouting

Author	Affiliation	Procedure	Type of tumor	Relevant cases	Postoperative facial nerve function[a]			Comments
					Short-term		Long-term	
Jenkins [56] 1980	University Hospital, Zurich, Switzerland	Transotic with long rerouting	Acoustic neuroma	4	4, grade VI	> 6 months:	4, grades I–II	-
Fisch [57] 1982	University Hospital, Zurich, Switzerland	ITFA	Glomus jugulare	23	23, paresis/ paralysis	> 2 years:	23, 85% avg. recovery	-
Kaye [58] 1984	Cleveland Clinic Foundation, Cleveland OH	Long rerouting	Varied	2	1, grades I–II; 1, paresis		2, grades I–II	-
Lambert [18] 1985	University of Virginia Medical Center, Charlottesville, VA; University of Washington Medical Center, Seattle, WA	ITFA/ infralabyrinthine	Varied	3	3, grade VI;	> 2 months:	I, grade I; 1, 80%–90% (postoperative RT); 1, > 80% recovery	c
Gardner [59] 1985	University of Tennessee, Center of Health Science Baptist Memorial Hospital, Memphis, TN	ITFA	Glomus jugulare	20	20, < 80% recovery	–	9, grade I; 11, < 80% recovery	
Bebear [60] 1985	Bordeaux, France	ITFA	Glomus jugulare	5	3, paresis; 2, grade VI	–	3, grade 1; 2, favorable	-

(continued on next page)

Table 1 (*continued*)

Author	Affiliation	Procedure	Type of tumor	Relevant cases	Postoperative facial nerve function[a]			Comments
					Short-term		Long-term	
Brammer [61] 1985	University of Michigan Medical School, Ann Arbor, MI	ITFA	Glomus jugulare	5	2, grade I; 2, paresis 1, grade VI	> 2 months:	4, grade 1; I, recovery with synkinisis	[c,d]
A1-Mefty [62] 1987	University of Mississippi; Medical Center, Jackson, MS George Washington University, Washington, DC King Faisal Specialist Hospital, Riyadh, Saudi Arabia	Combined infratemporal/ posterior fossa	Glomus jugulare, Chondro sarcoma	5	2, grades I–II; 3, paresis	–	-	
Brackmann [9] 1987	House Ear Clinic, Los Angeles, CA	ITFA with Brackmann SMF dissection	Glomus jugulare Meningioma, Varied others	23	10, grade I; 6, grade II; 2, grade III; 2, grade IV; 3, grade VI	> 1 year:	10, grade I; 7, grade II; 1, grade III; 2, grade IV (postoperative RT); 1, grade V (preoperative RT) I, grade VI (preoperative RT); I, died	

Hawthorne [63] 1988	University Hospital, Zurich, Switzerland	ITFA	Glomus jugulare	14	14, paresis/ paralysis	–	8, grade I;	c,d
Leonetti [64] 1989	House Ear Clinic, Los Angeles, CA	ITFA with Brackmann SMF dissection	Glomus jugulare, Varied others	15	14, grades I–II; 1, grades III–IV	–	6, good (preoperative RT) -	f
Poe [65] 1991	Otology Group, Nashville, TN	ITFA	Glomus jugulare, Varied others	32		> 2 years:	5, grade I; 13, grade II; 9, grade III; 3, grade IV; 2, grade V	b–d
Molony [66] 1992	House Ear Clinic, Los Angeles, CA	ITFA with Brackmann SMF dissection	Meningioma	7	2, grade I; 1, grade III; 2, grade IV; 2, grade VI	> 1 year:	3, grade I; 4, grade II	
Woods [67] 1993	Otology Group Nashville, TN	ITFA	Glomus jugulare, Glomus vagale	37		> 2 years:	6 grade h 16, grade II; 11, grade III; 3, grade IV; 1, grade V	b–d
Magliulo [68] 1994	University La Sapienza, Rome, Italy	ITFA	Glomus jugulare, Varied others	21	12, grade I–II; 4, grade III–IV; 8, grade V–VI	> 3 months:	16, grade I–II; 6, grade III–IV; 2, grade V–VI	b,d–f

(*continued on next page*)

Table 1 (*continued*)

Author	Affiliation	Procedure	Type of tumor	Relevant cases	Postoperative facial nerve function[a] Short-term		Long-term	Comments
Patel [69] 1994	University of Pittsburg Medical Center, Pittsburgh, PA; George Washington University Medical Center, Washington, DC	ITFA with Brackmann SMF dissection	Glomus jugulare	3	1, grade IV (I postoperative RT); 2, grade V	> 1 year:	1, grade II; 2, grade III (I postoperative RT)	[c,d,f]
Green [70] 1994	House Ear Clinic, Los Angeles, CA	ITFA with Brackmann SMF dissection	Glomus jugulare	40	25, grade I; 3, grade II; 2, grade III; 4, grade IV; 2, grade V; 1, grade VI	Average 3.4 years	27, grade I; 11, grade II; 2, grade III	[b,d,f]

Abbreviations: ITFA, infratemporal fossa type A; RT, radiation therapy.

* Unless otherwise indicated, based on data available, only patients with intact VII, rerouting indicated, and appropriate follow-up. Some overlap of patient population may exist between different studies from the same institution.

[a] Facial nerve function data provided using the six-point House-Brackmann grading format when possible.

[b] Some cases may not have only the method of rerouting described in this table.

[c] Some patients received preoperative and/or postoperative radiation therapy.

[d] All patients may not have had grade I facial function prior to surgery.

[e] Facial nerve may not have been preserved intact in all cases.

[f] Intraoperative facial nerve monitoring was utilized.

From Selesnick, SH, Abrahanm MT, Carew Jf Rerouting of the infratemporal facial nerve: an analysis of the literature Am J Otol 1996;17(5):793–805, Table 4; with permission.

Table 2
Facial nerve function after posterior rerouting

Author	Affiliation	Procedure	Type of tumor	Relevant cases[a]	Postoperative facial nerve function[b]		Comments
					Short-term	Long-term	
House [71] 1978	Otologic Medical Group, House Ear Clinic, Los Angeles, CA	Transcochlear	Cholesteatoma Meningioma	9	6, grade VI	> 6 months: 2–20% paresis; 3, some recovery 2, grade VI 2, died	[d]
Sekhar [72] 1986	Center for Cranial Base Surgery, Presbyterian University of Pittsburgh, Pittsburgh, PA	Combined transcochlear/ infratemporal	Varied	2	2, grade VI	> 6 months: 2, grades I–II (1 Postoperative RT) 2	
Pellet [73] 1988	Hopital St. Marguerite, Hopital de la Timone, Marseille, France	Combined transcochlear/ infratemporal	Glomus jugulare, varied others	7	7, grade VI	> 4 months: 1, grade I 1, regressive palsy 2, grade VI (I preoperative RT) 3, died (I postoperative RT)	[c,d]
Glasscock [74] 1989	Otology Group, Nashville, TN	Transcochlear	Cholesteatoma	4		> 1 year: 2, grade I 2, some recovery	[c]

(*continued on next page*)

Table 2 (*continued*)

Author	Affiliation	Procedure	Type of tumor	Relevant cases[a]	Postoperative facial nerve function[b]			Comments
					Short-term		Long-term	
Horn [75] 1991	Presbyterian Ear Institute, Neurological Associates, Albuquerque, NM	Transcochlear	Meningioma, Chordoma, varied others	7	7, grade VI	> 1 year:	7, recovery with mild synkinisis	f
Thedinger [76] 1992	Otology Group, Nashville, TN	Combined transcochlear/transtentorial	Meningioma	9		> 6 months:	6, grade III 2, grade IV (postoperative RT); 1, grade V (postoperative RT)	c,f
Arriaga [77] 1992	Otologic Medical Group, House Ear Clinic, Los Angeles, CA	Transcochlear	Meningioma	10		> 1 year:	3, grades I–II 4, grades III–IV 3, grades V–VI	d,f
Sanna [78] 1994	Gruppo Otologico, Ospedale Riuniti, Piacenza, Bergamo, Italy; Alexandria Univ., Egypt	Transcochlear	Meningioma, Chordoma, varied others	12	12, grade VI	> 1 year:	1, grade II 8, grade III 2, grade IV 1, grade V	c,f

Cass [79] 1994	Eye and Ear Institute, Pittsburgh, PA George Washington Univ., Washington, DC Hadassah Univ. Hospital, Jerusalem, Israel	Total petrosectomy	Meningioma, Chordoma, varied others	14	1, grade I; 1, grade III; 1, grade IV; 11, grade V	> 1 year:	2, grade I 1, grade II 7, grade III 3, grade IV 1, grades V–VI	c–f

Abbreviations: ITFA, infratemporal fossa type A; RT, radiation therapy.

[a] Unless otherwise indicated based on data available, only patients with intact VII, rerouting indicated, and appropriate follow-up. Some overlap of patient population may exist between different studies from the same institution.

[b] Facial nerve function data provided using the six-point House-Brackmann grading format when possible.

[c] Some patients received preoperative and/or postoperative radiation therapy.

[d] AI patients may not have had grade I facial function prior to surgery.

[e] Facial nerve may not have been preserved intact in all cases.

[f] Intraoperative facial nerve monitoring was utilized.

From Selesnick SH, Abrahanm MT, Carew Jf. Rerouting of the infratemporal facial nerve: an analysis of the literature Am J Otol 1996;17(5):793–805, Table 4; with permission.

Table 3
Facial nerve function after facial nerve rerouting (percentage with grades I–II facial nerve function)*

Type of rerouting	n	Short-term	Long-term
Short anterior	84	47% (27/58)	93% (78/74)
Long anterior	259	41% (77/190)	72% (175/242)
Posterior	74	2% (1/48)	26% (19/74)

* For facial nerve function data not provided in the six-point HouseBrackmann grading format, a best estimate of the House-Brackmann grade was made based upon the description of facial nerve function provided.

From Selesnick SH, Abraham MT, Carew JF. Rerouting of the intratemporal facial nerve: an analysis of the literature. Am J Otol 1996;17(5):793–805. Table 6; with permission.

surgery for nonmalignant tumors from 1970 to 1995. A lesser degree of rerouting correlated with better facial nerve outcomes. A worse post-operative HB score was associated with re-anastomosis, grafting, and 7-12 and 7-11 anastomosis. Average HB scores for mobilization were 1.65 for short mobilization, 2.74 for long mobilization, and 4.33 for grafting. Based on multivariate ANOVA analysis, this study also concluded that post-operative facial nerve function was most significantly dependent on type of CN 7 manipulation, then on preoperative facial function, and then on tumor staging.

In 1998, Sanna and colleagues [28] reported on their modified trans-cochlear approach for the management of central skull base lesions. In this retrospective review of 66 patients, 35 patients had extradural lesions, and 31 patients had intradural lesions. All patients were treated with the modified transcochlear approach. Total tumor removal was achieved in 58 cases, in either single or staged procedures. Subtotal tumor removal was performed in three patients. Two deaths occurred. In their description, the facial nerve was skeletonized from the SMF to the fundus of IAC. The greater superficial petrosal nerve was divided, and the facial nerve was anteriorly transposed. The authors reported a 67.5% recovery rate of facial nerve function to HB grade III or better 1 year after surgery.

In 2003, Russo and colleagues [29] published their results on 71 patients undergoing facial nerve rerouting from 1986 to 2001. The IFTA approach and the modified transcochlear approach were used for removal of glomus jugular tumors type C and for petroclival tumors, respectively. Facial nerve function was evaluated according to the HB grading system before surgery and at least 1 year postoperatively. Of the 54 patients undergoing anterior facial nerve rerouting, 51 had grade I facial nerve function preoperatively. Postoperatively, 33 patients (64.7%) had HB grade I/II function, 15 patients (29.4%) had grade III outcomes, 2 patients (3.9%) had grade IV function, and 1 patient (1.9%) had a grade VI outcome. All the 17 patients undergoing posterior facial nerve rerouting had HB grade I function preoperatively and HB grade VI function at discharge. At the 12-month follow-up, however, 12 patients (70.5%) had grade III function, 3 (17.6%) had grade IV function, 1 (5.8%) had grade V function, and 1 (5.8%) had grade VI function. The authors emphasize that anterior facial rerouting is indicated for resection of tympanojugular class C paragangliomas in the ITFA approach, and that this approach has an excellent function outcome of HB grade I to III in 94% of the cases. Furthermore, they conclude that posterior facial nerve rerouting using the transcochlear approach is expected to have recovery to HB grade III function in 70% cases at 1-year follow-up [29].

The data on facial nerve rerouting clearly indicate that facial nerve rerouting can be achieved safely with good outcomes in most cases, so that the excellent exposure gained by approaches requiring rerouting can be achieved with only limited added facial disability.

The facial nerve in acoustic neuroma surgery

The goal of acoustic neuroma surgery at the beginning of the twentieth century was to prolong life. Surgical treatment of these tumors now aims for total tumor removal with minimal mortality and morbidity, including hearing preservation and conservation of the facial nerve. Before the modern age of skull base surgery, many patients presented with a facial nerve palsy, and postoperative facial nerve weakness was considered routine. Now, with the use of MRI techniques and earlier detection, facial nerve function is intact in the most patients before surgery. With the evolution of anesthesia, microsurgical technique, and facial nerve monitoring, the facial nerve routinely is preserved anatomically and functionally.

Most studies published during the past half-century have reported facial nerve outcomes after surgical resection in both anatomic and functional terms, focusing on the facial nerve function at 1 year. Since the publication of the HB facial nerve grading system in 1985 [30], an objective, standardized scale has been used to communicate facial nerve outcomes more effectively and allowing a more accurate comparison of surgical outcomes. Factors that proved most prognostically important include preoperative facial nerve function, tumor size, and surgical approach.

Anatomic preservation

Although not equivalent with perfect facial nerve function, anatomic facial nerve preservation is an important aspect of acoustic neuroma surgery and thus is reported by most authors presenting their outcomes. It is considered the necessary first step in achieving postoperative facial nerve function. Recent large studies have reported an overall facial nerve preservation rate of greater than 90%, and some studies have even reached 96% [31–34]. Resection of tumors larger than 3 cm, however, is associated with significantly lower nerve preservation rates, ranging from 50% to 91% in studies with more than 50 patients [35–37]. This rate has greatly improved, to at least 78% in the post-1990 era of facial nerve monitoring. Notably, when segregating these studies dealing with large tumors by approach, reports of the translabyrinthine approach demonstrated preservation rates in the mid to high 90% range even in the 1960s and 1970s [38], whereas the suboccipital-retrosigmoid approaches achieved preservation rates of 88% [39]. These high rates of anatomic preservation for all tumors set the stage for the possibility of functional preservation.

Functional preservation and predictors of successful outcomes

The rates for preservation of facial nerve function have been favorable in the most recent era of acoustic neuroma surgery. In the literature, HB levels I and I are considered excellent or good outcomes, HB levels III and IV are considered intermediate or acceptable, and HB levels V and VI are considered poor. The discussion and reporting of functional preservation has often been examined preoperatively, immediately postoperatively, at hospital discharge, and at 1-year follow-up. As with anatomic preservation, facial function in influenced by variables including tumor size, approach, and era of surgery. Increasingly sophisticated surgical techniques and nerve monitoring also have allowed prognostication of function based on perioperative indicators.

Most often, patients with normal preoperative facial nerve function and a preserved nerve postoperatively have acceptable facial function postoperatively. More than 90% of these patients have an overall acceptable outcome at 1 year. Postoperative function can be characterized by early postoperative deterioration with improvement on long-term follow-up. In terms of prognosis, acceptable postoperative function predicts an acceptable result and poor postoperative function can be correlated with, but does not necessarily portend, a worse long-term outcome [39].

Analysis of specific trends in functional outcomes shows that better facial nerve function at 1-year follow-up is correlated with a lower HB grade immediately after surgery, a smaller tumor, and greater surgeon's experience. In the largest studies of more than 400 cases, tumors smaller than 2 cm had an excellent results, HB grade I and grade II, in the immediate and 1-year postoperative outcome in 85% and 95% of cases, respectively [39–41].

The discussion of large tumors and their outcomes is complicated by differences in the definition of tumor size (which in most studies varied between 2 and 3 cm), in whether the surgeries were performed before or after the era of nerve monitoring, and in technique. Four recent studies have reported more than 50 consecutive cases involving a large tumor (defined as > 2 cm in one study, > 3 cm in two studies, and > 4 cm in the final study). Three of the four studies used a translabyrinthine approach to the tumor. With the translabyrinthine approach in tumors larger than 2 cm, an excellent outcome (HB I and II) was achieved in 42% to 52% of the cases and acceptable function (HB grades I–IV) was found in 75% to 81% of operations at 1 year [31,37,38]. In one study, the retrosigmoid approach faired better, with an excellent result in 84% of cases at 1 year [42].

Several of the larger studies and several more recent studies have retrospectively and prospectively analyzed the three types of surgical approach—translabyrinthine, retrosigmoid, and middle fossa—in acoustic neuroma surgery. The various studies compared translabyrinthine versus retrosigmoid approaches and translabyrinthine versus middle fossa approaches. Although some decrease in immediate postoperative function was reported with the retrosigmoid approach as compared with the labyrinthine approach, outcomes at 1 year demonstrated no overall difference in facial nerve function [42–44]. In fact, in all studies tumor size is the major determinate in facial nerve function. The best approach is believed to be the one with which the surgeon has the most experience and is the most comfortable.

Intraoperative facial nerve monitoring (IFNM) has been used successfully to improve anatomic and physiologic preservation of the facial nerve. IFNM aids in detecting nerve location and is used to determine the stimulation thresholds of the nerve that predict long-term outcome. Since the use of facial nerve monitoring became widespread in the mid-1980s, there has been a steady increase in functional preservation of the facial nerve [45]. In studies using the constant voltage system, an electrical threshold of 0.2V or lower achieved an excellent result in 78% to 98% of patients at 1 year [46–48].

Several other variables have been investigated as further predictors of postoperative facial nerve function. One study found no significant correlation between patient age and facial nerve function [49]; another study demonstrated worse facial nerve outcomes in patients who had cystic tumors and who had undergone prior radiation therapy [34].

Technical aspects of facial nerve dissection

With tumor growth, the facial nerve is initially displaced from its anatomic position. It gradually is attenuated and then is splayed over the tumor. Accordingly, the larger the tumor, the more the nerve is stretched. Surprisingly, there are usually few disturbances of mimetic function during tumor growth, even in large tumors. In up to 10% of patients, however, facial twitching can be identified by careful examination or through electromyography [50]. As demonstrated in Fig. 3A, the facial nerve is most commonly compressed and stretched anteriorly. Less common, in decreasing order, are anterior superior compression (Fig. 3B), anterior inferior compression (Fig. 3C), directly superiorly compression (Fig. 3D), and compression posterior to the growing tumor (Fig. 3E). The surgeon

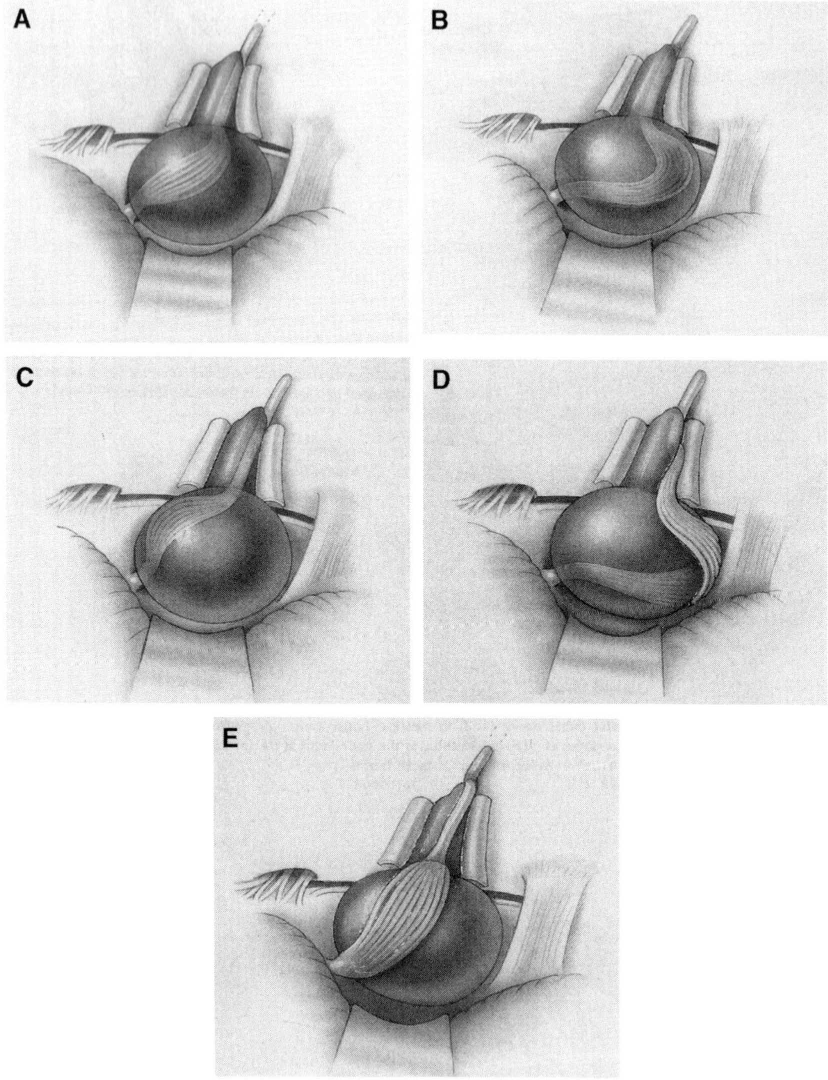

Fig. 3. Anatomic relationships between the facial nerve and acoustic neuromas in the left CPA. (*A*) Anterior displacement of the facial nerve, the most common course of the facial nerve. (*B*) Anterior superior displacement, the second most common course of the facial nerve. (*C*) Anterior inferior displacement, the third most common course. (*D*) Posterior superior displacement, a rarely seen course. (*E*) True posterior displacement, an extremely rare course. (*From* Jackler RK. Atlas of neurotology and skull base surgery. St Louis (MO): Mosby-Year Book; 1996. p. 11, 12 & 13; with permission.)

therefore cannot assume the path of the nerve in any operation. The tumor should not be stretched, twisted, or placed under unnecessary traction.

Several basic surgical principles and techniques should be followed when operating on tumors that displace the facial nerve. It is important to avoid disruption of attenuated fibers during dissection of the capsule off the nerve, and this precaution is facilitated by dissection parallel to the nerve to avoid transection. The surgeon may choose a round knife, sharp hook, or microscissors for sharp dissection or a microspatula for blunt dissection if only minimal adhesions are present. Hydrodissection is recommended as a less traumatic technique that may aid in developing a plane between the nerve and the tumor. More importantly, the nerve should not be allowed to dry, no matter what dissection technique is being used. A dry nerve, especially, in the IAC, makes the identification of a dissection plane difficult. When using bipolar cautery, local thermal injury should be minimized with effective suction irrigation techniques that dissipate the heat given off by the device. Bipolar cautery should never be used for hemostasis directly adjacent to the nerve. Thrombin-soaked gel foam may be used, even though the thrombin is sticky and may mask the plane of dissection. Additionally, when the tumor is resected, the core should be debulked initially to gain more space for inwardly reflecting the capsule being dissected off the nerve. If dissection becomes too precarious when nearing the nerve, the surgeon must consider leaving a thin veil of tumor capsule adjacent to the nerve as an alternative to possible nerve transaction [50]. A large amount of residual tumor, however, may maintain some of its blood supply and therefore carry a higher risk of recurrence [51]. The surgeon should also obtain feedback from the IFNM system, a guide during dissection. Trains of neurotonic discharges signify a risk of nerve injury; dissection should therefore be modified accordingly.

Approach-specific surgical techniques

The translabyrinthine approach has the advantage of defining the lateral end of the internal auditory and thus the distal portion of the facial nerve (Fig. 4A). Once the IAC and the labyrinthine portion of the facial nerve are defined, the superior and inferior vestibular nerves can be divided at the vestibule using a sharp hook. Beginning at Bill's bar, the plane of dissection is usually easy to develop, but some difficulty can be encountered at the porus acousticus. Dissection in this area can be hazardous because the nerve is particularly adherent at this site. Once the nerve is identified at the brainstem just ventral to the cochleovestibular nerve entry zone after tumor debulking, a medial plane can be established adding a second route for tumor dissection (Fig. 4B, C).

Dissection of the facial nerve by the suboccipital/retrosigmoid approach is similar to the translabyrinthine approach, but the cochleovestibular nerve is not divided. Also, during this hearing-preservation surgery, the exposure

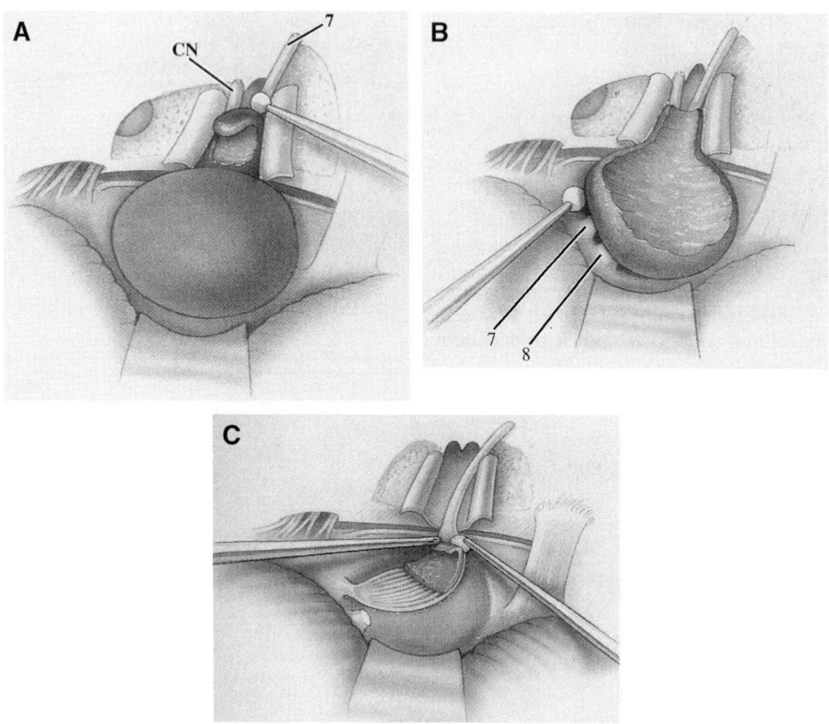

Fig. 4. Tumor removal off the facial nerve in left IAC and CPA. (*A*) The nerve is identified, and the tumor is removed beginning at the lateral end of the IAC. (*B*) The tumor is debulked in the CPA after identifying the facial and vestibular nerves. (*C*) The final portion of the tumor is removed at the porus acousticus. 7, facial nerve; 8, vestibular nerve. (*From* Jackler RK. Atlas of neurotology and skull base surgery. St Louis (MO): Mosby-Year Book; 1996. p. 14 & 15; with permission.)

of the IAC differs in that the overhanging posterior semicircular canal prevents drilling out the distal 3 to 4 mm of the internal IAC. The distal (lateral) tumor therefore can be removed only by using a blind, sweeping technique. Endoscopes can be used to assist in visualization but can be placed in the tight surgical field only between attempts at tumor removal.

In the middle cranial fossa approach, the IAC is approached superiorly, so the facial nerve lies in an extremely vulnerable position. Great care must be used when the bone is removed off of the roof of the IAC. Only 1-, 2-, or 3-mm diamond burrs should be used at this point. Once the dura is reached, it should be opened posteriorly and reflected anteriorly to avoid disturbing the facial nerve running anteriorly beneath the dura. Then the facial nerve should be visualized, and the dissection plane should be defined. Debulking of the tumor should be performed posteriorly to the nerve. This approach allows the surgeon to sweep underneath the facial nerve, thereby delivering additional tumor found anteriorly. Careful attention must be given to the nerve wrapping around medially at the cerebellopontine angle.

Intracranial facial nerve repair

Should the facial nerve be disrupted during skull base surgery, primary anastomosis is the preferred method of repair. This technique allows immediate attention to the injury and creates no new additional neurologic defects [50]. In the translabyrinthine approach, 5 to 10 mm of facial nerve in the mastoid can be mobilized or rerouted to provide additional length for primary re-anastomosis. Technically, the repair is complicated by the absence of epineurium around the intracranial portion of the facial nerve. Typically, only one 9-0 suture through the center of the nerve or fibrin glue is used to secure the anastomosis. Some consider sutureless repair with fibrin glue beneficial because of its technical simplicity and avoidance of neural trauma [52]. Most importantly, however, the anastomotic site must be stabilized, especially if the repair is in the cerebellopontine angle [50]. Stabilization can be accomplished by using fascia or packing with absorbable materials to support the repair. If an interposition graft is needed, the greater auricular nerve is used, primarily because of its availability and its comparable size to the facial nerve. Free nerve grafting is generally avoided, if possible, because two anastomoses are required. Overall, four studies that included more than 100 patients reported a satisfactory result of HB grade IV function in 44% to 100% of patients for all three intracranial facial nerve repairs [53–55].

In conclusion, facial nerve rerouting in skull base surgery has evolved in the last 50 years. Once inaccessible tumors are now regularly approached, and complete resections are accomplished with good outcomes of facial nerve rerouting.

References

[1] Fisch U, Mattox D. Microsurgery of the skull base. New York: Thieme; 1988. p. 468.

[2] Hall GM, Pulec JL, Rhoton AL. Geniculate ganglion anatomy for the otologist. Arch Otolaryngol Head Neck Surg 1969;90:568–71.

[3] Sheehy JL. The facial nerve in chronic otitis media. Otolaryngol Clin North Am 1969;7: 493–503.

[4] Balkany T, Fradis M, Jafek BW, et al. Intrinsic vasculature of the labyrinthine segment of the facial nerve; implications for site of lesions in Bell's palsy. Otolaryngol Head Neck Surg 1991; 104:20–3.

[5] Capps FCW. Glomus jugulare tumors of the middle ear. J Laryngol Otol 1952;66:302–14.

[6] Shapiro MJ, Neues DK. Technique for removal of glomus jugulare tumors. Arch Otolaryngol Head Neck Surg 1964;79:219–24.

[7] Glasscock ME III, Harris PF, Newsome G. Glomus tumors: diagnosis and treatment. Laryngoscope 1974;84:2006–32.

[8] Fisch U. Infratemporal fossa approach for extensive tumors of the temporal bone and base of the skull. In: Silverstein H, Norrel H, editors. Neurological surgery of the ear. Birmingham (AL): Aesculapius; 1977. p. 33–53.

[9] Brackmann DE. The facial nerve in the infratemporal approach. Otolaryngol Head Neck Surg 1987;97:15–7.

[10] Kinney SE. The facial nerve in skull base surgery. In: Graham MDF, House WF, editors. Disorders of facial nerve. New York: Raven Press; 1982. p. 407–12.

[11] Glasscock ME III, Miller GW, Drake FD, et al. Surgery of the skull base. Laryngoscope 1978;88:905–23.
[12] Jackson CG, Johnson GD, Poe DS. Lateral transtemporal approaches to the skull base. In: Jackson CG, editor. Surgery of skull base tumors. New York: Churchill Livingstone; 1991. p. 141–96.
[13] von Doerston P, Jackler RK. Anterior facial nerve rerouting in cranial base surgery: an anatomical study of three different techniques. Otolaryngol Head Neck Surg 1996;115: 82–8.
[14] Blunt MJ. The blood supply of the facial nerve. J Anat 1954;88:520–6.
[15] Cooper MH, Archer CR, Kveton JF. Correlation of high-resolution computed tomography and gross anatomic section of the temporal bone: part 1. The facial nerve. Am J Otol 1987;8: 375–84.
[16] Sheehy JL. The facial nerve in surgery of chronic otitis media. Otolaryngol Clin North Am 1974;7:493–503.
[17] Gantz BJ. Intratemporal facial nerve surgery. In: Cummings CW, Harker LA, editors. Otolaryngology—head and neck surgery. St. Louis: Mosby; 1986. p. 3353–66.
[18] Lambert PR, Johns ME, Winn RH. Infralabyrinthine approach to skull-base lesions. Otolaryngol Head Neck Surg 1985;93:250–8.
[19] Brackman DE. The facial nerve in the infratemporal approach. Otolaryngol Head Neck Surg 1987;97:15–7.
[20] Glasscock ME III, Steenerson RL. A history of acoustic tumor surgery 1961 to present. In: House WF, Luetje CM, editors. Acoustic tumors. Baltimore (MD): University Park Press; 1979. p. 33–41.
[21] House WF. Introductory remarks. Report of cases. Arch Otolaryngol Head Neck Surg 1964; 80:604–5, 617–67.
[22] House WF. History of the development of the translabyrinthine approach. In: Silverstein H, Norrel H, editors. Neurological surgery of the ear. Birmingham (AL): Aesculapius; 1977. p. 235–8.
[23] House WF, Hitselberger WE. The transcochlear approach to the skull base. Arch Otolaryngol Head Neck Surg 1976;102:L334–42.
[24] Pellet W, Cannoni M, Pech A. The widened transcochlear approach for jugular foramen tumors. J Neurosurg 1988;69:887–94.
[25] Horn KL, Hankinson HL, Erasmus MD, et al. The modified transcochlear approach to the cerebellopontine angle. Otolaryngol Head Neck Surg 1991;104:37–41.
[26] Selesnick SH, Abraham MT, Carew JF. Rerouting of the intratemporal facial nerve: an analysis of the literature. Am J Otol 1996;17:793–805.
[27] von Doersten PG, Jackson CG, Manolidis S, et al. Facial nerve outcome in lateral skull base surgery for benign lesions. Laryngoscope 1998;108(10):1480–4.
[28] Sanna M, Mazzoni A, Saleh E, et al. The system of the modified transcochlear approach: a lateral avenue to the central skull base. Am J Otol 1998;19:88–98.
[29] Russo A, Piccirillo E, De Donato G, et al. Anterior and posterior facial nerve rerouting: a comparative study. Skull base 2003;13(3):123–30.
[30] House JW, Brackmann DE. Facial nerve grading system. Otolaryngol Head Neck Surg 1985;93(2):146–7.
[31] Lanman TH, Brackmann DE, Hitselberger WE, et al. Report of 190 consecutive cases of large acoustic tumors (vestibular schwannoma) removed via the translabyrinthine approach. J Neurosurg 1999;90(4):617–23.
[32] Samii M, Matthies C. Management of 1000 vestibular schwannomas (acoustic neuromas): the facial nerve–preservation and restitution of function. Neurosurgery 1997;40(4):684–94.
[33] Arriaga MA, Chen DA, Fukushima T. Individualizing hearing preservation in acoustic neuroma surgery. Laryngoscope 1997;107(8):1043–7.
[34] Darrouzet V, Martel J, Enee V, et al. Vestibular schwannoma surgery outcomes: our multidisciplinary experience in 400 cases over 17 years. Laryngoscope 2004;114(4):681–8.

[35] Glasscock ME III, Kveton JF, Jackson CG, et al. A systematic approach to the surgical management of acoustic neuroma. Laryngoscope 1986;96(10):1088–94.
[36] Sluyter S, Graamans K, Tulleken CA, et al. Analysis of the results obtained in 120 patients with large acoustic neuromas surgically treated via the translabyrinthine-transtentorial approach. J Neurosurg 2001;94(1):61–6.
[37] Briggs RJ, Luxford WM, Atkins JS Jr, et al. Translabyrinthine removal of large acoustic neuromas. Neurosurgery 1994;34(5):785–90.
[38] Arriaga MA, Luxford WM, Atkins JS Jr, et al. Predicting long-term facial nerve outcome after acoustic neuroma surgery. Otolaryngol Head Neck Surg 1993;108(3):220–4.
[39] Ebersold MJ, Harner SG, Beatty CW, et al. Current results of the retrosigmoid approach to acoustic neurinoma. J Neurosurg 1992;76(6):901–9.
[40] Wiet RJ, Mamikoglu B, Odom L, et al. Long-term results of the first 500 cases of acoustic neuroma surgery. Otolaryngol Head Neck Surg 2001;124(6):645–51.
[41] Wiegand DA, Ojemann RG, Fickel V. Surgical treatment of acoustic neuroma (vestibular schwannoma) in the United States: report from the Acoustic Neuroma Registry. Laryngoscope 1996;106(1 Pt 1):58–66.
[42] Yamakami I, Uchino Y, Kobayashi E, et al. Removal of large acoustic neurinomas (vestibular schwannomas) by the retrosigmoid approach with no mortality and minimal morbidity. J Neurol Neurosurg Psychiatry 2004;75(3):453–8.
[43] Ho SY, Hudgens S, Wiet RJ. Comparison of postoperative facial nerve outcomes between translabyrinthine and retrosigmoid approaches in matched-pair patients. Laryngoscope 2003;113(11):2014–20.
[44] Colletti V, Fiorino F. Middle fossa versus retrosigmoid-transmeatal approach in vestibular schwannoma surgery: a prospective study. Otol Neurotol 2003;24(6):927–34.
[45] Esses BA, LaRouere MJ, Graham MD. Facial nerve outcome in acoustic tumor surgery. Am J Otol 1994;15(6):810–2.
[46] Selesnick SH, Carew JF, Victor JD, et al. Predictive value of facial nerve electrophysiologic stimulation thresholds in cerebellopontine-angle surgery. Laryngoscope 1996;106(5 Pt 1): 633–8.
[47] Lalwani AK, Butt FY, Jackler RK, et al. Facial nerve outcome after acoustic neuroma surgery: a study from the era of cranial nerve monitoring. Otolaryngol Head Neck Surg 1994; 111(5):561–70.
[48] Isaacson B, Kileny PR, El-Kashlan H, et al. Intraoperative monitoring and facial nerve outcomes after vestibular schwannoma resection. Otol Neurotol 2003;24(5):812–7.
[49] Oghalai JS, Buxbaum JL, Pitts LH, et al. The effect of age on acoustic neuroma surgery outcomes. Otol Neurotol 2003;24(3):473–7.
[50] Jackler RK. Acoustic neuroma (vestibular schwanoma). In: Jackler RK, Brackman DE, editors. Textbook of neurotology. St. Louis (MO): Mosby-Year Book, Inc; 1994. p. 729–85.
[51] Thedinger BS, Whittaker CK, Luetje CM. Recurrent acoustic tumor after a suboccipital removal. Neurosurgery 1991;29(5):681–7.
[52] Arriaga MA, Brackmann DE. Facial nerve repair techniques in cerebellopontine angle tumor surgery. Am J Otol 1992;13(4):356–9.
[53] Kanzaki J, Kunihiro T, O-Uchi T, et al. Intracranial reconstruction of the facial nerve. Clinical observation. Acta Otolaryngol Suppl 1991;487:85–90.
[54] Fisch U, Dobie RA, Gmur A, et al. Intracranial facial nerve anastomosis. Am J Otol 1987; 8(1):23–9.
[55] Jackler RK. Atlas of neurotology and skull base surgery. St Louis (MO): Mosby-Year Book; 1996.
[56] Jenkins HA, Fisch U. The Transotic approach to resection of difficult acoustic tumors of the cerebellopontine angle. Am J Otol 1980;2:70–6.
[57] Fisch U. Infratemporal fossa approach for glomus tumors of the temporal bone. Ann otol Rhinol Laryngol 1982;91:474–9.

[58] Kaye AH, Hahn JF, Kinney SE, Hardy RW, Bay JW. Jugular foramen schwannomas. J neurosurg 1984;60:1045–53.
[59] Gardner G, Cocke EW Jr, Robertson JH, Palmer RE IV, Bellott AL Jr, Hamm CW. Skull base surgery fro glomus jugular tumors. Am J Otol 1985;(suppl):126–34.
[60] Bebear JP, Stoll D, Francois JH. The facial nerine in the surgical approach to the subtemporal region and the jugular foramen (in surgery of the glumus tumors). In: Portmann M, editor. Proceedings of the fifth international symposium on the facial nerve. New York: Massson; 1985. p. 421–3.
[61] Brammer RE, Graham MD, Kemink JL. Glomus tumors of the temporal bone: contemporary evaluation and therapy. Otolaryngol Clin of North Am 1984;17:499–512.
[62] Al-Mefty O, Fox JL, Rifai A, Smith RR. A combined infratemporal and posterior fossa approach for the removal of giant glomus tumors nad chnodrosarcomas. Surg Neurol 1987; 28:423–31. Brackmann(9) (this reference is already present in the initial references.)
[63] Hawthorne MR, Makek MS, Harris JP, Fisch U. The histopathological and clinical features of irradiated and nonirradiated temporal paragangliomas. Layngoscope 1987;97:152–7.
[64] Leonetti JP, Brackmann DE, Prass RL. Imporved preservation of facial nerve function in the infratemporal approach to the skull base. Otolaryngol Head Neck Surg 1989;101:74–8.
[65] Poe DS, Jackson CG, Glasscock ME III, Johnson GD. Long-term results after lateral cranial base surgery. Laryngoscope 1991;101:372–8.
[66] Molony TB, Brackmann DE, Lo WWM. Meningiomas of the jugular foramen. Otolaryngol Head Neck Surg 1992;106:128–36.
[67] Woods CI, Strasnick B, Jackson CG. Surgery for Glomus tumors: the otology group experience. Laryngoscope 1993;103:65–70.
[68] Magliulo G, Vingolo GL, Cristofari P, Petti R, Ronzoni R. Post-operative complications in neoplasms of the skull base. In: Samii M, editor. Skull base surgery. First International Skull Base congress, Hannover, 1992. Basel: Karger; 1994. p. 1222–4.
[69] Patel SJ, Reckar LN, Cass SP, Hikrsch BE. combines approaches for resection of extensive glomus jugulare tumors. J Neurosurg 1994;80:1026–38.
[70] Green JD Jr, Brackmann DE, Nguyen CD, Arriaga MA, Telischi FE, De la Cruz A. Surgical Management of previously untreated glomus jugulare tumors. Laryngoscope 1994;104: 917–21.
[71] House WF, De La Cruz A, Hitselberger WE. Surgery of the skull base: transcochlear approach to the petrous apex and clivus. Otolaryngol Head Neck Surg 1978;86:770–9.
[72] Sekhar LN, Estonillo R. Transtemporal–infratemporal approach to the skull base. In: Scheunemann H, Shurmann K, Helms J, editors. Tumors of the skull base, extra-intracranial surgery of skull base tumors. New York: Walter de Gruyter; 1986. p. 199–207.
[73] Pellet W, Cannoni M, Peck A. The widened trancochlear approach for jugular foramen tumors. J Neurosurg 1988;69:887–94.
[74] Glasscock ME III, Woods CI III, Poe DS, Patterson AK, Welling DB. Petrous apex cholesteatoma. Otolaryngol clin North Am 1989;22:981–1001.
[75] Horn KL, Hankinson HL, Erasmus MD, Beauparalant PA. The modified transcochlear approach to the cerebellopontine angle. Otolaryngol Head Neck Surg 1991;104:37–41.
[76] Thedinger BA, Glasscock ME III, Cueva RA. Transcochlear transtentorial approach for removal of large cerbellopontine angle meningiomas. Am J otol 1992;13:408–15.
[77] Arriaga M, Shelton C, Nassif P, Brackmann DE. Selection of surgical approaches for meningiomas affecting the temporal bone. Otolaryngol Head Neck Surg 1992;107:738–44.
[78] Sanna M, Mazzoni A, Saleh EA, Taibah AK, Russo A. Lateral approaches to the median skull base through the petrous bone: the system of the modified transcochelar approach. J Laryngol Otol 1994;108:1036–44.
[79] Cass SP, Sekhar LN, Pmeneraz S, Hirsch BE, Snyderman CH. Excision of petroclival tumors by a total petrosectomy approach. Am J Otol 1994;15:474–84.

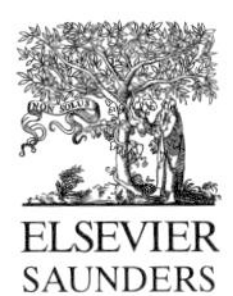

ELSEVIER
SAUNDERS

Otolaryngol Clin N Am
38 (2005) 711–722

OTOLARYNGOLOGIC
CLINICS
OF NORTH AMERICA

Iatrogenic Complications from Chronic Ear Surgery

Peter C. Weber, MD, MBA

The Cleveland Clinic Foundation, 9500 Euclid Avenue, A71, Cleveland, OH 44195, USA

Complications from ear surgery are many and varied, but fortunately, for the patient and surgeon, the major ones are relatively rare. In fact, the incidence of most complications is significantly less than 1% [1–3], in contrast to the actual risk involved to major structures caused by the sequelae of the disease itself, if the disease remains untreated [3]. This article discusses the essential complications to major structures: facial nerve injuries, tegmen dehiscence with or without cerebrospinal fluid (CSF) leak, bleeding from sigmoid or carotid artery, semicircular canal dehiscence, and ossicular disruptions. Because the article focuses on skull base complications incurred through ear surgery, it does not discuss the complications, such as seizure, stroke, intracranial bleeding, cerebral edema, or other cranial nerve deficits, that can arise from true skull base surgery. The article does not discuss infections or meningitis, because these complications normally are not immediate intraoperative complications. The author prefers to administer prophylactic antibiotics on call to the operating room to help prevent infections. The author also recommends not shaving any hair for any type of ear or lateral intracranial procedure, because without shaving the likelihood of a postoperative infection is extremely rare [4]. In fact, fewer infections have been noted with not shaving than with shaving, although the difference is not statistically significant.

Facial paralysis

No matter what type of ear surgery is performed, one of the most dreaded complications is facial paralysis. Therefore, before discussing what to do after the nerve has been injured, it is prudent to discuss how to avoid this particular injury in the first place.

E-mail address: weberp@ccf.org

doi:10.1016/j.otc.2005.01.007 **oto.theclinics.com**

The best way to avoid an injury to the facial nerve is to understand its anatomy thoroughly [5–7]. A preoperative CT scan of the temporal bones is recommended because the facial nerve can have an anomalous course in a small percentage of patients or be dehiscent within the horizontal or vertical segments; either naturally or by erosion from disease. A CT scan can demonstrate the course of the facial nerve and its relationship to known landmarks, alerting the surgeon to potential areas of danger. If the surgeon knows in advance that the nerve is located more anteriorly than usual, that disease goes deeply posteriorly and inferiorly, or that disease directly involves the facial nerve, the surgeon may be able to avoid any injury. Even in patients who may not be expected to be at risk for a facial nerve injury, such as those undergoing an operation for exostosis or keratitis obturans, a CT scan can help avert a facial nerve complication.

A mastoidectomy should always be performed in a systematic fashion. One should identify known landmarks from lateral to medial. Although not routinely done, the actual identification of the facial nerve during surgery can be beneficial (Fig. 1). If the surgeon intentionally identifies the nerve, unexpected injury to the nerve is less likely, especially if a thin bone layer is left over the nerve. Initially, the recommended procedure is to drill a wide mastoidectomy and to stay superiorly and anteriorly into the zygomatic root, that is, hugging the tegmen as one proceeds medially. This technique can significantly help in avoiding the facial nerve and lateral semicircular canal, especially in most chronically diseased mastoid bones, which resemble cue balls with no air cells until the antrum is reached. If the surgeon creates too low or too inferior a mastoidectomy in chronically diseased mastoids, there is a risk of injuring the lateral/horizontal semicircular canal or the facial nerve. Once the antrum, incus, and the lateral semicircular canal have been identified, a facial recess approach is the easiest method by which to

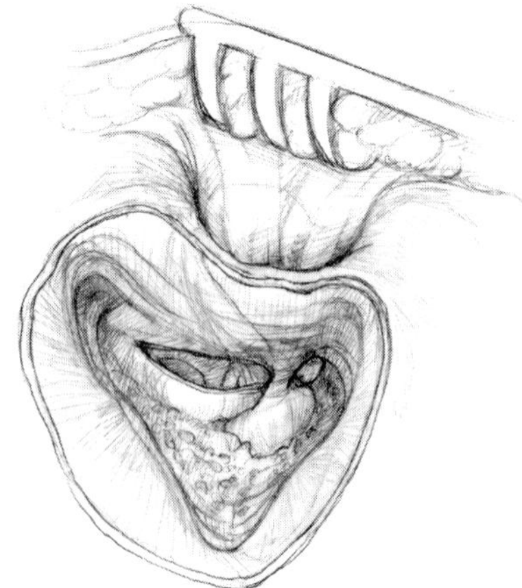

Fig. 1. Demonstrates the course of the facial nerve from the view of a mastoidectomy with a facial recess approach.

identify the facial nerve. Once the facial nerve is identified, it can be followed to the stylomastoid foramen as needed. The facial nerve rises somewhat from medial to lateral in the vertical segment. Another way to identify the facial nerve is to follow the digastric ridge to the stylomastoid foramen, which in turn leads to the facial nerve. Although the actual incidence of facial nerve injury is quite low for virgin ear surgery (less than 1%), it can be as high as 4% to 10% in revision cases [8].

Intraoperative monitoring of the facial nerve helps the surgeon protect the nerve, but it is not mandatory for ear surgery and cannot replace anatomic knowledge [9,10]. This anatomic knowledge should be obtained by many hours spent dissecting temporal bones in the temporal bone laboratory is also useful When severe disease has eroded the bony covering of the facial nerve, the facial nerve monitor can help the surgeon determine what is disease and what is normal nerve. In addition, up to 50% of normal temporal bones can have a small dehiscence (less than 0.4-mm in diameter) in the tympanic segment [11]. Other natural areas of dehiscence include the geniculate ganglion, facial recess, and the mastoid area (most commonly when the mucosa of an air cell covers the facial nerve) [12]. Using the stimulator or Prass probe associated with the facial nerve monitor, the surgeon can more readily identify the facial nerve.

The question remains as to what to do for an injured nerve. Ideally, the injury is recognized in the operating theater rather than when the patient awakes in the recovery room. If the injury is identified in the operating room, the surgeon must first determine the degree of injury. Exposing the nerve (ie, inadvertently removing bone from over the nerve) does not necessarily require any further action on the part of the surgeon. The same is true for a minor contusion of the facial nerve. The facial nerve is actually quite hardy and can be manipulated without significant effect [13,14]. If the bruising or contusion seems extensive, decompressing 5 to 10 mm of bone on either side of the dehiscence is recommended [15]. Opening the sheath of the nerve to allow expansion and to decrease any untoward effect of edema or hematoma is controversial, and the surgeon must make that decision when assessing damage to the nerve [16,17].

Occasionally, the injury is more extensive—either a partial or total transection of the nerve (Fig. 2). This type of injury can be devastating for both the surgeon and the patient. Even otologists who are fellowship trained may be too distressed to assess the true extent of the damage adequately. Consultation or referral is not a sign of defeat and in some cases might be in the best interest of the patient. The surgeon involved, however, is usually best equipped to treat the complication because he/she has intimate knowledge of the patient's surgery. One must guard against the natural tendency to underestimate the degree of injury to the facial nerve. Complete transection is easy to identify, but it is harder to tell if a partial injury or transection is slight (ie, less than one third of the nerve) or is greater than one third of the nerve. When less than one third of the nerve is cut,

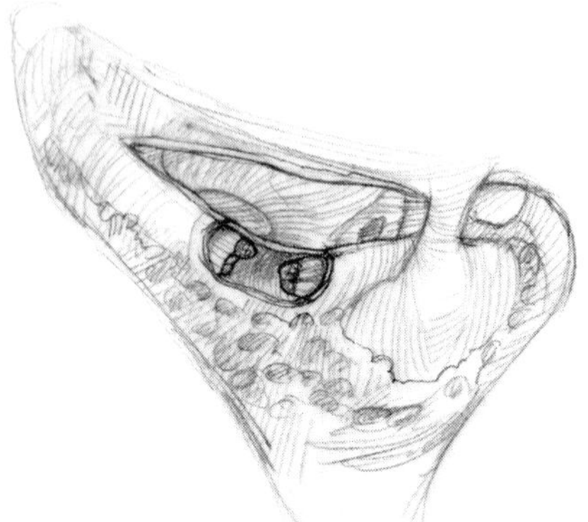

Fig. 2. Demonstrates a complete transection of the facial nerve in the vertical segment.

conventional teaching is to decompress on either side of the injury [18]. If more than one third of the nerve is cut, a nerve graft has a better chance of preserving facial nerve function at the level of grade 3 on the House-Brackman scale [19,20].

Fortunately, grafting the nerve back together does not require extensive equipment. If the nerve can easily be put back together primarily without tension, then this method is preferred because no graft is needed, and only one anastomosis is required. Sometime it is easier to make one clean cut of the damaged nerve, especially if half of the nerve is transected. If the damage seems to be more extensive, sometimes it is better to cut the nerve obliquely on either side of the damage so that there are two good, clean ends to reapproximate. If the two ends do not meet without tension, a graft is needed. An extra centimeter of length can be obtained from the facial nerve by drilling out the stylomastoid foramen. This technique, however, causes some disruption of the blood supply and can cause problems with healing. It has not been shown that one anastomosis, as opposed to two, causes any less synkinesis or better facial nerve function [16,21].

To repair the transected nerve, the nerve or the nerve graft can be sutured together using a 9-0 or 10-0 monofilament suture (Figs. 3, 4). In ear surgery,

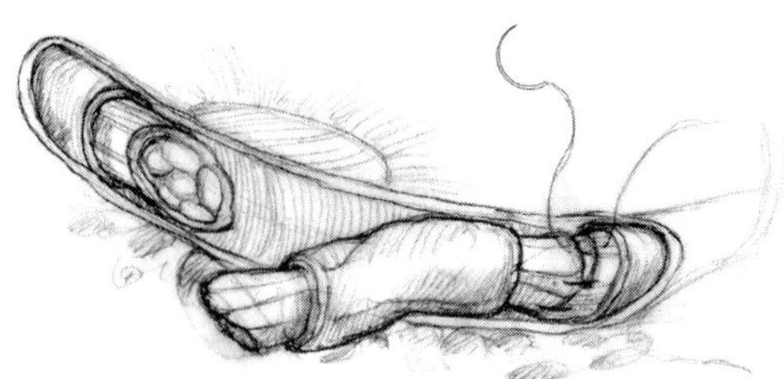

Fig. 3. Demonstrates the suturing in of a nerve graft. Note the beveled ends. Often sutures can not be placed, but laying the nerve graft next to each cut end may suffice or it can be sealed with fibrin glue.

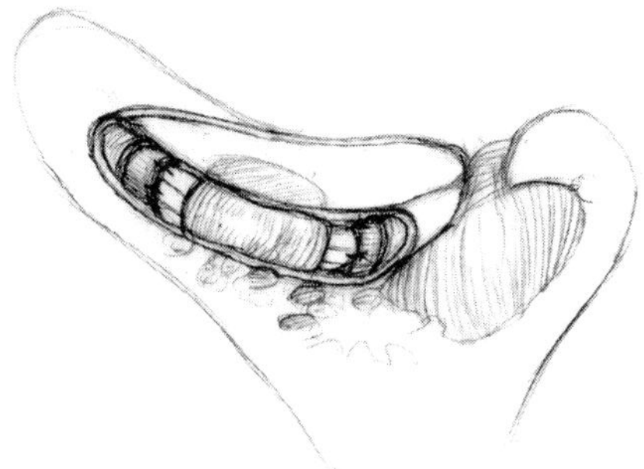

Fig. 4. Demonstrates the nerve graft in place.

however, it is very difficult to place a suture. Fortunately, the fallopian canal offers a suitable bed in which to place the nerve graft where it should not move. In this case, the ends can be reapproximated and then held in place using a sealant such as fibrin glue and Gelfoam or Cargile [16,17,22]. In placing the graft, it is important to cut the nerve graft and facial nerve obliquely to increase the surface area for axon regeneration [19,23]. Great care must be taken to assure that all bone spicules are removed from the nerve as well.

When a nerve graft is needed, the surgeon must know how to obtain one. Historically, two nerves have been used for facial nerve grafting: the great auricular nerve or the sural nerve. Because the length of nerve that is needed certainly should be less than 10 cm, which is about the length that can be obtained from the great auricular nerve, there is no reason to perform a sural nerve graft [16]. The great auricular nerve is readily available, and the incision needed has usually already been prepped and is in the field for any type of ear surgery. To access the auricular nerve, a line is drawn from the mastoid tip to the angle of the jaw and about two thirds away an incision is made down onto the sternocleidomastoid muscle where the great auricular nerve is usually found [19] (Fig. 5). The nerve can be mobilized, and a portion of the nerve can be transected and used for graft. To maximize healing and to maximize the area that can be used for the reapproximation, the ends are cut at a beveled angle. The nerve graft again is either sutured into place or placed next to the two ends of the facial nerve and held in place with the fibrin glue or other material.

The patient and the family must be appropriately counseled regarding the type of injury. If the nerve was grafted, they should understand that the final degree of facial function will not be known for at least 1 year and there will probably not be any type of activity in the fact for 6 to 9 months. The final outcome in grafting is about 75% of normal function, at best [21]. Synkinesis may be a problem and should be explained [24,25]. The use of high-dose steroids is certainly recommended; the dose usually given is about 60 to 80 mg/d for (prednisone) 7 to 10 days. For nerves that are only contused, recovery is usually quicker.

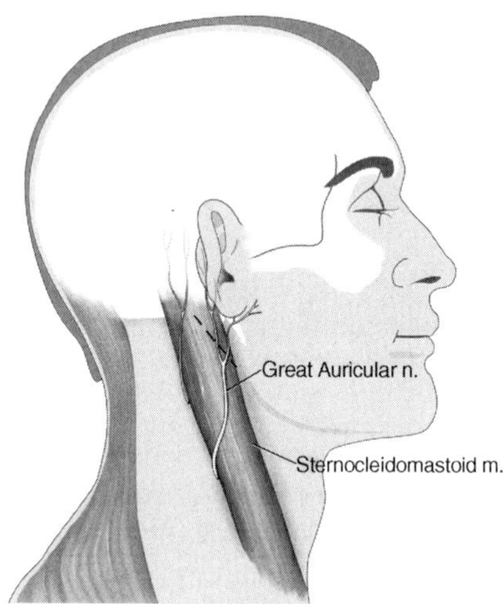

Fig. 5. Demonstrates the course of the great auricular nerve.

When the facial paralysis is discovered in the recovery room, rather than in the operating theater, a decision must be made as to the course of action. If the paralysis is not complete (ie, the patient has a good nasal sniff or has good reaction with grimacing), the nerve in all likelihood is not totally transected and has a less severe injury. In these cases, high-dose steroids are used, and the patient is monitored. If the injury does become a complete facial paralysis, electrical testing is performed, and a decision must be made whether any further surgical management (ie, facial nerve decompression) is warranted. Electroneurography (ENOG) is the preferred test. When degeneration is less than 95%, the possibility of decompression can be considered. One must be careful about relying on eye closure alone to assess facial function, because some eye closure is possible even with complete paralysis.

If a complete paralysis is noted in the recovery room, the surgeon must consider a few other possibilities besides surgical trauma. If the surgeon has placed a lot of packing in the mastoid cavity or even the middle ear, the packing may be too tight, especially in a dehiscent nerve, and may need to be loosened slightly. Another possibility is the effect of lidocaine, which can cause temporary paralysis in a dehiscent nerve for 3 to 12 hours. If the surgeon is reasonably sure that the nerve is actually injured and feels comfortable with re-exploration, then re-exploration should be done, usually as expeditiously as possible (ie, within 24–72 hours) [26,27]. The needed repair should be completed on this exploration as previously described. Some favor waiting 3 to 4 weeks to allow possible neurologic regrowth before undertaking any reanastamosis [16,28]. Most surgeons do not favor waiting 3 to 4 weeks. If the surgeon is certain that the nerve has not injured in any way and had identified it during surgery, it may be prudent to follow the patient with electrical testing. One must consider re-exploration or decompression only if a patient with a grade VI facial paralysis demonstrates more than 90% to 95% degeneration on ENOG studies.

The other issue to consider is whether a thermal injury has occurred, especially during facial recess surgery. The shaft of the bur spinning at a high rate of speed can produce enough heat to cause a thermal injury to the nerve if the nerve is slightly exposed or is covered with only a thin layer of bone. Thermal injuries usually get better with time, but 5 to 9 months may be needed to see a significant improvement in function. Steroids may help, but the role of decompression is unknown. Always, the best method for dealing with facial paralysis is to try to avoid it in the first place; should it occur, one must be calm and approach the injury in a systematic fashion to achieve the best result for the patient.

Vascular injuries

Sigmoid sinus

The sigmoid sinus is routinely identified during mastoid surgery. The sinus usually appears as a bluish hue under a thin plate of bone. It usually can be found more readily at its most lateral position, which usually corresponds to the center of the mastoid, where in most cases it forms a small arc. The most common anatomic variant, anterior displacement [8], can lead to injury, as can a lateralized sigmoid sinus. These locations, however, should be detected on any preoperative CT scan. Occasionally, the sinus obscures the view of the mastoid contents and requires decompression to visualize needed structures. Decompression is accomplished by removing bone around the sinus itself, usually leaving a bony island plate that can be pressed down on the sinus without significant risk for injury or tearing of the sinus.

Occasionally the sinus may be injured inadvertently, and profuse or mild bleeding may occur. Mild bleeding usually results from traumatized dural vessels that lie on the sinus [15]. These small vessels usually can be controlled quite easily with bipolar cautery. If there is a small laceration on the edge of the sinus with minimal bleeding, thrombin-soaked Gelfoam (Pharmacia Upjohn, Kalamazoo, MI), Gelfoam alone, or Surgicel may be used. More substantial bleeding or injury to the sinus usually requires some type of packing. Either Surgicel or Gelfoam can be held on the site of bleeding by gauze packing or other material for about 2 to 5 minutes. Fortunately, this technique is almost always successful, and the Gelfoam or Surgicel is then left in place. Once the bleeding has stopped, the surgeon can usually still work around these areas as needed. For large tears, the sinus bone is removed all around the sinus superiorly and inferiorly to the tear. The sigmoid sinus is packed distally and proximally to the laceration with large sheets of Surgicel or Gelfoam extraluminally to help prevent embolic events [29]. Intraluminal packing may be an option, but one must consider the risk of embolization of the packing material. Indeed, some physicians advocate ligation of the internal jugular vein in the neck to avoid an embolic complication if internal packing is used [15].

The anesthetist should be notified when this tear occurs so that anesthetist can monitor the patient and treat an air embolus quickly if necessary.

Jugular bulb

Like the sigmoid sinus, the jugular bulb is a low-pressure system but is one that can bleed profusely, with a significant amount of blood loss in a short time span. The bulb itself may be high (above the inferior annulus of the tympanic membrane) in up to 7% of people [30]. Occasionally, a high jugular bulb may be dehiscent, making it especially prone to injury when the surgeon is raising a tympanomeatal flap, cleaning out the hypotympanum, or performing a myringotomy.

Like sigmoid bleeding, jugular bulb bleeding may be controlled easily with pressure from Gelfoam or Surgicel. The Gelfoam or Surgicel is held in place, and, once the bleeding stops, it may be left there and even sealed slightly with bone wax. In the unlikely event that this treatment fails and the bleeding is profuse, it may be necessary to achieve control through ligation of the internal jugular vein in the neck followed by extraluminal or intraluminal packing of the sigmoid/jugular bulb. The inferior petrosal vein also drains around this area, so pressure on the bulb is essential. Therefore, the surgeon cannot expect to stop all bleeding by ligating the internal jugular vein and compressing the sigmoid sinus. Bleeding could still occur through back flow from the inferior petrosal vein out the jugular dehiscence.

If the bleeding occurs when the surgeon is raising the tympanomeatal flap, Surgicel and Gelfoam can be used to fill the middle ear, applying pressure onto the bulb. The tympanomeatal flap can be replaced and the external auditory canal packed for at least 1 week [15,30]. This technique should create enough pressure to allow the sinus/bulb to heal. Injury incurred during a myringotomy can usually be controlled with external auditory canal packing.

Carotid artery

Happily, injury to the carotid artery is exceedingly rare, because exposure of the carotid artery itself is very rare, occurring in less than 1% of cases [31]. The artery normally is covered by thick bone and lies medial to the eustachian tube orifice, anterior-medial to the cochlea, and anterior-inferior to the cochleariform process. Preoperative imaging studies can help identify a carotid artery anomaly. The knowledge that a dehiscence exists can help the surgeon to avoid any dissection in that area or, if dissection in that area is essential, to take extra care. One must also be vigilant when dissecting in the area because there may be a lack of pulsation within the petrous portion of the carotid artery, again making it more difficult to identify the artery [5].

Bleeding that occurs only from the wall of the artery usually is controlled adequately with Surgicel, because such bleeding usually originates in minor vessels along the wall. True carotid bleeding is a significant challenge. The bleeding must be controlled immediately, usually with packing and pressure. Once the hemorrhaging is controlled, decisions can be made whether to ligate and subsequently graft the artery, to balloon occlude the artery temporarily allowing suturing of the artery, to graft the artery, or to occlude the artery permanently with balloon occlusion or surgical ligation [15,32]. Balloon occlusion carries a risk of stroke, even in healthy persons, and the consequences of a stroke to a patient must be kept in mind when considering this option [33].

Tegmen injuries

During mastoid surgery, it is common to expose the tegmen or dura because the identification of the tegmen is one landmark used in performing safe mastoid surgery. The tegmen is identified to determine the actual superior limits during mastoid dissection [16]. Exposure of tegmen dura usually requires no further corrective action, because most often the dura of the tegmen is quite thick and can easily support the brain without causing any type of meningocele or encephalocele [17]. Over a long period, however, large defects may result in a meningoencephalocele. Nonetheless, because the incidence of meningoencephalocele is so low, the author would not treat an exposure of dura immediately but would wait until a problem actually develops. The repair of a tegmen dehiscence may require a middle cranial fossa approach to provide adequate support with bone, fascia, or cartilage.

Dural violation, on the other hand, whether by the drill, instruments, or cautery, does require corrective action. The site of the injury or leakage dictates some of the repair alternatives. Middle fossa tegmen dura is normally thick and is associated with a significant amount of arachnoid tissue. Arachnoid tissue helps form fibrous reactions and can assist in the sealing of a CSF leak. Normally, bone is removed all around the site of the leakage for at least ½ to 1 cm in diameter. This removal allows easy placement of a fascia or muscle plug or graft [15]. A piece of Gelfoam can be used to help hold the graft in place after it is tucked around the bony edges. For large defects, a middle cranial fossa craniotomy with a fascia–bone–fascia graft sandwich is usually most useful in repairing the CSF leak and the tegmen defect [5]. Antibiotic coverage is highly recommended in all CSF leaks.

CSF leakage in the posterior fossa dura is somewhat more challenging, because little arachnoid tissue is associated with this location. Thus, even though fascia grafts are tucked in and around the bone circumferentially, and Gelfoam is placed, the patient may require placement of a lumbar drain for a couple of days or bed rest to assure sealing [17]. Consultation with neurosurgery on a posterior fossa dura leak that does not seem to be abating is certainly recommended.

Canal dehiscences

During mastoid surgery, there are three chances of injuring a semicircular canal, because three canals—the horizontal (lateral), the posterior, and the superior—exist. Injury to the oval window, promontory, or round window can be equally as devastating, if not more so. It is more common to injure the semicircular canals when dissecting cholesteatoma off a dehiscent canal than to drill into a semicircular canal inadvertently. Indeed, a drilling accident probably occurs less than 0.1% of the time [34]. Drilling the canal open to expose the membranous portion of the semicircular canal or disrupting the membranous portion does not necessarily lead to permanent hearing loss. In fact, this process is done routinely to provide more exposure for some skull base surgery approaches or to plug the crystals associated with intractable benign positional vertigo. What creates a problem is not even significant violation of the membranous portion, but rather significant suction into the vestibular system. The suction in an open canal invariably results in sensorineural hearing loss and vertigo, with possible long-lasting disequilibrium resulting from a partial loss of vestibular function. Patients with a partial loss of vestibular function have more difficulty compensating than those who have a complete loss. Early identification of an iatrogenic injury is the key to minimizing symptoms. If the injury is noted immediately, the surgeon should not suction but rather should seal the fistula with bone wax, fascia, or muscle [35–37].

It is more common to encounter disease (cholesteatoma) that has eroded bone over the semicircular canal, causing a fistula. Preoperative CT scanning can usually identify this pathology. When it is identified, there are three options. One is removing the matrix while preserving the membranous canal and then sealing the dehiscence with muscle, fascia, or bone wax. The other is to leave a thin matrix covering the exposed fistula of the semicircular canal and then returning after 4 to 6 months to see if the matrix can be peeled off easily. Waiting may increase the chance of preserving the membranous portion, because the matrix is much easier to remove once the inflammation dissipates [15]. The third option is to complete a canal wall–down mastoidectomy and leave the matrix over the fistula providing an epithelial layer. Profound sensorineural hearing loss can occur in 3% to 22% of patients with a disease-induced canal fistula [1].

Fistulization of the oval window is a more common iatrogenic injury than injury of the semi-circular canals. The fistulization occurs not from drilling but usually from the dissection of disease, such as cholesteatoma, off the footplate or stapes. The other avenue for fistulization is an inadvertent stapes dislocation incurred when raising a tympanomeatal flap or with ossicular manipulations. If the footplate can be put back into position, it should be sealed with connective tissue, but one must make sure that it will not sink into the vestibule. If the footplate cannot be returned to its position, sealing the open window with fascia is recommended. If there is fistulization of the footplate, but the footplate is still in place and intact, sealing with a fascial muscle plug is recommended, as one would do for a perilymphatic fistula. Hearing loss and dizziness may occur in the short term, but these techniques are much less likely to cause indeterminate long-term problems. The possibility of a fistula or loss of stapes/stapes footplate is not to be taken lightly. It is better in cholesteatoma surgery to leave a little cholesteatoma and disease on the stapes and return in 6 to 9 months, when it should be easier to remove (it should form a small pearl), than to attempt total removal all at once [15].

Summary

Iatrogenic complications can and do occur in ear surgery. Whether the surgery is undertaken to treat chronic infectious disease or for other purposes (eg, for cochlear implants, shunts, or skull base approaches), the key to avoiding iatrogenic injuries and untoward events is attention to detail. Knowledge of what to do when the unexpected happens is the key to minimizing any negative outcome for the patient.

References

[1] Dawes PJD. Early complications of surgery for chronic otitis media. J Otolaryngol Otol 1999;(133):803–10.
[2] Kempf HG, Johann K, Lenarz T. Complications in pediatric cochlear implant surgery. Ear Arch Otorhinolaryngol 1999;(256):28–32.
[3] Greenberg MD, Jayson S, Manolidis MD, et al. High incidence of complications encountered in chronic otitis media surgery in a US metropolitan public hospital. Otolaryngol Head Neck Surg 2001;125(6):623–7.
[4] Miller J, Weber P, Patel S. Intracranial surgery: to shave or not to shave? Otol Neurotol 2001;(22):908–11.
[5] Bellucci R. Iatrogenic surgical trauma in otolaryngology. J Laryngol Otol 1983;8(Suppl): 13–7.
[6] May M, Wiet RJ. Iatrogenic injury—prevention and management. In: May M, editor. The facial nerve. New York: Thieme; 1986. p. 549–60.
[7] Wiert RJ. Iatrogenic facial paralysis. Otolaryngol Clin North Am 1982;15:773–88.
[8] Wiert RJ, Herzon GD. Surgery of the mastoid. In: Wiert RJ, Causse JB, editors. Complications in otolaryngology—head and neck surgery, vol. 1. Philadelphia: BC Decker; 1986. p. 25–31.
[9] Roland PS, Meyerhoff WL. Intraoperative electrophysiological monitoring of the facial nerve: is it standard of practice? Am J Otolaryngol 1994;15:267–70.
[10] Green JD, Shelton C, Brackman DE. Iatrogenic facial nerve injury [letter]. Laryngoscope 1995;105:444–5.

[11] Baxter A. Dehiscence of the Fallgren's canal. J Otolaryngol Otol 1971;85:487–94.
[12] Schuknecht HF, Guyle AJ. Anatomy of the temporal bone with surgical implications. Philadelphia: Lia and Feligren; 1986.
[13] Sheehy JL. Facial nerve in surgery of chronic otitis media. Otolaryngol Clin North Am 1974; 7:493–503.
[14] Neely JG. Surgery of acute infections and their complications. In: Brackmann DE, Shelton C, Arriaga MA, editors. Otologic surgery. Philadelphia: W.B. Saunders; 1994. p. 201–10.
[15] Wiet RJ, Harvet SA, Bauer GP. Management of complications of chronic otitis media. In: Brackmann DE, Shelton C, Arriaga MA, editors. Otologic surgery. Philadelphia: W.B. Saunders; 1994. p. 257–76.
[16] Smyth GD, Toner JG. Mastoidectomy: canal wall down techniques. In: Brackmann DE, Shelton C, Arriaga MA, editors. Otologic surgery. Philadelphia: W.B. Saunders; 1994. p. 225–39.
[17] Paparella MM, Meyerghoff WL, Morris MS, et al. Mastoidectomy and tympanoplasty. In: Paparella MM, Shumrick A, Gluckman JL, et al, editors. Otolaryngology, vol. 2. 3rd edition. Philadelphia: WB Saunders; 1991. p. 1405–39.
[18] May M, Schaitkin BM. Trauma to the facial nerve: external, surgical, iatrogenic. In: May M, Schaitkin BM, editors. The facial nerve. 2nd edition. New York: Thieme; 2000. p. 367–82.
[19] Adkins WY, Osguthorpe JD. Management of trauma of the facial nerve. Otolaryngol Clin North Am 1991;24:587–611.
[20] Brackmann D. Otoneurosurgical procedures. In: May M, editor. The facial nerve. New York: Thkieme; 1986. p. 589–618.
[21] Fisch U, Rouleau M. Facial nerve reconstruction. J Otolaryngol 1980;9:478 92.
[22] Fisch U. Facial nerve grafting. Otolaryngol Clin North Am 1991;7:691–708.
[23] Yamamoto E, Fisch U. Experiments on facial nerves suturing. ORL J Otorhinolaryngol Relat Spec 1974;36:193–204.
[24] Fisch U. Facial nerve grafting. Otolaryngol Clin North Am 1974;7:517–29.
[25] Johns M, Crumley R. Facial nerve injury, repair and rehabilitation (SIPac). 2nd edition. Alexandria (VA): American Academy of Otolaryngology; 1977. p. 9.
[26] Barrs DM. Facial nerve trauma: optimal timing for repair. Laryngoscope 1991;101:835–48.
[27] May M. Facial reanimation after skull base trauma. In: May M, editor. The facial nerve. New York: Thieme; 1986. p. 421–40.
[28] McQuarrie IG, Grafstein B. Axon outgrowth enhanced by previous nerve injury. Arch Neurol 1973;29:53–5.
[29] Moloy PJ, Brackmann DE. "How I do it." Control of venous bleeding in otologic surgery. Laryngoscope 1986;96:580–2.
[30] Graham MD. The jugular bulb: its anatomic and clinical considerations in contemporary otology. Laryngoscope 1977;87:105–25.
[31] Goldman NC, Singleton GI, Holly EH. Aberrant internal carotid artery. Arch Otolaryngol Head Neck Surg 1971;94:269–73.
[32] Andrews JC, Valavanis A, Fisch U. Management of the internal carotid artery of the skull base. Laryngoscope 1989;99:1224–9.
[33] DeVries EJ, Sekhar LN, Janecka IP, et al. Elective resection of the internal carotid artery without reconstruction. Laryngoscope 1988;98:960–6.
[34] Palva T, Karja J, Plva A. Immediate and short-term complications of chronic ear surgery. Arch Otolaryngol Head Neck Surg 1976;102:137–9.
[35] Jahrsdoerfer RA, Johns ME, Cantrell RW. Labyrinthine trauma during ear surgery. Laryngoscope 1978;88:1589–95.
[36] Canalis RF, Gussen R, Abemayor E, et al. Surgical trauma to the lateral semicircular canal with preservation of hearing. Laryngoscope 1987;97:575–81.
[37] Cullen JR, Kerr AG. "How I do it." Iatrogenic fenestration of a semicircular canal: a method of closure. Laryngoscope 1986;96:1168–9.

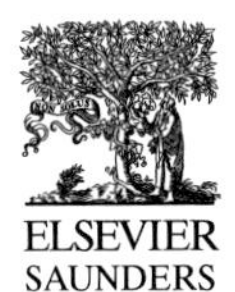

ELSEVIER
SAUNDERS

Otolaryngol Clin N Am
38 (2005) 723–735

OTOLARYNGOLOGIC
CLINICS
OF NORTH AMERICA

Endoscopic Transnasal Transsphenoidal Pituitary Surgery—Comparison with the Traditional Sublabial Transseptal Approach

Gady Har-El, MD, FACS[a,b,c,*]

[a]*State Univerisity of New York-Downstate Medical Center, Brooklyn, NY, USA*
[b]*Othmer Cancer Center, Brooklyn, NY, USA*
[c]*Department of Otolaryngology, Long Island College Hospital, 134 Atlantic Avenue, Brooklyn, NY 11201, USA*

The traditional transseptal, transsphenoidal hypophysectomy was introduced by Halstead [1] and then popularized and perfected by Cushing [2]. With the introduction of endoscopic sinus surgical instruments and techniques, the endoscopic transsphenoidal approach to the pituitary gland has been gaining increasing popularity [3–17]. Using rigid endoscopic techniques, with or without intraoperative computer-assisted navigation systems, the sphenoid sinus and pituitary gland may be approached transseptally, transethmoidally, or directly transnasally.

Surgical technique

A direct transnasal approach with superior turbinectomy is performed under general anesthesia by a team consisting of an otolaryngologist–head and neck surgeon and a neurosurgeon [5,6,8,9,18]. After appropriate intranasal vasoconstriction, the caudal aspect of the middle turbinate is gently displaced laterally under telescopic guidance. There is no need to manipulate the superior attachment of the middle turbinate, and doing so may result in skull base injury. The superior meatus and the superior turbinate are now exposed. Additional vasoconstriction may be achieved by inserting neurosurgical cottonoids soaked with the appropriate solution

* Correspondence. Department of Otolaryngology, Long Island College Hospital, 134 Atlantic Avenue, Brooklyn, NY 11201.

doi:10.1016/j.otc.2005.01.004 *oto.theclinics.com*

medial to the superior turbinate. A long, self-retaining nasal speculum or the Hardy transsphenoidal pituitary speculum is inserted. (The author has found, however, that with increasing experience and confidence, the entire procedure may be performed without a speculum.) A long, bipolar forceps is introduced into the superior meatus. The forceps jaws are placed on both sides of the superior turbinate, thus hugging the turbinate as superior as possible and as posterior as possible. The bipolar cautery is activated (Fig. 1). For this maneuver, the author currently uses the newer endoscopy coaxial bipolar cautery unit, which is easier to maneuver within the nasal cavity and the superior meatus than the conventional bayonet bipolar forceps. Next, endoscopic scissors are used to transect the superior turbinate, close to its skull base attachment, through the coagulated area (Fig. 2). The anterior-inferior tip of the turbinate is gently pulled down, and with the combination of bipolar forceps and endoscopic scissors, the posterior attachment of the superior turbinate to the anterior sphenoid wall is removed (Fig. 3). An upturned 90° bipolar forceps may be used to control bleeding from the transected attachment of the superior turbinate on the anterior sphenoid wall (Fig. 4). If the sphenoid ostium has not been identified, it is usually apparent now (Fig. 5). A sphenoidotomy is performed using fine Kerrison rongeurs or a sphenoid punch (Fig. 6). It is safer to begin from the natural ostium, moving laterally, superiorly, and inferiorly. If the ostium is difficult to identify, the sphenoid sinus may be penetrated medially about half way between the skull base and the choana. Rarely, a drill may be required to penetrate a thick anterior sphenoid wall.

The surgeon must remember that the posterior division of the sphenopalatine artery (the nasoseptal division) traverses the anterior wall of the sphenoid sinus from lateral to medial. It then makes a 90° turn and becomes the posterior septal artery [19,20]. Depending on the extent of

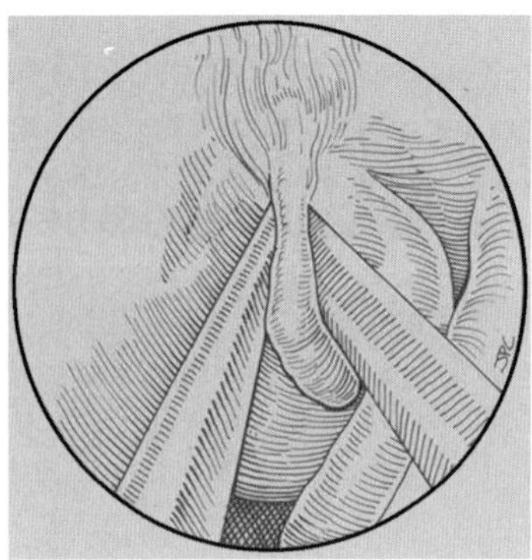

Fig. 1. Endoscopic bipolar cauterization of the superior turbinate. (*From* Har-El G. Approaches to the sphenoid sinus. In: Bluestone CD, Rosenfeld RM, editors. Surgical atlas of pediatric otolaryngology. 2nd edition. Hamilton [Ontario, Canada]: BC Decker; 2002. p. 359; with permission.)

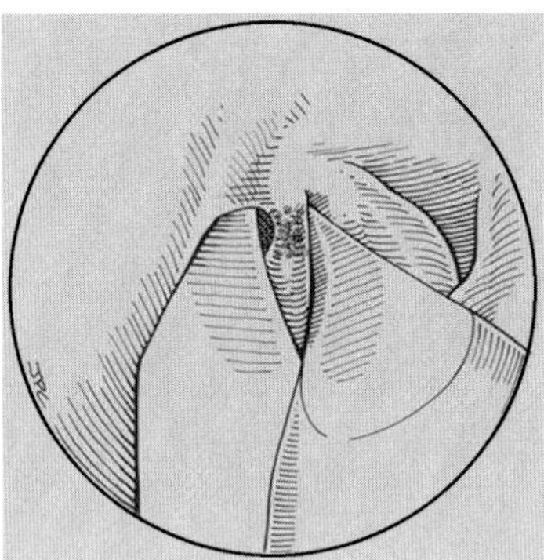

Fig. 2. Endoscopic anterior-to-posterior transection of the superior turbinate. (*From* Har-El G. Approaches to the sphenoid sinus. In: Bluestone CD, Rosenfeld RM, editors. Surgical atlas of pediatric otolaryngology. 2nd edition. Hamilton [Ontario, Canada]: BC Decker; 2002. p. 361; with permission.)

sphenoidotomy required, it is safer to cauterize the inferior aspect of the anterior sphenoid wall before using the rongeurs to remove it.

In about 20% of cases, the size or orientation of the middle turbinate or nasal septum may not allow sufficient exposure of the superior meatus. In these cases, the author recommends limited middle turbinectomy. Only the anterior and caudal aspect of the middle turbinate is removed. The ethmoid complex is not entered. This procedure can be done with the same endoscopic bipolar cautery and endoscopic scissors (Fig. 7).

By approaching the sphenoid sinus after superior turbinectomy, there is usually a wide exposure of the anterior sphenoid wall, allowing a large sphenoid sinus opening. If a wider exposure is required, the surgeon may extend the sphenoidotomy laterally or medially. Lateral exposure is

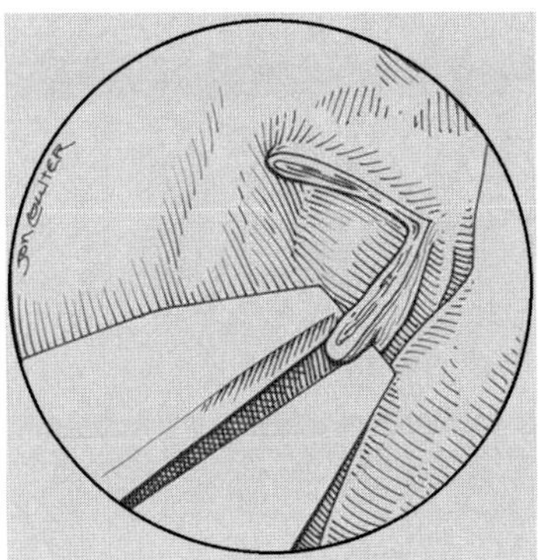

Fig. 3. Removal of the superior turbinate. (*From* Har-El G. Approaches to the sphenoid sinus. In: Bluestone CD, Rosenfeld RM, editors. Surgical atlas of pediatric otolaryngology. 2nd edition. Hamilton [Ontario, Canada]: BC Decker; 2002. p. 361; with permission.)

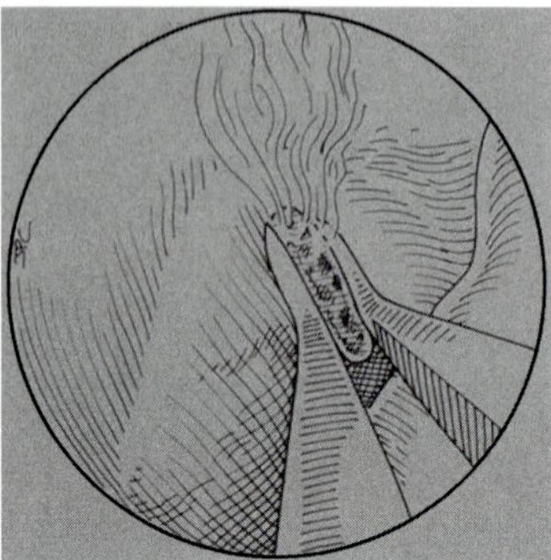

Fig. 4. If there is bleeding, the posterior insertion of the superior turbinate is cauterized. (*From* Har-El G. Approaches to the sphenoid sinus. In: Bluestone CD, Rosenfeld RM, editors. Surgical atlas of pediatric otolaryngology. 2nd edition. Hamilton [Ontario, Canada]: BC Decker; 2002. p. 361; with permission.)

achieved by performing limited posterior ethmoidectomy through the superior meatus. This procedure is followed by anterior sphenoid wall removal in a medial-to-lateral direction. This technique will not affect the anterior ethmoid region, the frontal sinus outflow tract, or the maxillary sinus opening. Before lateral bone removal, it is safer to insert an up-biting forceps or a neurosurgical nerve hook to palpate within the sinus behind the segment of bone about to be removed (Fig. 8). The surgeon may also introduce a 70° telescope into the sphenoid sinus and examine the lateral aspect of the sinus to determine how much anterior wall can be removed laterally without risking injury to the optic nerve or the carotid artery (Fig. 9).

For extended medial exposure and for exposure of the contralateral sphenoid sinus, the author uses one of two maneuvers. The surgeon may

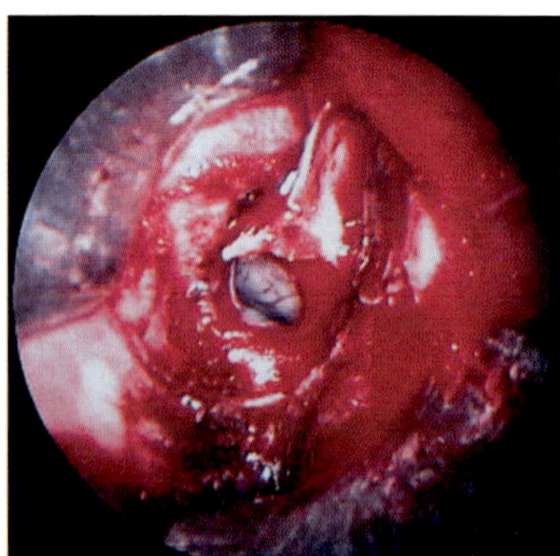

Fig. 5. Wide exposure of the sphenoid ostium. (*From* Har-El G, Swanson RM. The superior turbinectomy approach to isolated sphenoid sinus disease and to the sella turcica. Am J Rhinol 2001;15:154; with permission.)

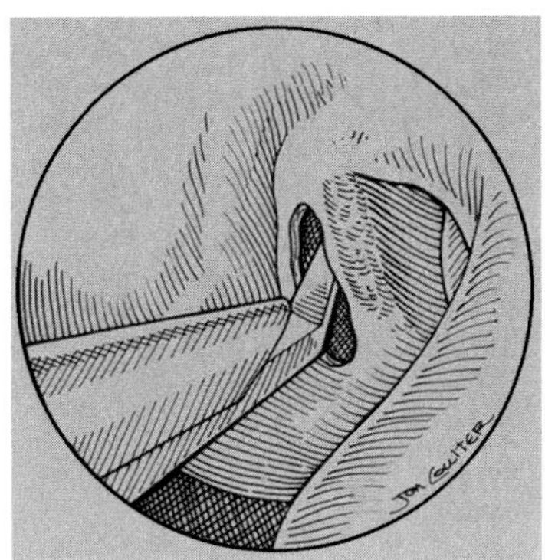

Fig. 6. Kerrison rongeurs are used to enlarge the sphenoidotomy. (*From* Har-El G. Approaches to the sphenoid sinus. In: Bluestone CD, Rosenfeld RM, editors. Surgical atlas of pediatric otolaryngology. 2nd edition. Hamilton [Ontario, Canada]: BC Decker; 2002. p. 361; with permission.)

insert a backbiting bone punch into the sphenoid sinus and then remove the posterior aspect of the nasal septum in a posterior-to-anterior direction. Alternatively, especially when the intrasphenoidal septum is thick and does not allow the use of the backbiting forceps, the author uses the sharp blade of a Freer elevator to penetrate through the posterior septum, about 3 to 5 mm anterior to the sphenoid sinus, into the contralateral posterior nasal cavity (Fig. 10). Heavy straight forceps are used to remove the remaining strut of nasal septum. The surgeon can then proceed into both sphenoid sinuses by removing the sphenoid rostrum and the intrasphenoidal septum (Fig. 11). If needed, the use of both lateral and medial extension techniques will result in an extremely wide exposure of the sphenoid sinus and sella turcica.

The intrasphenoidal septum is removed with straight-biting forceps, and the sella turcica is identified. A preoperative CT scan is essential for this part of the operation. The surgeon should evaluate the direction and the orientation of the intrasphenoidal septum. Occasionally, it will attach to the carotid canal. In this situation, great care must be taken in removing the septum.

The bulging pituitary tumor usually makes the identification of the sella turcica quite easy (Fig. 12). Nevertheless, the exact location of the sella may be confirmed by using the C-arm image intensifier or with computed-assisted technology. If not eroded by the pituitary tumor, the bony wall of the sella turcica is removed, and the dura is exposed. Fine Kerrison rongeurs are used to remove the sellar floor (Fig. 13). The distal blade is introduced gently between the dura and the bone, and the bony opening is enlarged cautiously with small bites. Occasional epidural bleeding may be encountered at this time and can be effectively controlled with thrombin-soaked Gelfoam pledgets (Johnson & Johnson, Somerville, New Jersey).

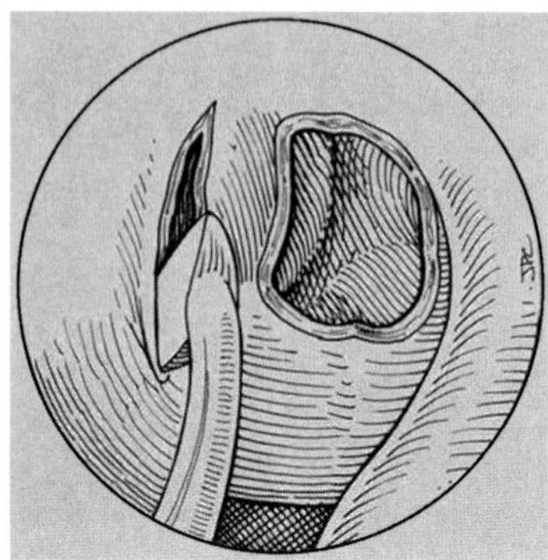

Fig. 10. For medial/contralateral extension, the posterior septum is incised to enter the contralateral posterior nasal cavity. (*From* Har-El G. Approaches to the sphenoid sinus. In: Bluestone CD, Rosenfeld RM, editors. Surgical atlas of pediatric otolaryngology. 2nd edition. Hamilton [Ontario, Canada]: BC Decker; 2002. p. 363; with permission.)

the intranasal use of moisturizing sprays. If there is no evidence of significant diabetes insipidus, the patient may be discharged home in 24 to 48 hours.

The recent introduction of intraoperative MRI may be of significant benefit in pituitary surgery. Unlike computer-assisted technology, intraoperative MRI images are updated for changes in tumor volume and in the location of the dura and the normal pituitary. Because these structures shift after tumor removal, the use of intraoperative MRI may be safer than computer-assisted navigation systems.

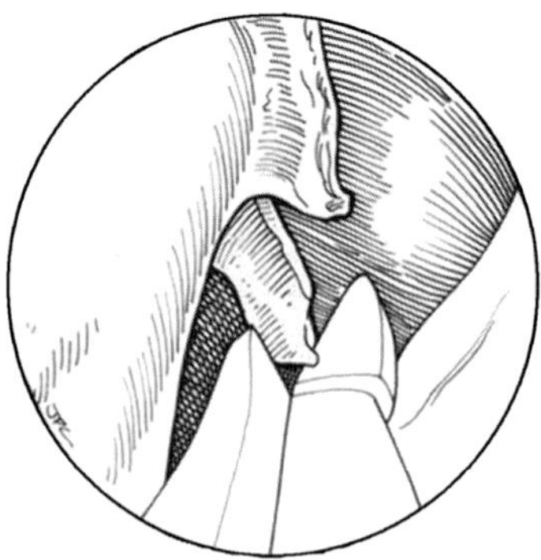

Fig. 11. The contralateral sphenoid sinus is entered. (*From* Har-El G. Approaches to the sphenoid sinus. In: Bluestone CD, Rosenfeld RM, editors. Surgical atlas of pediatric otolaryngology. 2nd edition. Hamilton [Ontario, Canada]: BC Decker; 2002. p. 363; with permission.)

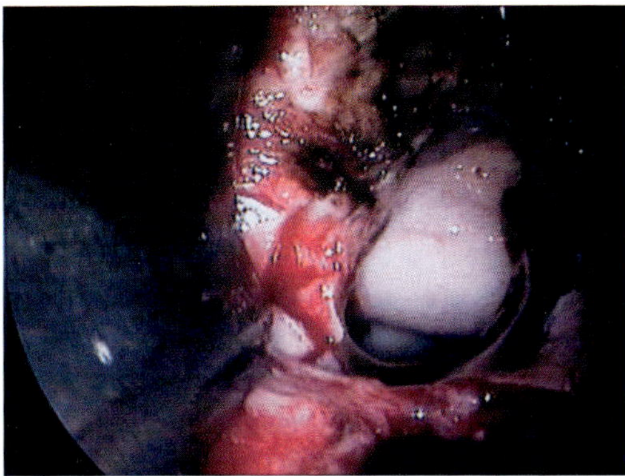

Fig. 12. The bulging sellar tumor is seen in the sphenoid sinus. (*From* Har-El G, Swanson RM. The superior turbinectomy approach to isolated sphenoid sinus disease and to the sella turcica. Am J Rhinol 2001;15:155; with permission.)

Discussion

The number of new reports describing endoscopic pituitary surgery has been increasing significantly [3–17,21]. As surgeons' confidence and comfort levels increase, they have used the endoscopic technique more frequently. Since 1997, the author and colleagues have used only the endoscopic direct, transnasal, nontransseptal approach for management of all pituitary surgical cases.

Advantages of the endoscopic technique: otolaryngologic aspects

The author and colleagues have found that the endoscopic transnasal approach is significantly quicker than the traditional sublabial transseptal

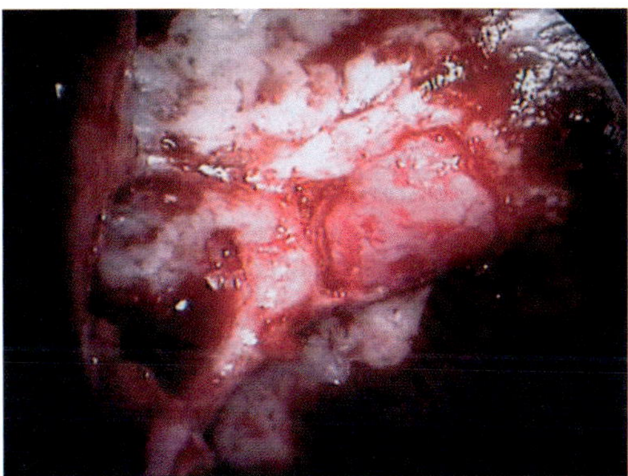

Fig. 13. The bony sellar floor is removed and the dura is exposed. (*From* Har-El G, Todor R. Endoscopic transnasal transsphenoidal pituitary surgery. Op Tech Otolaryngol Head Neck Surg 2003;14:205; with permission.)

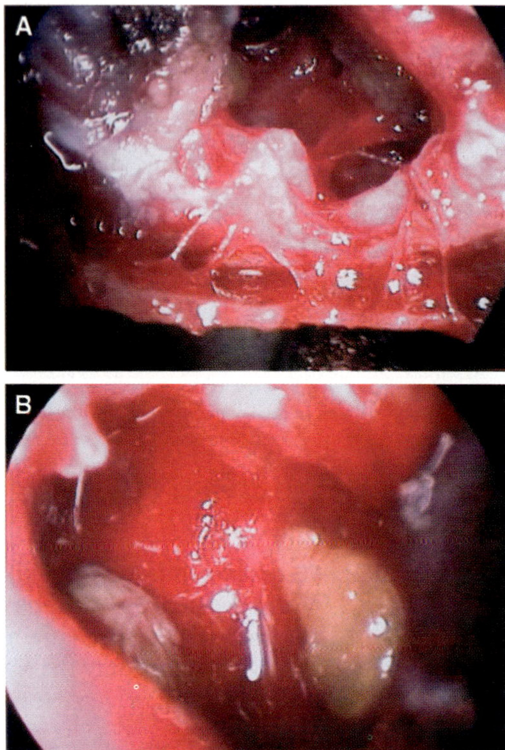

Fig. 14. Surveillance at the conclusion of the procedure. (*A*) 0° telescope within the sphenoid sinus showing the bony and dural opening into the sella. (*B*) 70° telescope within the sella showing residual tumor. (*From* Har-El G, Todor R. Endoscopic transnasal transsphenoidal pituitary surgery. Op Tech Otolaryngol Head Neck Surg 2003;14:206; with permission.)

approach. In an uncomplicated case, the sella turcica can be exposed in 10 to 20 minutes. The procedure is safe, both in the nasal cavity and the sphenoid sinus. Within the nasal cavity, the endoscopes provide excellent view of the bony and soft tissues about to be manipulated. Direct control of any possible vessels on the anterior face of the sphenoid sinus is easy. Within the sphenoid sinus, the use of the angled telescopes allows direct visualization of the carotid arteries and optic nerves before proceeding with surgery on the sella turcica itself. The microscope does not offer this ability to inspect around the corner. The endoscopic approach avoids the possible complications and sequelae that may be associated with the transseptal approach, such as perforation, septal deformity, saddle nose deformity, nasal obstruction, and long-term epistaxis and crusting. The endoscopic approach also avoids possible dental complications from the sublabial approach, including hypoesthesia or anesthesia of the incisor teeth, which is common after the sublabial approach. The endoscopic approach avoids the complications and sequelae that may accompany the transethmoidal approach, including ethmoid or frontal sinusitis, synechiae, crusting, chronic pain, and maxillary sinus obstruction. The endoscopic approach provides as wide an exposure as needed, from limited widening of the natural ostium to a subtotal removal of the anterior sphenoid face on both sides.

At the end of the procedure, only a few minutes are needed to inspect the sphenoid sinus and nasal cavity for possible bleeding. Compared with the septal and sublabial closure required in sublabial transseptal approach, surgical time is reduced significantly. Recovery from the otolaryngologic aspect of the surgery is rapid. There is no swelling or oral wounds that may contribute to postoperative pain and discomfort. Therefore, normal oral food intake is immediate. These factors contribute to a shorter hospital stay.

Advantages of the endoscopic technique: neurosurgical aspects

The endoscopes allow direct visualization of the sella turcica, bone, and dura, at the site of surgery. Using the endoscopic technique, the author and colleagues make a smaller opening into the bony sellar floor, because they can use angled telescopes to inspect within the sella. A smaller bony opening makes the reconstruction quicker and easier at the conclusion of the surgery. A smaller bony opening is especially important when CSF leakage is noted, because tight closure is much easier with a smaller bony opening. Within the sella turcica, endoscopic surgery is less aggressive and more precise than traditional surgery. The endoscopes allow direct visualization of the tumor to be removed, the surrounding dura, and the shifting normal pituitary gland. With the endoscopic technique, blind curettage can be avoided. The author and colleagues use angled 30° and 70° telescopes to visualize the intrasellar cavity for possible residual tumor posteriorly, superiorly, inferiorly, and laterally. If identified, residual tumor can be removed under direct visualization.

The author and colleagues have previously studied the incidence of diabetes insipidus after pituitary surgery and compared the results of traditional and the endoscopic approaches [7]. They found that although the intermediate and long-term incidences are similar, the incidence of immediate diabetes insipidus and of immediate electrolyte imbalance were reduced by more than 50% with the endoscopic approach [7]. The lower incidence of diabetes insipidus may contribute to the shorter hospital stay, as well as to decreased concerns about the potential cardiac effects of DAAVP treatment.

Disadvantages of the endoscopic technique

The main problem the author and colleagues have encountered in implementing the endoscopic pituitary surgical technique has been making their neurosurgical colleagues familiar and comfortable with the endoscopic technique and endoscopic instruments. Because most otolaryngologists have significant experience with endoscopic sinus surgery, they are comfortable with extending its indications. To familiarize their neurosurgical colleagues, the author and colleagues have worked closely with them. After the approach is completed and the sella turcica is exposed, the otolaryngologist remains in the room as an assistant. During the first few cases, the otolaryngologist may hold the telescope, provide irrigation and cleaning, and assist with maneuvering the different instruments. After only a few cases, most neurosurgeons become comfortable with the technique and do not require the otolaryngologist's presence for actual tumor removal.

Unlike microscopic pituitary surgery, the endoscopic technique is two-dimensional. Some neurosurgeons consider this two-dimensionality a significant disadvantage. For this reason, and because of lack of endoscopic experience, some surgical teams perform a combined approach. After the otolaryngologist exposes the sella turcica using the endoscopic approach, the neurosurgeon inserts a Hardy speculum and performs the actual tumor removal using the microscope. This operation may be difficult in patients with a small nose or tight nostril. The exposure may be limited, and the speculum may traumatize the nostril. This problem can be solved by performing a low columellar (external rhinoplasty) incision or an alotomy incision.

A theoretic disadvantage of the endoscopic technique is that the anterior wall of the sphenoid sinus is removed. When there is CSF leakage at the end of the procedure, tight reconstruction and packing of the sphenoid sinus may be more difficult than after the transseptal technique, because the anterior wall of the sphenoid sinus is not available to buttress the reconstruction. In the author's experience, this situation has not been a problem. In more than 120 cases, only one patient had persistent CSF leakage that required return to the operating room.

Summary

The technique of endoscopic transnasal, nontransseptal, transsphenoidal pituitary surgery is gaining increasing popularity. Many pituitary surgical teams consider it the procedure of choice. It provides a rapid and safe approach to the sella turcica. Within the sella turcica, the endoscopes give the surgeon the ability to inspect around the corner and to remove residual tumor. The procedure avoids the complications related to the sublabial transeptal approach. Hospital stay is shorter.

References

[1] Halstead AE. Remarks on the operative treatment of tumors of the hypophysis. Trans Am Surg Assoc 1910;28:73–93.

[2] Cushing H. Surgical experiences with pituitary disorders. JAMA 1914;63:1515–25.
[3] Jankowski R, Auque I, Simon C. Endoscopic pituitary tumor surgery. Laryngoscope 1992; 102:198–202.
[4] Jho HD, Carrau RL. Endoscopic endonasal transsphenoidal surgery: experience with 50 patients. J Neurosurg 1997;87:44–51.
[5] Har-El G, Swanson RM. The superior turbinectomy approach to isolated sphenoid sinus disease and to the sella turcica. Am J Rhinol 2001;15:149–56.
[6] Har-El G. Approaches to the sphenoid sinus. In: Bluestone CD, Rosenfeld RM, editors. Surgical atlas of pediatric otolaryngology. 2nd edition. Hamilton (Ontario, Canada): BC Decker; 2002. p. 353–65.
[7] Shah S, Har-El G. Diabetes insipidus after pituitary surgery: incidence after traditional versus endoscopic transsphenoidal approaches. Am J Rhinol 2001;15:377–9.
[8] Har-El G, Todor R. Endoscopic pituitary surgery—the direct transnasal transsphenoidal approach. In: Har-El G, Weber PC, editors. Skull base medicine and surgery. Alexandria (VA): American Academy of Otolaryngology – Head and Neck Surgery; 2004. p. 114–30.
[9] Har-El G, Todor R. Endoscopic transnasal transsphenoidal pituitary surgery. Op Tech Otolaryngol Head Neck Surg 2003;14:204–6.
[10] Gamea A, Fathi M, el-Guindy A. The use of rigid endoscopy in transphenoidal pituitary surgery. J Laryngol Otol 1994;108:19–22.
[11] Sethi PS, Pillay PK. Endoscopic management of lesions of the sella turcica. J Laryngol Otol 1995;109:956–62.
[12] Helal MZ. Combined microendoscopic trans-sphenoid excisions of pituitary macroadenomas. Eur Arch Otorhinolaryngol 1992;252:186–202.
[13] Carrau RL, Jho H, Ko Y. Transnasal-transsphenoidal endoscopic surgery of the pituitary gland. Laryngoscope 1996;106:914–8.
[14] Sheehan MT, Atkinson JL, Kasperbauer JL, et al. Preliminary comparison of the endoscopic transnasal vs. the sublabial transseptal approach for clinically nonfunctioning pituitary macroadenomas. Mayo Clin Proc 1999;74:661–70.
[15] Nasseri SS, McCaffrey TV, Kasperbauer JL, et al. A combined, minimally invasive transnasal approach to the sella turcica. Am J Rhinol 1998;12:409–16.
[16] Moses RL, Keane WM, Andrews DW, et al. Endoscopic transseptal transsphenoidal hypophysectomy with three-dimensional intraoperative localization technology. Laryngoscope 1999;109:509–12.
[17] Gopal HV. Endoscopic transnasal transsphenoidal pituitary surgery. Curr Opin Otolaryngol Head Neck Surg 2000;8:43–8.
[18] Har-El G. Endoscopic direct transnasal sphenoidotomy: the superior turbinectomy approach. Op Tech Otolaryngol Head Neck Surg 2003;14:185–7.
[19] Har-El G. The anterior wall of the sphenoid sinus. Ear Nose Throat J 1994;73:446–8.
[20] Schwartz JS, Har-El G. Posterior septal perforation after nontransseptal sphenoid sinus surgery. Op Tech Otolaryngol Head Neck Surg 2003;14:221–2.
[21] Aust MR, McCaffrey TV, Atkinson J. Transnasal endoscopic approach to the sella turcica. Am J Rhinol 1998;12:283–7.

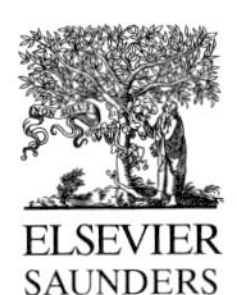

ELSEVIER
SAUNDERS

Otolaryngol Clin N Am
38 (2005) 737–771

OTOLARYNGOLOGIC
CLINICS
OF NORTH AMERICA

Vascular Lesions of the Skull Base: Endovascular Prospective for the Otolaryngologist

David H. Robinson, MD

Vascular Center, Section of Interventional Radiology, Department of Radiology, Virginia Mason Medical Center, 1100 Ninth Avenue, Seattle, WA 98101, USA

With continually advancing device technology and endovascular techniques, endovascular procedures are playing an increasing role in the multidisciplinary management of vascular lesions of the skull base. This article reviews the concepts and techniques of embolization and endovascular management of vascular lesions of the skull base, with the objective of providing the practicing otolaryngologist with a brief review of current techniques and general concepts in the endovascular management of these lesions and facilitating interactions with the neuroendovascular operator in the multidisciplinary management of these patients.

Skull base vascular anatomy and dangerous anastomoses

A thorough understanding of the vascular anatomy of the head and neck is essential to the performance of diagnostic angiography and intervention by either embolization or revascularization. Although a detailed discussion of the vascular anatomy of the skull base is beyond the scope of this article, this body of knowledge is well covered in several excellent review articles and basic neuroangiography texts [1–6]. Arterial branches that most commonly come into consideration in the treatment of lesions of the skull base include the ascending pharyngeal artery, the transmastoid and meningeal branches of the occipital artery, and branches of the internal maxillary artery including middle meningeal artery, accessory meningeal artery, and sphenopalatine artery. Direct meningeal branches of the vertebral artery and internal carotid artery may also contribute significantly to the arterial

E-mail address: raddhr@vmmc.org

doi:10.1016/j.otc.2005.03.008 **oto.theclinics.com**

supply of skull base lesions. Therefore, a comprehensive, four-vessel diagnostic cerebral angiogram, including bilateral external carotid artery injections, bilateral internal carotid injections, and at least an ipsilateral vertebral artery injection, is generally warranted when investigating arterial supply to a suspected hypervascular lesion of the skull base. Of primary concern during embolization of skull base lesions is the possibility of the passage of embolic material through the so-called "dangerous anastomoses," which are well-characterized embryonic collateral connections between external carotid artery branches and eloquent neurovascular territory, including the internal carotid artery, vertebral-basilar system, the retina, and the anterior spinal artery. These channels can provide a critical back-up system for arterial supply to neurovascular territory in the event of major neurovascular stenosis or occlusion. Although in a normal patient they are frequently too small to appreciate angiographically, in patients with occlusive atherosclerotic disease they are commonly identified as a hypertrophied arterial network connecting the extracranial circulation to the intracranial circulation. A thorough understanding of the dangerous anastomoses for the specific territory being investigated is therefore prerequisite for any consideration of therapeutic embolization, and it should be assumed that these small arterial collaterals are present in all cases, whether or not they are visualized on the initial diagnostic angiogram.

Nontarget embolization of normal arteries supplying cranial nerves is another cause of morbidity with neurologic dysfunction after embolization of skull base arteries. These arteries are not dangerous anastomoses but instead are normal arterial supply to cranial nerves of the skull base through small arterial pedicles that may be inseparable from the arterial supply to the target lesion and therefore are subjected to embolization. The resulting cranial nerve dysfunction, if any, is nearly always incomplete and temporary, although more permanent cranial nerve dysfunction can be experienced with liquid embolic agents such as liquid tissue adhesive, described later.

Concepts and techniques of embolization

A number of embolic agents are commonly used in current approaches to therapeutic embolization [7]. In general, there is an inverse relationship between the physical size of the embolic agent and the degree of end-organ devascularization, ranging from mild reduction in tissue perfusion pressure to complete and permanent microvascular devascularization with resultant tissue necrosis. Therefore, the size of embolic agent chosen directly influences the efficacy, safety, and extent of tissue devascularization, and the choice of embolic agent depends on the objectives of the particular case (Fig. 1). Deposition of fibered microcoils into medium-sized arteries typically results in a modest decrease in tissue perfusion pressure, a strategy that may be appropriate to promote hemostasis in the setting of traumatic

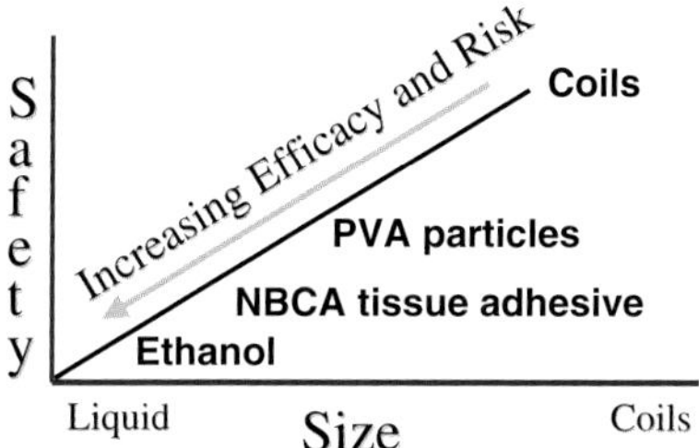

Fig. 1. Theoretical qualitative relationship between size of embolic material, risk of necrosis or nontarget embolization, and efficacy of tissue devascularization. Larger embolic materials, such as coils, are generally safer but less effective at target lesion devascularization. Liquid agents can result in complete devascularization and are therefore relatively dangerous. Particulate agents represent a compromise between these extremes and are the most commonly used embolic agents in the head and neck. NBCA, *N*-butyl cyanoacrylate; PVA, polyvinyl alcohol.

vascular injury. On the other end of the spectrum, liquid embolic agents, such as tissue adhesive and ethanol, may result in complete tissue devascularization, a strategy that may be appropriate for permanent devascularization of a vascular tumor or a vascular malformation.

Specific embolic agents used in the head and neck

Fibered platinum microcoils

The physically largest embolic agent commonly used in the head and neck is the fibered microcoil, which occludes mid- to small-caliber arteries with coils of specific size chosen according to the diameter of the target artery. These coils are composed of a complex of wound filaments of platinum wire, usually interwoven with polyester fibers to promote thrombosis (Fig. 2A). Each coil has a preshaped diameter that it tends to assume after it is ejected from the microcatheter. Arteries ranging from less than 1 mm to several millimeters in diameter can be effectively occluded with coils designed to conform to the diameter of the artery. Even the largest arteries in the head and neck, the common and internal carotid arteries, which range from 4 to 10 mm in diameter, can be effectively occluded with fibered microcoils. For most vascular beds, including virtually all territories in the extracranial head and neck (the brain is a notable exception), existing collateral pathways are sufficient to maintain adequate tissue perfusion distal to these small and mid-sized arterial occlusions, so that tissue necrosis does not occur. The most common goal of embolization with fibered microcoils is the reduction of tissue perfusion pressure to promote hemostasis in the setting of trauma or for preoperative occlusion before tumor resection. Coil embolization is also performed to protect a specific vascular bed from the effects of a subsequent more proximal embolization with a smaller agent such as polyvinyl alcohol (PVA) particles, by directing the

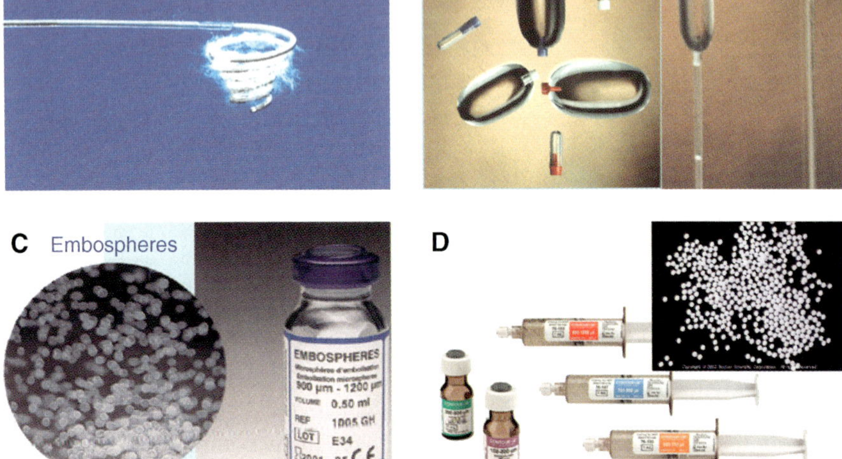

Fig. 2. Embolic agents. (*A*) Fibered microcoil (Target Therapeutics, Freemont CA). (*B*) Detachable silicone balloons (Target Therapeutics, Freemont CA). (*C*) Particulate agent (Embospheres, Biosphere Medical, Rockland MA). (*D*) Polyvinyl alcohol microspheres (Contour SE Microspheres, Boston Scientific, Natick, MA).

particles away from the territory occluded by coils and into the target territory.

Particulate embolic agents

PVA particles, the most commonly used embolic agent, are available in diameters from 1000 μm (too large for most microcatheters) to 100 μm (small enough to risk tissue necrosis). The ability to select a specific range of particle diameter for a particular situation is a major advantage of PVA particles. The operator can take into account the desired depth of penetration into the target lesion (or degree of devascularization) on one hand and the likelihood of presence of significant dangerous collateral channels or significant cranial nerve supply on the other hand. Traditional PVA particulate agents are composed of shredded PVA, which is irregular in shape and variable in diameter within a specified range. This variability in shape and size predisposes PVA to particle clumping and more proximal occlusion than the nominal particle size would suggest. A newer, spherical PVA (Contour SE Microspheres, Boston Scientific, Natick, MA) is composed of uniform spheres of PVA. These uniform spheres have less tendency to clump proximally, theoretically resulting in a more uniform embolization and a more precise diameter of vessel occlusion when compared with the standard shredded PVA particles (Fig. 2D). A newer agent, which has a scope of use similar to that of PVA but with the possible advantage of more uniform particle diameter, trisacryl gelatin microspheres, or Embospheres (Biosphere Medical Rockland, MA; Fig. 2C) may provide a more controlled level of arterial occlusion and more distal arterial occlusion than is achieved with traditional PVA. (Spherical PVA has a similar theoretical advantage.)

Silk suture and liquid coils

Segments of 6-0 silk suture, cut into lengths from 1 to 4 cm and injected by a microcatheter, provide an inexpensive alternative to other commercial products for flow-directed embolization of small to mid-sized arteries such as those supplying arteriovenous malformations. In these high-flow lesions, the suture segments are carried distally toward the nidus of the lesion by flow. Once the segments are lodged, thrombosis and an inflammatory reaction are incited, resulting in permanent arterial occlusion. One disadvantage of silk suture is its lack of visibility on fluoroscopy. Although PVA is not radio-opaque, its course is usually tracked by the contrast in which it is suspended. The so-called "liquid" coils (Target Therapeutics, Fremont, CA) are commercially available segments of a thread of finely wound platinum filament that are intended to be carried by flow to a target lesion, similar to silk suture segments. Liquid coils have the advantage of being visible on fluoroscopy and the disadvantage of increased cost.

Absorbable gelatin sponge

One cm × 1 mm pledgets or torpedoes of absorbable gelatin sponge (Gelfoam, Pharmacia Upjohn, Kalamazoo, MI) can be rolled from a sheet of Gelfoam, and delivered through a microcatheter, providing temporary occlusion of a mid-sized artery (1–2 mm). This temporary agent is used most commonly in the setting of trauma or to protect a distal vascular bed before a more proximal embolization with a smaller agent such as PVA particles. Gelfoam slurry provides a quick and effective temporary embolic agent that can establish hemostasis in small to medium-caliber arteries. It is prepared by placing thin strips cut from sheets of Gelfoam into a syringe containing contrast and then repeatedly forcing the mixture back and forth through a three-way stopcock, shredding the strips of Gelfoam into a radio-opaque slurry that can be delivered through a microcatheter. One disadvantage of this technique is the uncertain particle size obtained with this shredding technique, which produces a mixture of particles with a wide range in diameter.

Tissue adhesive

N-butyl cyanoacrylate (NBCA) is liquid tissue adhesive that has been used for years as a convenient liquid embolic agent. This material was originally marketed as a liquid suture and is commonly referred to as "glue." For intra-arterial embolization, this tissue adhesive is mixed with a lipid-soluble contrast agent such as ethiodized oil in a ratio ranging from 1:1 to one part NBCA: four parts ethiodized oil. The more dilute the concentration of glue, the longer the polymerization time. A longer polymerization time has the practical benefits of a longer infusion time before occlusion occurs and a more distal embolization, when desired. In very high-flow arteriovenous malformations, a more concentrated ratio may be used, which will polymerize rapidly and solidify before passing through the nidus into the recipient venous system. In slow-flow lesions, or when there is some distance between the tip of the microcatheter and the target lesion, more dilute mixtures are preferred. Care must be taken not to allow the tissue adhesive to be exposed to ionic solutions such as saline or blood, because contact with ionic solutions initiates polymerization. Once the microcatheter is in position, and after contrast injections have been performed to gauge the rate of flow, the microcatheter is thoroughly flushed with D5-water solution before the slow infusion of the NBCA tissue adhesive opacified with ethiodized oil, which is well visualized fluoroscopically. Precisely predicting the behavior of this moderately viscous liquid can be tricky. There is the unique risk of gluing the microcatheter in place (less of a concern with current-generation hydrophilic-coated catheters). Also, clumps of glue can adhere to the tip of the microcatheter and become dislodged when the microcatheter is withdrawn, resulting in the embolization of a clump of polymerized glue into a nontarget vessel. In certain territories, this embolization can be disastrous. Once the injection is completed, the microcatheter is removed and discarded; the target vessel may need to be selectively catheterized again with a new catheter, so this process can be a tedious. Tissue adhesive can be used for tumor embolization in a safe feeding pedicle (an artery is safe if it does not supply cranial nerves and has no anastomoses with the internal carotid artery, vertebral artery, anterior spinal artery, or ophthalmic artery). Only recently has an NBCA product (Trufill, Cordis Endovascular, Miami Lakes, FL) gained Food and Drug Administration approval for intravascular use in the United States, with an indication for use in the embolization of brain arteriovenous malformations.

Ethanol

Concentrated ethanol (ethyl alcohol) is an effective and therefore dangerous liquid embolic agent that penetrates to the microvascular level. When injected into an artery, ethanol denatures proteins within the endothelium lining cells, precipitating protoplasm and effectively stripping the endothelium, and resulting in a permanent devascularization. Although still frequently used for direct percutaneous sclerotherapy of low-flow vascular malformations (veno-lymphatic malformations or hemangiomas), ethanol is rarely used intra-arterially today, especially in the head and neck.

Detachable balloons

Detachable silicone balloons, are delivered transarterially or transvenously mounted on a microcatheter in the collapsed state (Fig. 2B). They then are filled with an isotonic contrast solution to a volume sufficient to occlude the target artery, detached, and left permanently in position with contrast inflation maintained by a microvalve mechanism. These balloons (previously marketed by Target Therapeutics, Fremont, CA) have been widely used for the permanent closure of large vessels and larger fistulas, including direct carotid cavernous fistulas, and for permanent occlusion of vertebral and carotid arteries. At present, however, no detachable balloon system is commercially available in the United States. In situations in which balloons were previously used, the most common endovascular strategy is to perform occlusion by deploying multiple fibered coils, pending reintroduction of a detachable balloon system into the United States market.

Arteriovenous fistulas

Introduction/definition

Dural arteriovenous fistulas (DAVF) are acquired arteriovenous shunts located within the dura matter in close association with a dural sinus. They have also been widely referred to as dural arteriovenous malformations, but because these lesions are acquired, not congenital, malformations, dural arteriovenous fistulas has become the preferred designation. Although the pathophysiology of DAVF is not fully understood, the prevailing theory is that a predisposing thrombosis of a dural sinus results in the in-growth and hypertrophy of normally microscopic dural arterioles that extend into the occluded sinus [7]. This process is followed by some degree of antegrade or retrograde recanalization of the sinus, establishing the arteriovenous shunt physiology. Although no predisposing factor is identified in more than 50% of cases, etiologic factors associated with the pathogenesis of DAVF include a number of conditions predisposing to dural sinus thrombosis. These conditions include dural sinus thrombophlebitis (otitis, sinusitis, phlebitis of the lower extremity), cranial trauma including neurosurgical procedures, general surgery (particularly gynecologic), and hypercoagulable conditions [8]. It is also well known that venous thrombosis may be clinically silent, so the incidence of asymptomatic dural sinus thrombosis is probably underestimated, and only a small minority of patients with sinus thrombosis ultimately develops symptomatic DAVF.

The arterial supply of dural venous fistulas may arise from any of the meningeal branches of the external carotid arteries, internal carotid arteries, vertebral arteries, or, rarely, from parasitized cortical branches. Symptoms are related to the arterialization of the recipient venous system, that is, of a dural sinus (resulting in tinnitus or intracranial hypertension), of ophthalmic veins (producing ocular symptoms), or of cortical veins (causing headaches, focal neurological deficits, seizures, or hemorrhage). Although any dural sinus can be involved, the transverse sinus is the one most commonly involved and encountered by the head and neck surgeon.

Classification of dural arteriovenous fistulas

It is now understood that the natural risk of DAVF may be estimated for each patient according to the pattern of venous drainage. A useful general classification of DAVF, correlating the pattern of venous drainage with symptoms has been elaborated by Djindjian and Merland [9] and later validated and refined by Cognard et al [10]. A similar classification has been proposed by Borden [11]. The aim of these classification schemes is to predict the natural history risk of a particular DAVF lesion to make a better-informed decision regarding treatment. The configuration of venous anatomy, as reflected by both the Cognard [10] and Borden [11] classifications, has been found to be a strong predictor of intracranial DAVFs that will present with intracerebral hemorrhage or nonhemorrhagic neurologic deficit [12,13]. The anatomic considerations of the Cognard classification are summarized in Fig. 3, and therapeutic implications based on this scheme are discussed later. In general, DAVFs draining freely and antegrade into a sinus produce only benign symptoms, whereas cortical venous drainage predisposes more aggressive neurologic symptoms and possible hemorrhage. Direct leptomeningeal venous drainage, variceal dilation of the venous recipient, and central drainage to the vein of Galen correlate with neurologic risk. The most common locations of DAVFs in Cognard's large series [12] were the transverse sinus (50%), the cavernous sinus (16%), the tentorium cerebelli (12%), and the superior sagittal sinus (8%).

Type I dural arteriovenous fistulas

Type I DAVFs drain into a sinus with a normal, antegrade flow direction (Fig. 3). These lesions have benign behavior and present with functional symptoms such as tinnitus, with retroauricular pain, or with ocular symptoms. Treatment of these DAVFs may be justified by the level of functional symptoms, which can be disturbing to the patient, but the lesions themselves do not place the patient at neurologic risk. Objective (ie, heard by the examiner on auscultation), pulse-synchronous, pulsatile tinnitus in a middle-aged patient suggests DAVF of the transverse sinus and warrants further evaluation with diagnostic angiography. Type I fistulas may not need treatment if the functional symptoms are not disturbing and if the cerebral venous drainage is normal. The patient must be made aware that any change in symptoms, such as increased or decreased tinnitus, headaches, otalgia, retroauricular pain, vertigo, or visual disturbance, requires reevaluation.

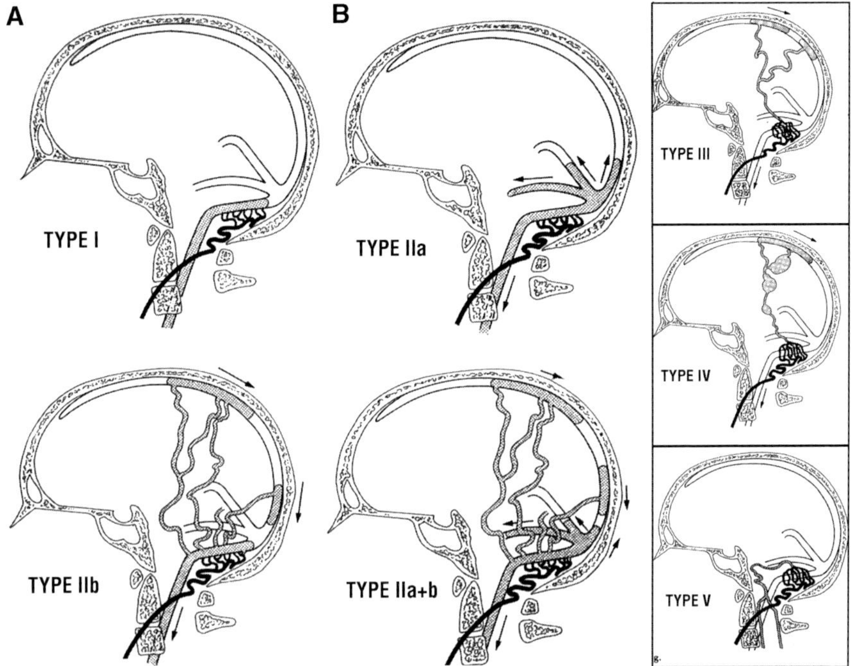

Fig. 3. (*A,B*) Classification of dural arteriovenous fistulas. Type I fistulas drain antegrade to ipsilateral sinus and jugular vein. Type II fistulas drain retrograde into the sinus. In type IIb fistulas, there is also some retrograde flow within cortical veins. Type III lesions drain into cortical veins directly, and venous varicosities are present in type IV lesions. Type V fistulas drain into spinal veins. Neurologic risk by natural history progresses from type I (benign) to type IIb (neurologic dysfunction from focal venous congestion) and type IV (high risk for hemorrhage). Type V fistulas present with myelopathic symptoms of venous congestion of the spinal cord. (*From* Cognard C, Gobin Y, Pierot L, et al. Neurological symptoms of intracranial dural arteriovenous fistulas: clinical and angiographic correlation in 205 cases. A revisited classification of the venous drainage. Radiology 1994;194:671–80; with permission.)

Type IIa dural arteriovenous fistulas

Type II fistulas have retrograde venous drainage within the draining dural sinus, predisposing to intracranial hypertension and its complications. Type IIa DAVFs drain into a sinus with insufficient or absent antegrade venous drainage because of stenosis or thrombosis downstream to the fistula, resulting in reflux into other sinuses but without reflux into cortical veins. Symptoms of intracranial hypertension, such as headaches, transient visual disturbances, decreased visual acuity, and diplopia (caused by cranial nerve VI palsy), were present in 20% of the type IIa fistulas in Cognard's series [12], along with either bilateral papilledema or optic disc atrophy seen on fundoscopic examination. It is theorized that the increase in sinus pressure lowers resorption of cerebrospinal fluid, which in turn leads to increased intracranial pressure, restoring the gradient across the arachnoid granulation villi [12]. Neurologic deterioration following lumbar puncture or shunting has been described in the setting of intermediate-grade DAVF. The mechanism of the deterioration in these cases is believed to be a rapid decrease in intraspinal cerebral spinal fluid pressure inducing acute herniation. In the long-term, type IIa DAVFs may result in significant visual loss from sustained intracranial hypertension, and these lesions therefore deserve strong consideration for definitive treatment, if treatment is practical.

Type IIb, III, and IV dural arteriovenous fistulas

DAVFs of types IIb to IV drain into cortical veins and thus are associated with a higher risk of focal neurologic deficits or hemorrhage. This risk increases from type IIb to type IV. Type IIb fistulas drain into a sinus with insufficient or absent antegrade flow and thus reflux into cortical veins as well as other sinuses. A complete and durable cure of these fistulas is required, because a subtotal occlusion may result in symptomatic recurrence. In type III fistulas, venous outflow is restricted to the cortical veins only, with no direct communication with a dural sinus. In type IV fistulas cortical venous varicosities are present.

Type V dural arteriovenous fistulas

Type V DAVFs drain into spinal veins. The pathophysiologic mechanism of the spinal symptoms is spinal cord venous hypertension with venous congestion, resulting in cord swelling and edema, as seen in the much more common but unrelated thoracolumbar spinal DAVF [14].

Endovascular treatment, techniques, risks, and efficacy

The treatment strategy for any particular DAVF should take into account (1) the estimated risk to the patient by natural history of the lesion, using the classification scheme discussed previously, (2) the patient's ability to tolerate symptoms such as tinnitus, which may be produced by a lesion that in itself does not pose significant neurologic risk to patient, and (3) the perceived safety and efficacy of the proposed treatment. Treatment possibilities include conservative management, manual compression of the ipsilateral carotid artery (performed by the patient with the contralateral hand), arterial embolization with particles or glue, sinus or cortical venous occlusion with coils, and open surgical obliteration of the fistula, alone or in combination with endovascular therapy. Radiosurgical therapy has also proved useful in lesions that may be difficult to treat by either endovascular or surgical means, and the strategy of combined radiosurgery before embolization has been proposed [15]. A multidisciplinary approach to treatment of DAVFs, considering the appropriate role of endovascular, open surgical, and radiosurgical treatment, is therefore recommended.

Before embolization of the middle meningeal artery, the ophthalmic arterial supply must be carefully assessed for a common variant in which the ophthalmic artery arises directly from the middle meningeal artery and for the presence of potentially dangerous arterial anastomoses to the orbit. As always in head and neck embolization procedures, for any arterial pedicle under consideration for embolization, assessment of potential dangerous collaterals to the internal carotid artery or vertebrobasilar system must be made before and during embolization. Anastomoses between the occipital and vertebral arteries may appear and enlarge during embolization. The presence of anastomoses between the ascending pharyngeal artery, middle meningeal, and/or internal maxillary artery and the internal carotid artery should be excluded by coil embolization, if possible, before attempting particulate embolization of these branches. It is important to maintain antegrade flow within the pedicle being embolized, to avoid inducing spasm in the feeding pedicle, and to avoid injections when there is stasis within the pedicle, all of which may reverse flow through dangerous collateral channels. Although transient cranial nerve dysfunction can be encountered, longer-term cranial nerve palsies are extremely rare after embolization with particles greater than 150-μm in size. Transient nerve dysfunction can occur after embolization with NBCA tissue adhesive, however.

In treating type I and type IIa fistulas, the aim is to achieve a complete cure. If a complete cure is not practical, therapy can be aimed at reducing the flow to decrease or eliminate functional symptoms. Arterial embolization with particles is frequently attempted before consideration of coil occlusion of the recipient segment of sinus. If possible, all external carotid artery feeders are embolized to obtain the most complete devascularization. The more complete the embolization, the greater is the probability of a durable cure. A truly isolated sinus segment, which does not serve a route of venous drainage of any portion of the brain, may be safely occluded with coils, often combined with particulate embolization of the major arterial feeding pedicles (Fig. 4). A durable cure can be expected in such cases. It is not necessary to embolize the meningeal feeders arising from the internal carotid artery or vertebral artery. This embolization is relatively dangerous, and the expected benefit does not justify the risk.

Arterial embolization with tissue adhesive

The aim of arterial embolization with tissue adhesive is to obtain a complete, definitive cure by creating a glue cast of the arterial feeders at the level of the fistula, including the origin of the recipient sinus segment draining the fistula (Fig. 5). This cast may be extremely difficult to accomplish when there are fistulas with multiple feeding pedicles. Several procedures may be required, each associated with a significant risk of cranial nerve deficits or neurologic sequelae, as described previously. Proximal

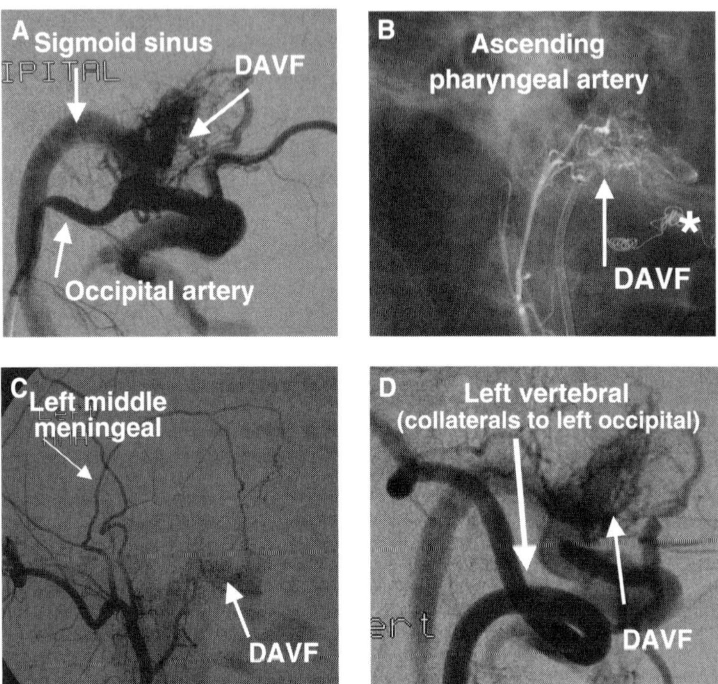

Fig. 4. Lower-grade dural arteriovenous fistula. Lateral views from a diagnostic cerebral angiogram performed on a 56-year-old woman who presented with objective, pulse-synchronous, pulsatile tinnitus. Study confirms low-grade dural arteriovenous fistula of the left sigmoid sinus, with multiple feeding arteries, including (*A*) occipital artery, (*B*) ascending pharyngeal artery, (*C*) middle meningeal artery, and (*D*), and left vertebral artery. Each of these feeding arteries was embolized to stasis using polyvinyl alcohol particles. Coils were placed in the distal occipital artery to protect the cutaneous branches from the effects of the proximal embolization (*, seen in B). DAVF, dural arteriovenous fistula. Following transarterial embolization of the feeding arteries, transvenous embolization was performed for a combined transarterial-transvenous approach, resulting in complete obliteration of the fistula. (*E*) Microcatheter advanced into recipient sigmoid sinus using arterial injections to guide placement (performed before arterial embolization). (*F*) Unsubtracted and (*G*) subtracted angiograms after embolization of arterial feeders and the venous recipient show the fistula is obliterated. This combined transarterial and transvenous treatment results in durable cure of this fistula without open surgery.

injection in the feeding pedicle that does not reach the shunt is to be avoided, because it increases the risk of late recanalization and makes further treatment more difficult. Direct sinus occlusion with NBCA, on the other hand, can achieve a cure in one session. Coil embolization can accomplish the same result, without the concerns of inadvertent embolization of glue into the systemic venous system or unintended reflux of glue into cortical veins. Glue injection is more dangerous than particulate injection; the main risk is forcing glue through an anastomosis between the internal

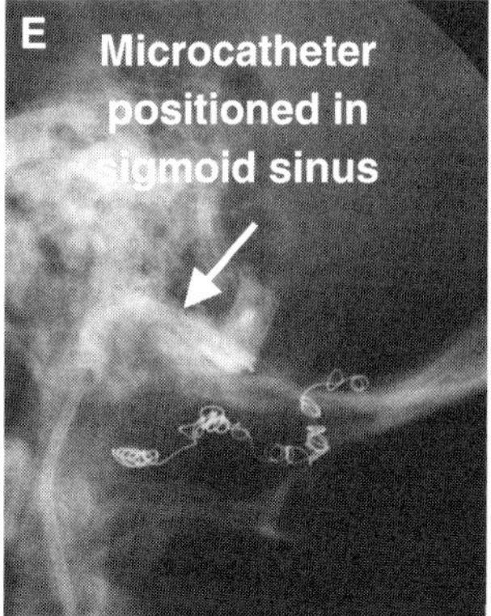

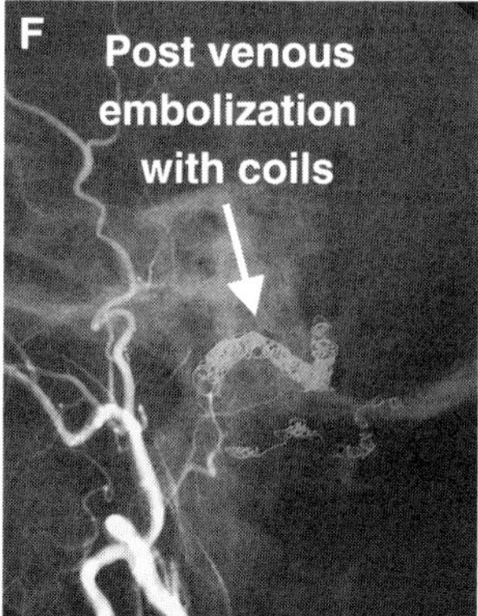

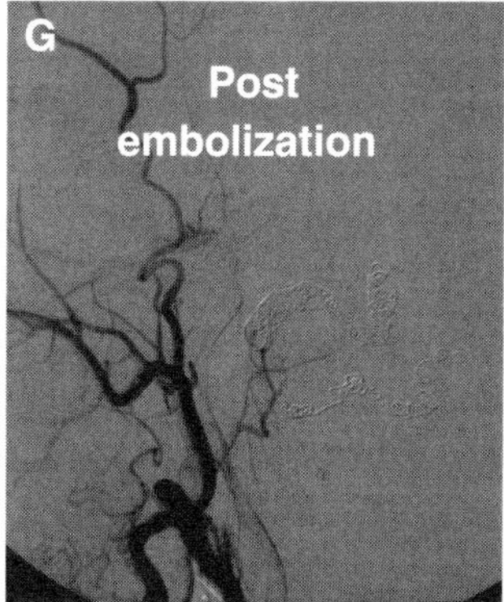

Fig. 4 (*continued*)

and external carotid arteries, most of which are not visible on pre-embolization angiograms. Thus, one must know the anatomy and potentially dangerous anastomoses of the vessel in which one is working. Glue should be injected slowly and at low pressure to reduce the risk of opening these anastomoses.

Sinus occlusion with coils

Sinus occlusion provides the most definitive endovascular means of occluding the fistula. The aim of venous embolization is to occlude the draining sinus with coils. Done properly, sinus occlusion allows a complete cure of the fistula [16–18]. To adopt the strategy of sinus occlusion for a particular case, the endovascular operator must first conclude that sinus occlusion is safe and then successfully access the recipient segment of sinus with a microcatheter; such assessment may be tedious, if not impossible. A complete angiogram must be obtained to analyze the precise extension of

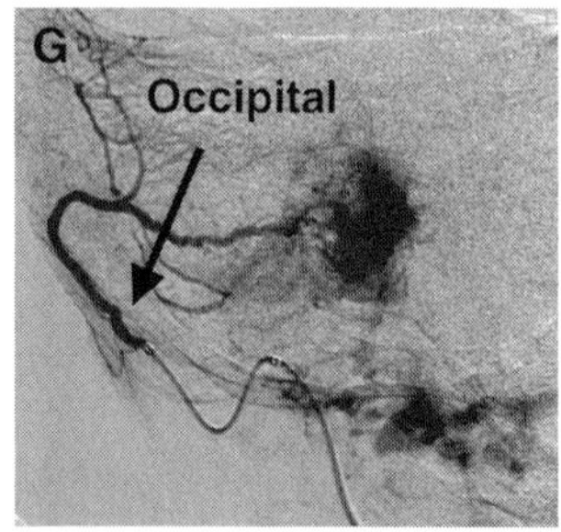

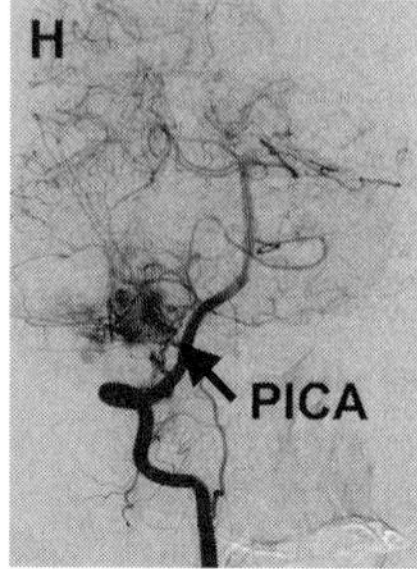

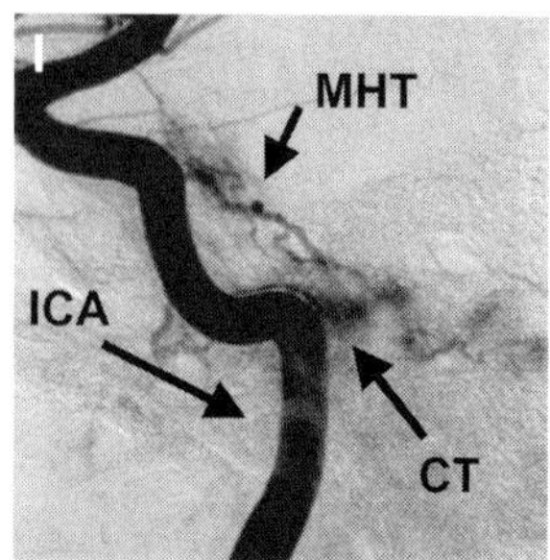

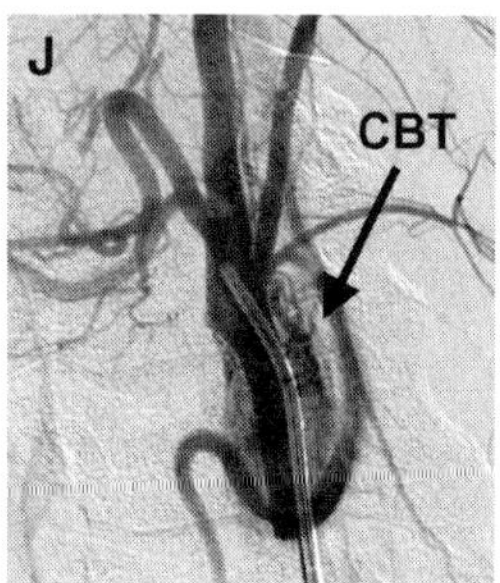

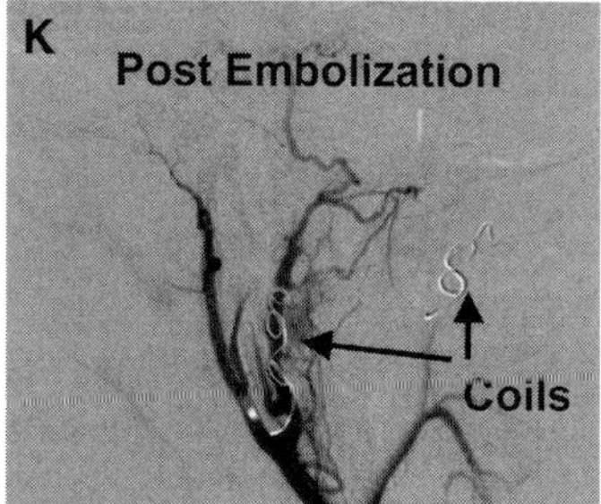

Fig. 7 (*continued*)

Juvenile nasopharyngeal angiofibromas

Juvenile nasal angiofibroma is a histologically benign fibrovasclar tumor with the potential for locally aggressive behavior. Most occur in males near puberty [38]. These tumors typically arise near the sphenopalatine foramen and from there may spread to involve paranasal sinuses, infratemporal fossa, skull base, middle cranial fossa, and orbit. Presenting symptoms are usually nasal obstruction and epistaxis of variable severity, with additional symptoms depending on the pattern of tumor spread.

Classification of juvenile nasal angiofibroma

A classification scheme for these tumors devised by Fisch [39] is summarized in Box 4.

A widely used surgical staging system proposed by Radkowski et al [40] is given in Box 5.

The treatment of choice for these lesions is preoperative embolization followed by complete surgical removal if possible. Thin-section CT and MRI with contrast are essential imaging studies for planning angiographic work-up, embolization strategy, and surgical resection. Before the routine application of preoperative embolization, patients who underwent surgery for juvenile nasal angiofibroma were at significant risk for intraoperative exsanguination [41]. Without embolization, the average blood replacement

Box 4. Fisch classification

Class I: Limited to the nasopharynx and nasal cavity, without significant bony destruction
Class II: Involvement of paranasal sinuses, with bony destruction
Class IIIa: Invasion of pterygopalatine fossa, infratemporal fossa, or orbit
Class IIb: Intracranial extradural extension lateral to cavernous sinus
Class IVa: Involvement of cavernous sinus
Class IVb: Intradural extension, or into pituitary fossa

was reported to be about 2000 cm^3. With routine preoperative embolization, the risk of exsanguination has almost disappeared; blood loss during surgery is reduced to less than 1000 cm^3, and endoscopic resection has become a more common approach [42]. The embolization procedure itself, if properly performed, carries low risk. Angiographic findings include intense, slightly heterogeneous tumor blush with arteriovenous shunting, an appearance that distinguishes these lesions from angiomatous polyp, hemangioma, angiosarcoma, and hemangiopericytoma (Fig. 8). As with glomus tumors, the strategy of angiographic evaluation and embolization of juvenile nasal angiofibroma is dictated by the pattern of spread determined by cross-sectional imaging.

Meningioma

Meningiomas are usually slow-growing tumors originating from the arachnoid cells of the dural coverings of the brain. Meningiomas account

Box 5. Radowski surgical staging system

Stage IA: Limited to nose and nasopharyngeal area
Stage IB: Extension into one or more sinus
Stage IIA: Minimal extension into pterygopalatine fossa
Stage IIB: Occupation of the pterygopalatine fossa without orbital erosion
Stage IIC: Infratemporal fossa extension without cheek or pterygoid plate involvement
Stage IIIA: Erosion of the skull base (middle cranial fossa, or pterygoids)
Stage IIIB: Erosion of skull base with intracranial extension with or without cavernous sinus involvement

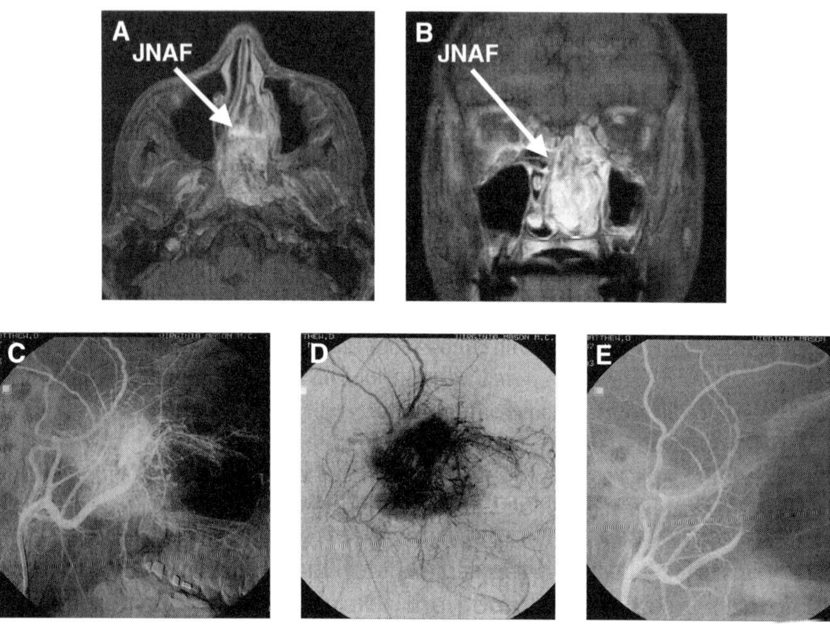

Fig. 8. Juvenile nasal angiofibroma. A 15-year-old male presented with symptoms of nasal obstruction without epistaxis. Examination revealed an expansile mass in the left nasal cavity, with septum displaced rightward. CT (not shown) revealed remodeling and erosion of left posterior ethmoid sinuses, left sphenoid sinus, and nasal septum. (*A*) Axial and (*B*) coronal T1-weighted MRI with contrast confirms the intensely enhancing mucosal mass in left nasal cavity, with rightward displacement of the nasal septum, consistent with juvenile nasal angiofibroma (JNAF) (*arrows*). (*C*) Unsubtracted and (*D*) subtracted cerebral angiogram demonstrates intense tumor blush in nasal cavity during internal maxillary artery. (*E*) Postembolization angiogram of the sphenopalatine artery shows no residual tumor blush. The tumor subsequently was resected endoscopically, with an estimated total blood loss of 75 cm^3.

for 15% of all primary intracranial tumors [43,44]. Treatment objectives for meningiomas of the cranial base include relief of neurologic disability and prevention of clinical progression or recurrence with the least morbidity. Because significant morbidity may be incurred during surgical resection of these tumors, especially in terms of cranial nerve dysfunction, the value of aggressive surgical resection must be weighed against the often-indolent natural history of these lesions. Advances in the clinical management of tumors of the skull base have had perhaps the greatest impact for patients with meningiomas. Although most have benign histologic features, skull base meningiomas can present a formidable challenge because of their proximity to vital structures, surgical inaccessibility, and occasional aggressive features. In recent years, the combination of advances in skull base surgical techniques, adjuvant therapy, and rehabilitation methods has dramatically improved the outcome for patients treated for these tumors [44]. In patients with typical benign meningiomas, completeness of resection is the major prognostic indicator for length of survival, risk of recurrence, and neurologic disability. Various means of predicting the growth potential of a given tumor are being investigated, but none has yet been confirmed for its predictive value in typical, histologically benign meningiomas. The role of external beam radiotherapy has not been subject to adequately controlled, prospective studies, and there is currently insufficient follow-up to assess the risks and benefits of stereotactic radio surgery [45].

Preoperative embolization

Meningiomas exhibit a characteristic angiographic pattern of dilated feeding meningeal arteries, converging toward the dural site of attachment, with radiating intratumoral arteries (producing a spoked-wheel appearance) and a fairly homogeneous tumor blush that persists late into the venous phase.

Dural vascular supply to skull base meningiomas by tumor location is typically as follows:

- Sphenoid wing tumors derive supply from the middle meningeal artery and meningohypophyseal trunk of the internal carotid artery.
- Tentorial and cerebellar pontine angle masses are supplied by the tentorial marginal artery branch of the meningohypophyseal trunk and posterior branches of the ipsilateral middle meningeal artery.
- Foramen magnum tumors typically receive supply from dorsal meningeal branches of the occipital or vertebral artery and posterior (neuromeningeal) trunk of the ascending pharyngeal artery.

Each location may also have a component of parasitized pial supply, which may even dominate. In such cases, surgical resection can be anticipated to be more difficult, because the tumor adheres to the pial surface with multiple bridging arteries. Tumors that display this tendency for pial arterial parasitization generally have a more aggressive behavior and carry a worse prognosis than more indolent tumors [46].

Endovascular devascularization of meningiomas has been shown to decrease blood loss and reduce the incidence of intraoperative transfusions [47]. The degree of devascularization can be assessed with postprocedure contrast-enhanced CT or MRI, which show absent enhancement in successfully embolized portions of the tumor [48]. The goals and techniques for preoperative embolization of skull base meningiomas are similar to those described for paragangliomas. With proper angiographic analysis before embolization and proper embolization technique, embolization of skull base meningiomas should result in effective temporary preoperative arterial stasis within the tumor in almost all hypervascular tumors; the expected incidence of significant morbidity is less than 1%. In a large series of meningioma embolizations beginning as early as 1987, the overall incidence of permanent neurologic deficits was reported to be 1.6%; the incidence of mortality was

0%; and the incidence of minor or transient complications was 2.7% [49]. Limitations of embolization include tumors in which significant supply is derived from pial branches and short, small-diameter feeding pedicles that can arise directly from the carotid, vertebral, or ophthalmic artery. In these cases, risk–benefit considerations frequently do not warrant attempted catheterization. The success of preoperative embolization depends largely on the extent of dural supply; little benefit may be gained from preoperative embolization of a tumor with primarily pial supply. Fortunately, the internal carotid and vertebral arterial branch supply to meningiomas is usually a minor component, with the majority of supply derived from external carotid artery branches. Exceptions are olfactory groove or planum sphenoidale meningiomas, which often derive the majority of their supply from small ethmoidal branches of the ophthalmic artery, frequently precluding safe preoperative embolization.

Trisacryl gelatin microspheres may be effective in the preoperative embolization of meningiomas. In one series, their use produced significantly less blood loss at surgery than seen with PVA particles of equal size, possibly because of the significantly more distal vascular penetration of the microspheres [50]. Embolization with 50- to 150-μm PVA particles may improve surgical treatment of meningiomas when compared with larger-particle embolization and also may be the only treatment required in older or high-risk patients [51]. Whether all patients with meningiomas should undergo preoperative embolization is a subject of debate [52]. This decision should remain at the discretion of the operating neurosurgeon, taking into account the size and location of the tumor, the degree of enhancement seen on preoperative cross-sectional imaging, and imaging findings suggesting significant pial arterial supply. Embolization without subsequent surgery has been shown to reduce tumor bulk and symptoms in nonoperative cases [53].

Other vascular lesions

A number of vascular tumors of the skull may warrant further evaluation by angiography and, if deemed appropriate, preoperative embolization. These less commonly embolized tumors include primary carcinoma, metastasis (including renal, melanoma, lung, choriocarcinoma, thyroid), hemangioma, fibrosarcoma, hemangiopericytoma, hemangioblastoma, chordoma, esthesioneuroblastoma, osteoblastoma, osteosarcoma, and lymphoma. The decision to proceed to angiographic evaluation in these cases is based on the degree of enhancement seen on cross-sectional imaging.

Elective, presurgical carotid occlusions and preoperative test occlusions

For extensive tumors with known arterial invasion, the surgeon may request elective, presurgical internal carotid artery occlusion. This occlusion can be accomplished by endovascular means, with detachable silicone balloons, fibered platinum coils, or a combination of these techniques. Temporary test occlusion can also performed when open surgical sacrifice of the carotid or vertebral artery sacrifice may be required [54–56].

Aneurysmal disease, pseudoaneurysms, and dissecting aneurysms

Skull base level intracranial aneurysmal disease is a rare cause of lower cranial nerve deficits, including facial nerve dysfunction, tinnitus, hearing

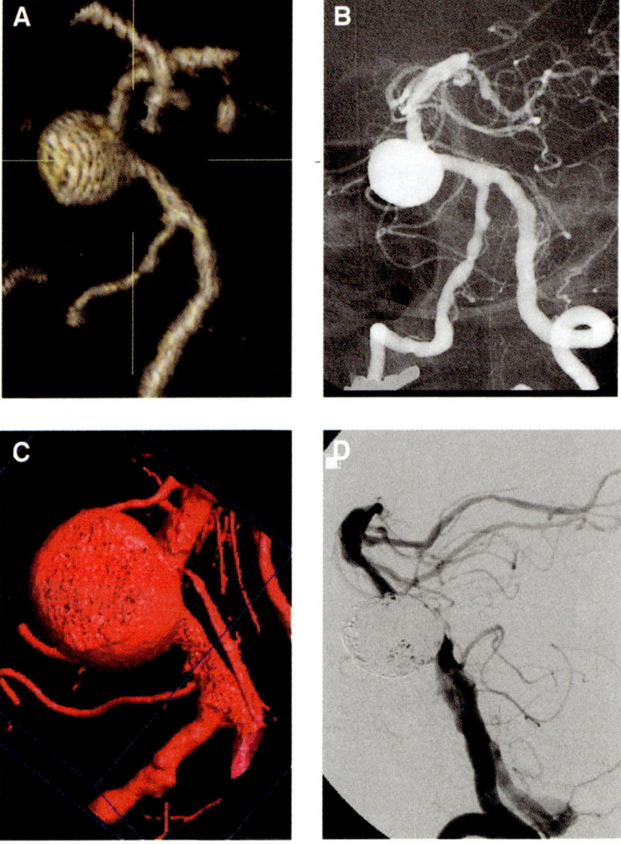

Fig. 9. Symptomatic mid-basilar aneurysm. A 69-year-old woman referred to an otolaryngologist for complaints of vertigo, right otalgia, and hearing loss was found to have a large mid-basilar aneurysm with involvement of 360° of the basilar artery wall (no aneurysm neck). (*A*) 3-D reconstructions from magnetic resonance angiography. (*B*) Diagnostic cerebral angiogram, anteroposterior projection from (*C*) 3-D rotational angiography. (*D*) Lateral projection from cerebral angiogram obtained after endovascular treatment with a combination of endovascular stents for reconstruction of the arterial lumen, followed by coiling. Patient's symptoms resolved following this treatment.

loss, otalgia, and dysphagia. Current advanced imaging techniques, including MR angiography, and CT angiography, generally reveal these lesions and in most cases also provide adequately accurate three-dimensional (3-D) imaging to assist in determining the most appropriate treatment strategy. The newer and more precise technique of 3-D rotational angiography (3-D images produced during a conventional angiogram) is now also available at some centers, providing highly detailed morphologic characterization of these lesions (Fig. 9). At present, approximately 80% of intracranial aneurysms can be treated effectively by endovascular means (aneurysm coiling, including use of more advanced balloon or stent assisted techniques). The recently published International Subarachnoid Aneurysm Trial showed significantly better outcomes in patients with ruptured aneurysms treated by endovascular means than in patients treated with open surgical clipping, in aneurysms that were considered treatable by either

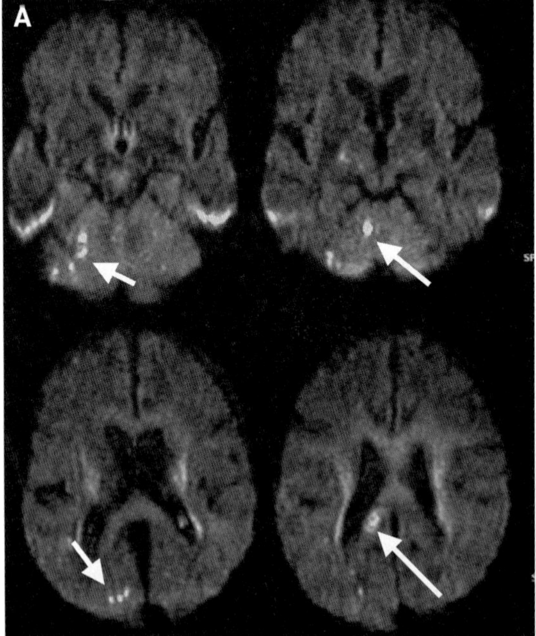

Fig. 10. (*A*) Symptomatic left vertebral artery stenosis in a 56-year-old male house painter, who was referred to an otolaryngologist for recurrent, disabling vertiginous spells. Diffusion-weighted MRI shows multiple, small foci of hyperintensity indicating multiple posterior circulation embolic infarcts. MRA (not shown) and (*B*) diagnostic angiogram confirmed high-grade narrowing of the distal aspect of left vertebral artery at level of penetration through the dura (*arrow*) and isolated posterior circulation (no posterior communicating arteries). (*C*) Endovascular treatment of the symptomatic stenosis was performed by deployment of a balloon expandable stent (*arrow*). (*D*) Posttreatment angiogram shows no residual stenosis (*arrow*). The patient's symptoms resolved with this therapy, and he was able to return to work.

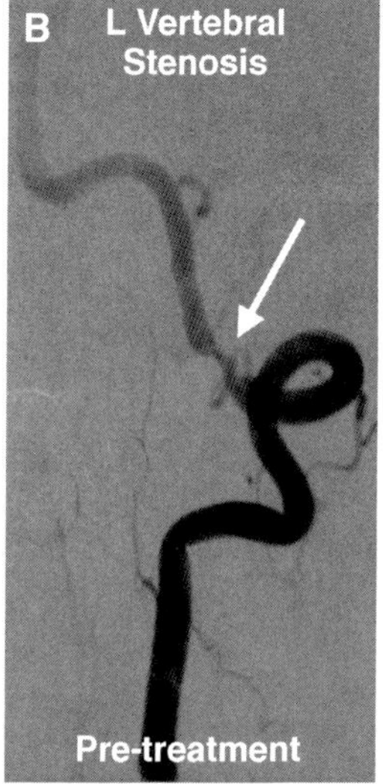

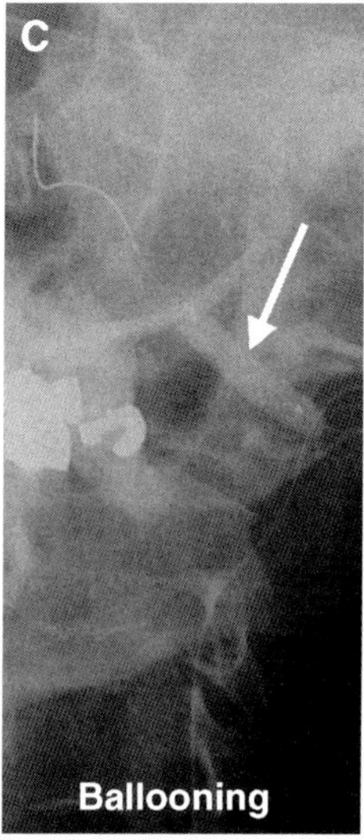

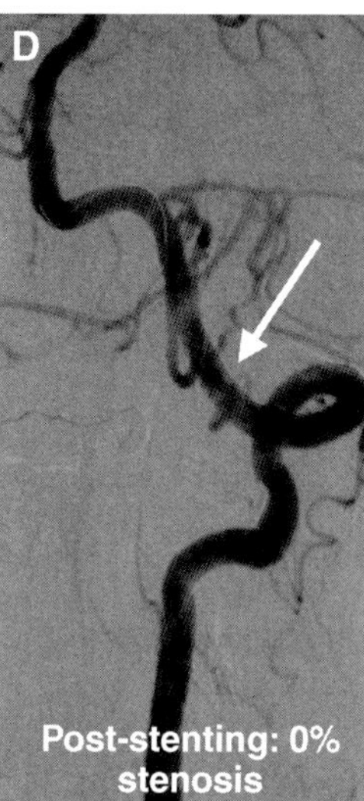

Fig. 10 (*continued*)

method [57]. It is therefore appropriate that both endovascular and surgical treatment options be considered in all such patients.

Symptomatic atherosclerotic disease and arterial dissections

Continued advances in stent technology, with more flexible and deliverable neurovascular stents, as well as covered stents (stent-grafts) suitable for smaller vessels, are now emerging as endovascular options for techniques that spare the parent-vessel in the treatment of skull base pseudoaneurysms, dissections of symptomatic disease, and dissecting aneurysms [58–64]. Accompanied by advances in periprocedural medical management, endovascular revascularization (angioplasty and stenting) of symptomatic extracranial and intracranial atherosclerotic stenosis or symptomatic arterial dissection at the skull base level is also becoming more widely practiced in capable centers worldwide. Implantable bioactive devices are also on the horizon and are expected to affect significantly the scope and efficacy of endovascular treatment options. An ongoing trial, funded by the National Institutes of Health, is comparing endovascular treatment with surgical endarterectomy in the treatment of atherosclerotic disease at the carotid bifurcation (Carotid Revascularization Endarterectomy vs Stent Trial [CREST]). Two industry-supported, randomized trials of carotid bifurcation treatment in surgical higher-risk patients (SAPPHIRE and ARCHER) have been completed with very encouraging results [65,66]. At present, however, there are no randomized trials comparing endovascular treatment with medical management or surgical treatment of neurovascular

[30] Weber PC, Patel S. Jugulotympanic paragangliomas. Otolaryngol Clin North Am 2001; 34(6):1231–40.
[31] Wasserman PG, Savargaonkar P. Paragangliomas: classification, pathology, and differential diagnosis. Otolaryngol Clin North Am 2001;34(5):845–62.
[32] Zanella FE, Valavanis A. Interventional neuroradiology of lesions of the skull base. Neuroimaging Clin N Am 1994;4(3):619–37.
[33] Valavanis A. Preoperative embolization of the head and neck: indications, patient selection, goals, and precautions. AJNR Am J Neuroradiol 1986;7(5):943–52.
[34] Connors JJ, Wojak JC. Paragagliomas. In: Connors JJ, Wojak JC, editors. Interventional neuroradiology: strategies and practical techniques. Philadelphia: W.B. Saunders; 1999. p. 130–41.
[35] Casasco A, Herbreteau D, Houdart E, et al. Devascularization of craniofacial tumors by percutaneous tumor puncture. AJNR Am J Neuroradiol 1994;15(7):1233–9.
[36] Casasco A, Houdart E, Biondi A, et al. Major complications of percutaneous embolization of skull-base tumors. AJNR Am J Neuroradiol 1999;20(1):179–81.
[37] Valavanis A. Embolization of intracranial and skull base tumors. In: Berenstein A, Valavanis A, editors. Interventional neuroradiology. Berlin: Springer-Verlag; 1993. p. 63–92.
[38] Lasjuanias P, Berenstein A. Nasopharyngeal tumors. In: Surgical neuroangiography, vol. 2: endovascular treatment of craniofacial lesions. New York: Springer-Verlag; 1987. p. 101–26.
[39] Fisch U, Fagan P, Valavanis A. The infratemporal fossa approach for the lateral skull base. Otolaryngol Clin North Am 1984;17(3):513–52.
[40] Radowski D, McGill T, Healy GB, et al. Angiofibroma. Changes in staging and treatment. Arch Orolaryngol Head Neck Surg 1996;122:122–9.
[41] Cummings BJ. Relative risk factors in the treatment of juvenile nasopharyngeal angiofibroma. Head Neck Surg 1980;3(1):21–6.
[42] Wormald PJ, Van Hasselt A. Endoscopic removal of juvenile angiofibromas. Otolaryngol Head Neck Surg 2003;129(6):684–91.
[43] Halbach VV, Hieshima GB, Higashida RT, et al. Endovascular therapy of head and neck tumors. In: Vineula F, Halbach V, Dion JE, editors. Interventional neuroradiology: endovascular therapy of the central nervous system. New York: Raven; 1992. p. 17–28.
[44] Desai R, Bruce J. Meningiomas of the cranial base. J Neurooncol 1994;20(3):255–79.
[45] Connors JJ, Wojak JC. Meningiomas. In: Connors JJ, Wojak JC, editors. Interventional neuroradiology: strategies and practical techniques. Philadelphia: W.B. Saunders; 1999. p. 100–20.
[46] Alvernia JE, Sindou MP. Preoperative neuroimaging findings as a predictor of the surgical plane of cleavage: prospective study of 100 consecutive cases of intracranial meningioma. J Neurosurg 2004;100(3):422–30.
[47] Dean BL, Flom RA, Wallace RC, et al. Efficacy of endovascular treatment of meningiomas: evaluation with matched samples. AJNR Am J Neuroradiol 1994;15(9):1675–80.
[48] Rodesch G, Lasjuanias P. Embolization and meningiomas. In: Al-Mefty O, editor. Meningiomas. New York: Raven; 1991. p. 285–97.
[49] Lasjuanias P, Berenstein A. Dural bony tumors. In: surgical neuroangiography, vol. 2: endovascular treatment of craniofacial lesions. New York: Springer-Verlag; 1987. p. 57–99.
[50] Bendszus M, Klein R, Burger R, et al. Efficacy of trisacryl gelatin microspheres versus polyvinyl alcohol particles in the preoperative embolization of meningiomas. AJNR Am J Neuroradiol 2000;21(2):255–61.
[51] Wakhloo AK, Juengling FD, Van Velthoven V, et al. Extended preoperative polyvinyl alcohol microembolization of intracranial meningiomas: assessment of two embolization techniques. AJNR Am J Neuroradiol 1993;14(3):571–82.
[52] Bendszus M, Rao G, Burger R, et al. Is there a benefit of preoperative meningioma embolization? Neurosurgery 2000;47(6):1306–11 [discussion: 1311–2].

[53] Bendszus M, Martin-Schrader I, et al. Embolisation of intracranial meningiomas without subsequent surgery. Neuroradiology 2003;45(7):451–5.

[54] Adams GL, Madison M, Remley K, et al. Preoperative permanent balloon occlusion of internal carotid artery in patients with advanced head and neck squamous cell carcinoma. Laryngoscope 1999;109(3):460–6.

[55] Connors JJ. Temporary test occlusion of the internal carotid artery. In: Connors JJ, Wojak JC, editors. Interventional neuroradiology: strategies and practical techniques. Philadelphia: W.B. Saunders; 1999. p. 377–89.

[56] Connors JJ. Permanent occlusion of the internal carotid artery. In: Connors JJ, Wojak JC, editors. Interventional neuroradiology: strategies and practical techniques. Philadelphia: W.B. Saunders; 1999. p. 390–3.

[57] Molyneux A, Kerr R, Stratton I, et al. International Subarachnoid Aneurysm Trial (ISAT) Collaborative Group. International Subarachnoid Aneurysm Trial (ISAT) of neurosurgical clipping versus endovascular coiling in 2143 patients with ruptured intracranial aneurysms: a randomised trial. Lancet 2002;360(9342):1267–74.

[58] Redekop G, Marotta T, Weill A. Treatment of traumatic aneurysms and arteriovenous fistulas of the skull base by using endovascular stents. J Neurosurg 2001;95(3):412–9.

[59] Fischer B, Palkovic S, Wassmann H, et al. Endovascular management of tandem extracranial internal carotid artery aneurysms with a covered stent. J Endovasc Ther 2004;11(6):739–41.

[60] Auyeung KM, Lui WM, Chow LC, et al. Massive epistaxis related to petrous carotid artery pseudoaneurysm after radiation therapy: emergency treatment with covered stent in two cases. AJNR Am J Neuroradiol 2003;24(7):1449–52.

[61] Liebman KM, Rosenwasser RH, Heinel LA. Endovascular management of aneurysm and carotid-cavernous fistulae from gunshot wounds to the skull base and oropharynx. J Craniomaxillofac Trauma 1996;2(2):10–6.

[62] Simionato F, Righi C, Scotti G. Post-traumatic dissecting aneurysm of extracranial internal carotid artery: endovascular treatment with stenting. Neuroradiology 1999;41(7):543–7.

[63] Butterworth RJ, Thomas DJ, Wolfe JH, et al. Endovascular treatment of carotid dissecting aneurysms. Cerebrovasc Dis 1999;9(4):242–7.

[64] Biggs KL, Chiou AC, Hagino RT, et al. Endovascular repair of a spontaneous carotid artery dissection with carotid stent and coils. Vasc Surg 2004;40(1):170–3.

[65] Yadav JS, Wholey MH, Kuntz RE, et al. Stenting and Angioplasty with Protection in Patients at High Risk for Endarterectomy Investigators. Protected carotid-artery stenting versus endarterectomy in high-risk patients. N Engl J Med 2004;351(15):1493–501.

[66] Gray WA. Acculink for Revascularization of Carotids In High Risk Patients (ARCHER) Trials final one year results. Presented at American College of Cardiology Annual Scientific Sessions. New Orleans, March 7, 2004.

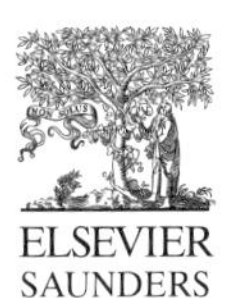

ELSEVIER
SAUNDERS

Otolaryngol Clin N Am
38 (2005) 773–794

OTOLARYNGOLOGIC
CLINICS
OF NORTH AMERICA

Diagnostic and Surgical Challenges in the Pediatric Skull Base

Scott C. Manning, MD[a,b,*], David C. Bloom, MD[a,b], Jonathan A. Perkins, DO[a,b], Joseph S. Gruss, MD[c,d], Andrew Inglis, MD[a,b]

[a]*Department of Otolaryngology–Head and Neck Surgery, University of Washington, 4800 Sand Point Way NE, Seattle, WA 98105, USA*

[b]*Division of Pediatric Otolaryngology, Children's Hospital and Regional Medical Center, 4800 Sand Point Way NE, Seattle, WA 98105, USA*

[c]*Department of Plastic and Reconstructive Surgery, University of Washington, 4800 Sand Point Way NE, Seattle, WA 98105, USA*

[d]*Division of Pediatric Plastic and Reconstructive Surgery, Children's Hospital and Regional Medical Center, 4800 Sand Point Way NE, Seattle, WA 98105, USA*

Pediatric skull base lesions are relatively unusual and are generally managed with a team approach at tertiary pediatric institutions. Pediatric skull base issues run the gamut from relatively simple and localized, such as unilateral choanal atresia in a nonsyndromic child, to extremely complex and difficult, such as a parameningeal rhabdomyosarcoma involving the middle cranial fossa (Box 1). The role of the pediatric otolaryngologist in management of pediatric skull base pathology varies by institution. Usually, the otolaryngologist member of the skull base team is involved primarily in airway management and in excision of benign lesions that present as nasal masses, such as teratomas, gliomas, and nasopharyngeal angiofibromas. The otolaryngologist also plays a primary role in the transnasal or transfacial biopsy of suspected skull base neoplasms. Increasingly, otolaryngology is assuming a more direct role in management of cerebrospinal fistulas and in excision of sellar lesions. Much of the increased involvement of otolaryngology in the management of skull base pathology has resulted from the natural evolution of experience with endoscopic techniques in sinus surgery for inflammatory disease and of experience with management of chronic ear disease. The skull base represents one of the last frontiers in the

* Corresponding author. Division of Pediatric Otolaryngology, Children's Hospital and Regional Medical Center, 4800 Sand Point Way NE, Seattle, WA 98105.

E-mail address: scott.mannng@seattlechildrens.org (S.C. Manning).

doi:10.1016/j.otc.2005.03.001 ***oto.theclinics.com***

Box 1. Differential diagnosis of pediatric skull base lesions

A. Anterior cranial fossa lesions
- Sinonasal
  - Epithelial
    - Inverted papilloma
    - Mucocele
    - Nasal Polyposis
  - Nonepithelial
    - Olfactory neuroblastoma
    - Rhabdomyosarcoma
    - Juvenile nasopharyngeal angiofibroma
    - Large cell lymphoma
- Bony
  - Fibrous dysplasia
  - Chondrosarcoma
  - Ossifying fibroma
  - Osteoblastoma
  - Aneurysmal bone cyst
- Intracranial
  - Meningioma
- Developmental
  - Nasal glioma
  - Nasal dermoids
  - Encephaloceles/meningoceles
    - Nasofrontal
    - Nasoethmoidal
    - Nasoorbital

B. Middle cranial fossa lesions
- Sellar and suprasellar
  - Pituitary microadenoma
  - Craniopharyngioma
- Clivus and petro-occipital fissure
  - Chordoma
  - Chondrosarcoma
  - Ewing's Sarcoma
  - Osteosarcoma
  - Lymphoma
  - Rhabdomyosarcoma
- Developmental
  - Teratoma
- Dura (extending down)
  - Meningioma

C. Posterior cranial fossa lesions
- Jugular foramin
  - Paraganglioma

- Nerve sheath tumors
  - Schwannoma
  - Neurofibroma
- Meningioma

Petroclival
- Meningioma
- Schwannoma
- Chordoma
- Chondrosarcoma

D. Temporal bone lesions

Benign
- Otitis externa
- Cholesteatoma
- Eosinophilic granuloma
- Exostosis or osteoma
- Paraganglioma

Intermediate
- Langerhans' cell histiocytosis

Malignant
- Rhabdomyosarcoma
- Lymphoma
- Malignant paraganglioma

E. Orbital lesions

Primary orbit
- Hemangioma
- Fibrous dysplasia
- Hemangiopericytoma
- Schwannoma
- Dermoid cysts
- Neurofibroma
- Lymphatic venous malformation

Lacrimal
- Benign mixed adenoma
- Lymphoma
- Idiopathic inflammatory
- Minor salivary lesions (adenoid cystic carcinoma)

F. Cerebral spinal fluid leaks

Congenitall
- Encephalocele

Traumatic
- Skull fracture
- Iatrogenic

development of surgical approaches. Generally speaking, advances in surgical techniques have been developed first in adults and then applied to progressively younger children, who present special management challenges.

Airway

Infants are obligate nasal breathers, and congenital skull base pathology often presents as airway distress because of nasal obstruction. The pediatric otolaryngologist is often called on for both airway management and establishment of a diagnosis in an infant with a nasal mass and with airway symptoms. Fiberoptic nasopharyngoscopy-laryngoscopy and imaging studies are the primary tools for initial airway and diagnostic assessment. Initial airway management options run the spectrum from prone positioning to establishing an oral or nasopharyngeal airway with placement of a nasogastric tube, to tracheotomy. Infants generally learn to become mouth breathers by age 4 months, but otherwise normal babies with nasal obstruction often learn sooner. At Children's Hospital and Regional Medical Center in Seattle, the preferred initial management of airway distress caused by nasal obstruction is placement of a nasopharyngeal tube. The authors use a segment of endotracheal tube placed through the nose with the distal edge positioned (by palpation with a finger in the mouth or by use of a small fiberoptic scope within the tube) just beyond the soft palate. Some trial and error is usually required to determine the optimal position allowing relief of airway obstruction and, it is hoped, ability to feed. In an infant, the free edge of the soft palate is close to the laryngeal inlet. The distal edge is cut so that a few millimeters of tube project beyond the nostril. A small safety pin through the tube is attached to the face with tape to hold the tube in place.

Case 1

A healthy term female baby was referred for management of airway distress after biopsy of a congenital left temporal mass and imaging studies revealed a large sphenoid wing teratoma involving the nasopharynx. Fiberoptic nasopharyngoscopy demonstrated significant mass effect along the left nasopharyngeal wall with obstruction of about 80% of the nasopharyngeal airway. Initial management consisted of placement of a nasopharyngeal tube (Fig. 1). After several weeks, the patient developed further obstruction, confirmed by sleep study, associated with weight loss. A tracheotomy was performed, and the patient is now growing well. The plan is for surgical excision with a combined craniotomy and lateral orbitotomy approach after age 1 year. The assessment of the skull base team was that the advantages of further growth and development on subsequent surgical morbidity potential (especially blood loss) outweighed the concerns related to the tracheotomy and the very small risk of malignant degeneration of the teratoma.

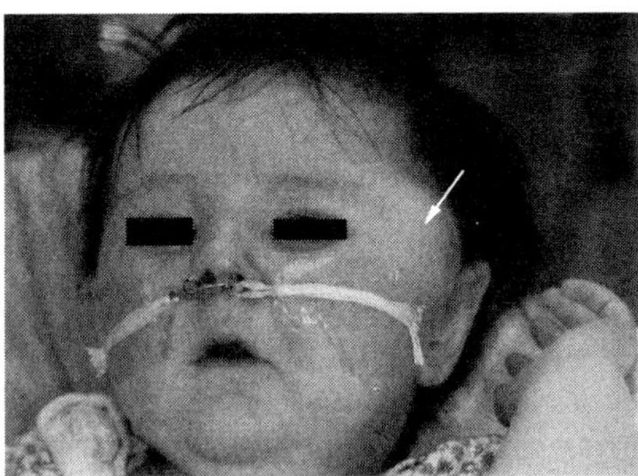

Fig. 1. Infant girl with biopsy-proven teratoma of sphenoid (*arrow*). A nasopharyngeal airway was placed for treatment of airway obstruction caused by tumor involvement of the nasopharynx and pharynx.

Other developmental issues

Depending on the age of the child, the surgeon must recognize the anatomic and developmental constraints that influence treatment options for pediatric patients with skull base pathology. In considering surgical approaches, one must keep in mind the importance of primary growth centers such as tooth buds, nasal septum and palate, and the zygomatic process of the maxilla. The cranial vault is fairly well developed at birth, but the basicranium and facial skeleton are relatively undeveloped and undergo rapid growth in the first few years of life. The distance from the cranial base to cervical flexure increases rapidly after birth (but remains relatively flat in certain conditions such as Down and Turner syndromes) [1].

The sinuses are relatively undeveloped at birth and do not afford surgical access to the skull base in the first few years of life (although improving technology is pushing back the minimum age for endoscopic approaches). The ethmoid cells are recognizable by the fifth fetal month and may provide some surgical access to the anterior cranial fossa (with 2.8-mm endoscopes) by age 1 year. Sphenoid pneumatization is highly variable, but the minimum age for an endoscopic optical environment to the middle cranial skull base is probably about age 3 years, on average. To assess the feasibility of a sphenoid sinus approach to a sellar or suprasellar lesion, both axial and coronal imaging with CT are necessary to determine whether pneumatization has reached the area of surgical interest. The frontal sinuses are usually not radiographically apparent before age 6 to 8 years, and approximately 8% of the population has no significant frontal pneumatization in adulthood. Maxillary sinus approaches to the pterygomaxillary fossa and middle cranial fossa may be limited by small sinus size and by presence of molar tooth buds before the teenage years.

Approximately 8% of pediatric craniotomies are performed to treat skull base pathologies, and neurosurgeons and craniofacial surgeons confront special anatomic and developmental concerns in children [2,3]. The thinner bone of the pediatric cranium has implications for pin fixation and the option of using split calvarial grafts for reconstruction. The orbital dissection landmark of the supraorbital notch is often absent before age 8 years, as is the pterion, an important landmark for burr hole placement. The pediatric brain may be more sensitive to retraction ischemia, an especially important issue in deep midline skull base lesions. The brain itself may be firmer and less physically retractable in young children than in adults, and blood loss is less well tolerated [3]. A tenet of pediatric neurosurgical approaches to skull base lesions is that more extensive removal of bone for better access is preferable (when possible) to extensive or prolonged brain retraction. Also, the incidence of diabetes insipidus and vision loss may be greater in younger children with traditional neurosurgical approaches to sellar and suprasellar lesions. All these factors make the development of improved transnasal, transfacial, or transoral approaches to the pediatric skull base important, with the goal of minimizing or avoiding the craniotomy approach in children.

Radiotherapy is an important treatment option for treatment of many malignant skull base lesions, but the long-term effects on facial and cranial growth, vision, and cognitive function can be devastating. In addition, the long-term risk of inducing a secondary malignancy with radiation therapy in a child is a significant concern. Strategies to conform high-dose radiation better to the specific tumor areas seem to be resulting in better tumor control with fewer long-term side effects [4,5].

Technologic innovations

From the perspective of the otolaryngologist, advances in technology for endoscopic sinus surgery techniques have been the principle drivers pushing the frontier of skull base approaches. Better endoscopes, including the 2.8-mm sizes for small spaces, have enhanced visualization. Compared with microscopic view, depth perception is limited, but the gain in magnification and the ability to see in a nonlinear fashion confer large potential advantages. In particular, the recent advent of the 45° telescope has allowed comfortable off-axis views that are particularly helpful in endoscopic resection of angiofibromas with lateral extension and of large sellar lesions. Equipment combining dissection with suction, such as suction Freer elevators, has allowed more function to be placed in one hand. The development of long, tapered drills and bipolar cautery instruments has also facilitated endonasal approaches to skull base lesions. Switching from a microscopic to an endoscopic method of visualization has allowed use of more direct instrumentation without need for a bayonet design.

The application of microdebrider techniques has greatly added to the armamentarium of the endoscopic surgeon. The growing range of sizes, angles, and tips (from aggressive cutting to diamond burr) has greatly increased the applicability of microdebrider techniques for skull base pathology. Also, the microdebrider has resulted in a conceptual shift regarding treatment of benign lesions from en bloc excision to piecemeal resection with careful removal of tissue margins at the sites of origin. This perceptual change is probably the most difficult aspect of adapting to new techniques in skull base surgery for many clinicians but has the potential for greatest improvement in reduced morbidity and improved cosmesis versus traditional approaches.

General advances include improvements in intravascular embolization techniques, which are necessary for endoscopic approaches to most vascular tumors, and the development of image guidance systems for precise intraoperative localization. Repair of cerebral spinal fluid (CSF) fistulas is a required skill for skull base surgery, and the development of better fibrin glues and collagen-based substrate graft materials has increased the range of endoscopic applicability. Absorbable fixation materials have improved the management of pediatric craniotomy sites. Better imaging techniques, such as helical CT with three-dimensional reconstruction software, have simplified preoperative planning.

Surgical approaches for specific pathologies

Choanal atresia

Although perhaps more nasal than skull base, transnasal repair of choanal atresia requires attention to skull base anatomy and familiarity with some skull base techniques. Choanal atresia is rare, occurring in about 1 in 7000 live births. Unilateral cases are often isolated, but up to 50% of bilateral cases are syndromic, and CHARGE syndrome (coloboma, heart defects, atresia choanae, retardation of growth and development, genitourinary disorders, and ear abnormalities) should be considered. Patients may present with airway distress because infants are obligate nasal breathers, and initial treatment may involve establishment of an oral airway. Preoperative evaluation should include axial CT (after nasal suctioning to improve air contrast) including the face and skull base. Most cases of choanal atresia involve bony overgrowth of the distal nasal septum medially and pterygoid plates laterally with thin bone or mucous membrane centrally [6]. The anatomy of the nasopharynx and skull base should be carefully noted before surgery. Patients with CHARGE syndrome may have extremely small nasopharyngeal spaces with close proximity of the atretic area to the clivus, making transnasal repair more problematic. It is better to address the airway initially with tracheotomy in these patients, especially if they have also significant heart disease.

The prevailing philosophy regarding surgical approach has shifted during the past 2 decades from transpalatal to transnasal because of the benefits of shorter operative time and less risk of future effect on dental or facial growth [7,8]. More recently, transnasal approaches are shifting from microscopic to endoscopic. Typical current approaches involve initial blunt puncture of the central thin area with a urethral sound or suction under endoscopic guidance with subsequent removal of posterior septum using backbiting forceps or drills. Some authors also remove a portion of the pterygoids laterally. Small 2.8-mm telescopes are usually necessary for visualization with infants, and 2.9-mm microdebrider cutters and drills are useful for a less traumatic removal of soft tissue and bone, respectively. A useful landmark for avoiding skull base injury during transnasal repair of choanal atresia is the posterior tip of the middle turbinate, which should stay superior to the field of dissection.

Unresolved issues in choanal atresia repair include whether to stent, to try to develop mucosal flaps, or to use fibroblast inhibitor therapy (mitomycin-C). Most retrospective reviews demonstrate a significant recurrence rate with need for repeat dilations in a large percentage of patients, especially those with bilateral disease. A recent review from Great Ormond Street Hospital did not show any outcome differences, with various surgeons using different approaches [9]. The literature does indicate a trend toward better outcomes with larger initial openings (older patients, unilateral atresia), less overall trauma (mucosal flaps, more atraumatic technique), and nonsyndromic patients.

Nasal dermoids, gliomas, encephaloceles, and teratomas

At about 8 weeks' gestation, a diverticulum of dura extends through the fonticulus frontalis into the prenasal space. If regression and involution of this projection is incomplete, an embryologic fusion anomaly, such as a dermoid, glioma, or encephalocele, can result. As mentioned previously, congenital nasal masses often present with airway obstruction in an infant. Initial biopsy might result in a rapid diagnosis but might also result in a cerebrospinal fistula. Therefore, nasal masses should be evaluated first with imaging.

CT, with its ability to define bone, is the image modality of first choice, but positioning for true coronal images is difficult in infants and young children, and determination of skull base defects can be difficult. Helical scanning with image acquisition overlap combined with three-dimensional imaging software can allow much better evaluation of potential communications of nasal masses through the skull base [10]. The clinician must keep in mind that the infant skull base is incompletely ossified, and determining meningeal intracranial connections can be difficult even with excellent images. True nasal encephaloceles usually have connections in the region of the cribiform plate anterior to the crista galli. MRI (usually requiring general anesthesia in infants and young children) can be a useful adjunct to CT in the evaluation of potential encephaloceles. Ruling out a significant intracranial connection initially allows an endonasal approach and avoidance of a craniotomy.

Nasal dermoids account for approximately 10% of all head and neck dermoids and usually present as noncompressible masses over the nasal dorsum with an associated midline pit. Masses and pits may appear laterally on the nasal dorsum or distally down to the nasal tip. Only a small percentage of nasal dermoids retain a connection to the subarachnoid space, usually through a tract extending through the nasal septum between the nasal bones. If imaging studies fail to demonstrate a definite intracranial connection, these lesions are approached externally. For lesions that do not extend above the glabela, most surgeons prefer an external rhinoplasty approach [11]. For high lesions, or those with a small suspected intracranial extension based on imaging studies, a midline incision over the dorsum is preferred. For lesions with a stalk extending superiorly, the nasal bones are displaced laterally, and the stalk is dissected from inside the nasal septum. Microscopic visualization and otologic instruments can be of great value in dissection of these lesions. Small CSF leaks can be managed directly, without a craniotomy. A craniotomy is required for a lesion with extensive intracranial connection, often in a dumbbell configuration with an intracranial cyst above the stalk (Fig. 2). With craniotomy approaches to these lesions, however, olfaction must be sacrificed at least on one side.

Case 2

A 1-year-old boy presents with a history of a congenital pit over the midline nasal dorsum with recent surrounding infection. CT imaging demonstrated a possible small stalk extending superiorly toward the foramen cecum. An elliptical incision was outlined around the pit, and the underlying dermoid was noted to extend through the nasal bones. The bones were gently divided in the midline with a Freer elevator, and the deep portion of the dermoid was excised from a pocket within the nasal septum. With final delivery of the mass, a brisk CSF leak resulted from the superior aspect of the dissection field. The area was inspected with a microscope, and a small dural opening was noted. After consultation with neurosurgery, the

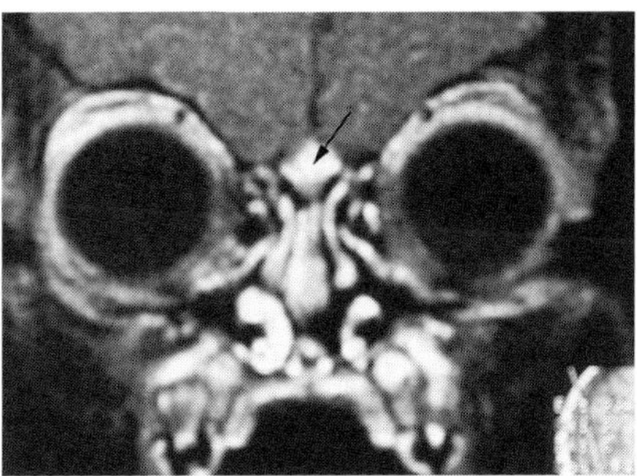

Fig. 2. Coronal CT scan of nasal dermoid with intracranial extension (*arrow*).

area was packed with a small amount of frontalis muscle taken from the superior aspect of the incision and with hemostatic collagen. The patient had an uneventful recovery.

Nasal gliomas are benign glial heterotopias that present as noncompressible masses [12]. Nasal gliomas may be intranasal, extranasal, or combined intra- and extranaxal (Fig. 3). As with dermoid cysts, a small percentage retains a connection to the subarachnoid space. Approach for surgical excision is based on imaging diagnosis of possible CSF connection, location of the pathology, and surgeon experience. Recent reports in the literature support an endoscopic intranasal approach for intranasal gliomas even if a central connection is possible, assuming surgeon experience with endoscopic repair of small CSF leaks [13–15].

Encephaloceles are defined clinically by evidence of a significant connection to the central nervous system. They tend to be soft and compressible and may enlarge with crying or with cervical compression of the jugular veins (Furstenberg sign). Sincipital (anterior or frontoethmoidal) encephaloceles have a facial component and typically require a combined approach with craniotomy for repair and reconstruction. The rare basal encephaloceles present as a nasal mass with the potential for airway obstruction or meningitis. The two most common imaging findings with basal encephaloceles are foramen cecum defects with variable extension into the ethmoid roof and cribiform or isolated ethmoid roof defects with low-lying funnel-shaped anterior skull base anatomy [16].

Traditional approaches to basal encephaloceles involved an anterior craniotomy with repair of the skull base defect with pericranial flaps. Management is shifting in many centers to endoscopic nasal approaches even for large encephaloceles in young patients [17]. The encephalocele itself tends to create more intranasal space by deflecting the septum and middle turbinate, although angled telescopes, possibly including 70° scopes, may be necessary to visualize anterior connections. Generally, the intranasal portion of the encephalocele is ablated progressively with bipolar cautery until

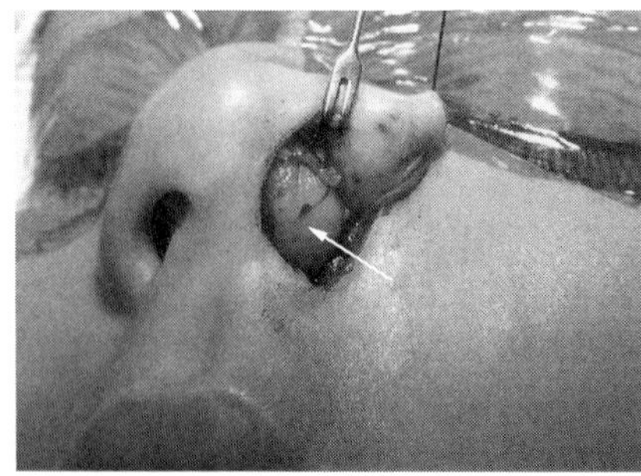

Fig. 3. Five-year-old boy with large nasal glioma (*arrow*) approached with an alar incision.

the skull base defect is seen. The mucosal cuff is removed circumferentially around the bony defect, which is then repaired endoscopically.

Teratomas are defined histologically by the presence of differentiated tissue from three germ layers. The clinical presentation of head and neck teratomas is highly variable, ranging from intraoral or nasopharyngeal well-circumscribed masses with small pedicled attachments to large masses extending into the middle cranial fossa. Head and neck teratomas can be associated with maternal polyhydramnios and other congenital anomalies. Most commonly, patients present with airway obstruction in the neonatal period [18]. The usual treatment approach for isolated teratomas with no intracranial extension is directly transnasal or transoral with endoscopic or microscopic visualization. Some authors have described endoscopic approaches even for lesions with limited intracranial involvement [19]. Large teratomas with intracranial extension present special management dilemmas balancing airway issues with concerns for surgical morbidity. Some authors have advocated aggressive early craniofacial resection for these lesions, but the potential for malignant degeneration seems to be low [20,21].

Case 3

An infant boy is found to have a large left nasopharyngeal mass on flexible endoscopy for evaluation of airway difficulty. CT and MRI demonstrate a large mass with extension through the greater wing of the sphenoid and middle cranial fossa involvement adjacent to the carotid artery and optic chiasm (Fig. 4). Nasopharyngeal biopsy demonstrated teratoma, and the nasopharyngeal portion of the mass was excised by a midline palate splitting incision up to the medial pterygoid and eustachian tube. The patient is now 2.5 years old and is asymptomatic except for left middle-ear effusion (managed with a tympanostomy tube). The plan is for neurosurgical excision using a lateral craniotomy approach if and when the mass progresses radiographically or becomes significantly symptomatic.

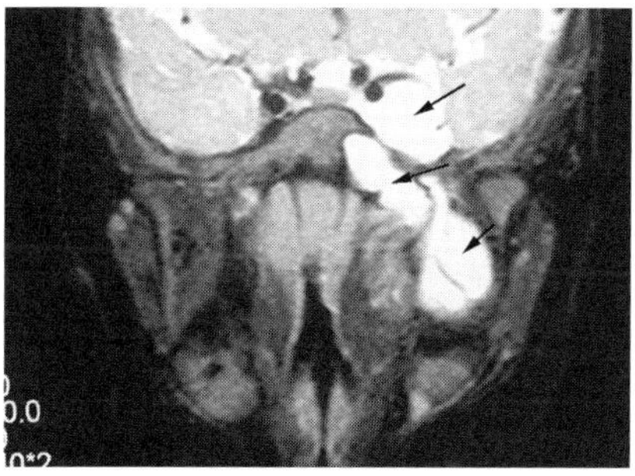

Fig. 4. Infant boy with large nasopharyngeal, infratemporal fossa teratoma with extension through the greater wing of the sphenoid into the middle cranial fossa (*arrows*).

Angiofibroma

Angiofibromas are rare benign tumors typically presenting in adolescent males as epistaxis and nasal airway obstruction. The management of angiofibromas is complex, involving many facets of skull base surgery. The diagnosis of angiofibroma is usually suspected on the basis of imaging findings of a vascular lesion involving the skull base in the anterior lateral nasopharyngeal vault. The tumors can extend along lines of least resistance into the nasal cavity, paranasal sinuses, pterygomaxillary fissure, infratemporal fossa, orbit, or cranial cavity [22]. Pterygomaxillary extension with anterior bowing of the posterior wall of the maxillary sinus (Homan Miller sign) is a common finding on imaging studies. Twenty percent to 36% of patients present with intracranial extension, usually extradural and limited. A small percentage presents with extensive intracranial extension, usually involving the cavernous sinus and carotid arteries; these patients are often managed with radiotherapy. The clinical and imaging diagnosis of angiofibroma is often confirmed with angiography demonstrating intense vascularity with most feeders arising from the terminal branches of the external carotid system. Angiography is generally scheduled within 48 hours of planned surgery so that the tumor can be embolized if the diagnosis is confirmed. Lesions are usually not biopsied before planned surgical excision.

Angiofibromas are staged according to degree of extension at initial presentation. Classically, tumors confined to the nasal cavities and nasopharynx with little lateral extension (stage I or IIA) (Box 2) [23] were approached through transpalatal or external transnasal (lateral rhinotomy) approaches. Tumors with more lateral extension (stage IIB and IIC) were approached with combinations of lateral rhinotomy, Caldwell–Luc, or facial degloving techniques. More recently, with the development of better microplate technology, many authors have advocated Le Fort 1 approaches for large tumors without extensive lateral or intracranial involvement [24]. Osteotomies are outlined high above dental roots, and plate screw holes are

Box 2. Staging system for juvenile nasopharyngeal angiofibromas [23]

I A Midline, nose, and nasopharynx
I B Extension into sinuses
II A Minimal involvement of the pterygopalatine fossa
II B Filling the pterygopalatine fossa
II C Infratemporal fossa
III A Skull base, pterygoid, or middle cranial fossa
III B Skull base with intracranial extension

drilled before bone cuts to guarantee precise realignment. Advantages over traditional techniques include better exposure to the nose and central skull base (with potentially less intraoperative blood loss), avoidance of facial or palatal incisions, and more rapid recovery. Potential complications include loss of tooth buds, enophthalmus, and tooth hypesthesia. Large tumors with lateral extracranial extension into the infratemporal fossa (stage III) have been managed with transmaxillary approaches, whereas lateral intracranial involvement has required some form of lateral skull base craniofacial resection approach.

Endoscopic techniques were first described for stage I tumors, but more recent reports are steadily expanding endoscopic resection to endonasal approaches or in combination with other approaches [25]. Endoscopic approaches to angiofibromas require arranging for possible transfusion (autologous when possible), preoperative embolization within 48 hours before surgery, and discussion with anesthesia personnel regarding arterial lines and maintenance of some degree of hypotensive anesthesia. Coordinated management also involves preoperative planning with appropriate neurosurgical and other craniofacial colleagues to formulate a back-up plan should endoscopic exposure prove too limited.

Adding to the difficulty of angiofibroma surgery in general is the dense, fibrous nature of the tumor, which makes compression for exposure impossible. Also, the tumors recruit blood supply easily and tend to become densely adherent to contact points in adjacent areas such as the posterior septum. They are notorious to surgeons for their tendency to act more like arteriovenous malformations than vascular neoplasms in their propensity to bleed intraoperatively, especially if not embolized. Descriptions of endoscopic approaches often begin with injection of the greater palatine foramen and then complete endoscopic ethmoidectomy, sphenoidotomy, and middle meatus antrostomy for initial tumor exposure [26]. Resection of posterior portions of the middle or inferior turbinates may be necessary. The general approach is to perform dissection initially in areas of best visualization, hoping to reduce blood supply to the tumor progressively. Some authors recommend starting with endoscopic or mirror transoral cautery dissection of the posterior inferior nasopharyngeal portion and proceeding to endoscopic transnasal takedown of the posterior septal attachments. Lateral extensions can be followed into the pterygomaxillary fissure by taking down the posterior wall of the maxillary sinus through the antrostomy with forceps, Kerrison rongeurs, or drills [27]. The 45° telescope is helpful for visualization of lateral disease.

Coagulation of the central tumor bulk with laser or cautery followed by microdebrider piecemeal removal of the resulting devascularized tissue is one strategy for decompressing the tumor and gaining exposure [28]. Strategies for combining function with endoscopic techniques include use of suction instruments such as suction Freer elevators. Having assistants hold the telescope or suction allows the operator to use two hands [29]. Areas of tumor attachment are cleaned up with microdebrider cutting tips and drills. Angled microdebrider tips are often necessary for access to the most superior limits of tumor extension. Frozen section analysis of margins is used to help ensure adequate resection.

Increasingly, authors are reporting endoscopic resection combined with other approaches, such as midface degloving or Caldwell–Luc operation, to approach lateral disease [30]. The endoscopes provide better illumination, magnification, and panoramic views of otherwise difficult-to-see areas deep in the dissection field where residual tumor is most likely to result in clinical recurrence. The development of new technologies such as optical dissectors may allow more direct endoscopic approaches to lateral extensions in the temporal fossa with significant reduction in surgical morbidity [31].

Case 4

An 11-year-old boy presented with a history of complete nasal obstruction and with CT findings of a vascular tumor involving nasopharynx, left nose, left maxillary sinus, left pterygomaxillary fissure with extension into the infratemporal fossa, left sphenoid, and left infrarorbital fissure (stage III, Figs. 5 and 6). The day before surgery, the patient underwent angiography with embolization of feeding vessels from the distal external carotid system. The patient was noted to have a few internal carotid feeders in the region of the sphenoid sinus, which could not be embolized. At surgery, the tumor was initially visualized by nasopharyngoscopy with an oral 120° telescope, and a combination of microdebrider and insulated monopolar cautery was used to dissect the posterior inferior margin of the tumor as much as possible. The intranasal portion was then removed with monopolar cautery and straight microdebrider dissection back to the level of the sphenopalatine foramen using endoscopic guidance. An endoscopic ethmoidectomy and middle meatus antrostomy was performed followed by a Caldwell–Luc approach. The posterior wall of the maxillary sinus was removed, and the most lateral portion of the tumor

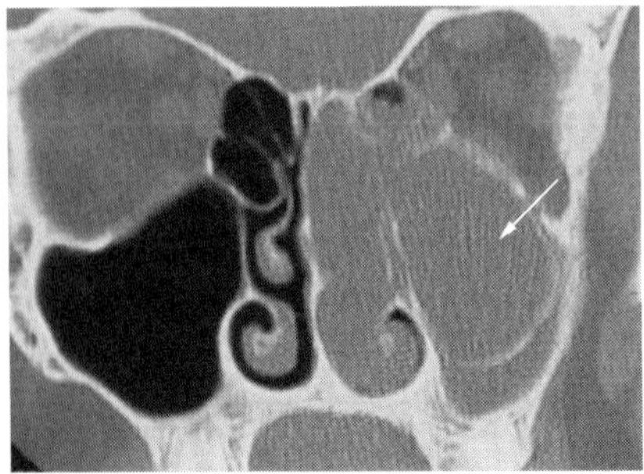

Fig. 5. Coronal CT of an angiofibroma with lateral extension into the maxillary sinus (*arrow*).

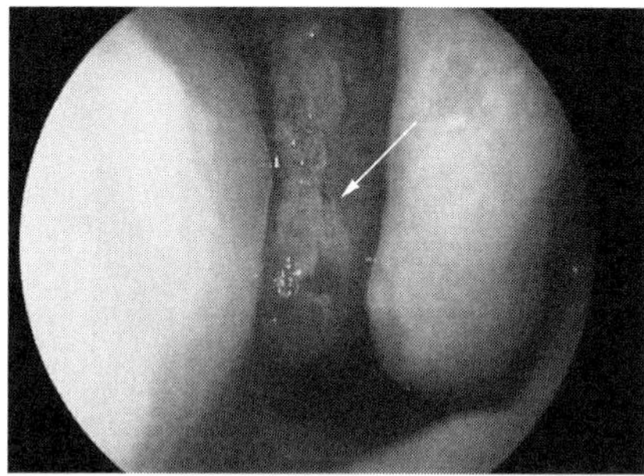

Fig. 6. Same patient as shown in Fig. 5. Endoscopic view of the left nasal cavity showing the nasal extension of the angiofibroma (*arrow*).

was removed with bipolar cautery, suction Freer, and microdebrider dissection with the transmaxillary approach. A curved Allis clamp was used to grab the nasopharyngeal tumor mass from a transoral approach, and further dissection with downward posterior traction allowed delivery of the tumor into the oral cavity. Brisk bleeding was controlled with direct pressure followed by bipolar cautery. Subsequent frozen section of tissue from the bleeding site was positive for tumor, and further endoscopic inspection demonstrated a small residual tumor lobulation involving the lateral sphenoid and inferior orbital fissure. The residual tumor was removed using a transnasal endoscopic view with the suction Freer and bipolar cautery. Imaging studies 1 year after surgery show no residual tumor.

Fibro-osseous lesions

Fibro-osseous lesions comprise a wide range of poorly understood pathologies ranging from clinically benign to histologically benign but clinically aggressive to frankly malignant. Benign osteomas in the head and neck have a predilection for the frontoethmoid sinus region and usually present in adult patients with frontal headache or sinusitis. Increasingly, these lesions are approached endoscopically [32]. Fibrous dysplasia is a rare disorder of unknown origin that may involve the skull base in pediatric patients. Eighty percent of fibrous dysplasia presents as isolated monostotic disease; the remaining 20% of polyostotic cases present with the McCune–Albright syndrome of café-au-lait spots and endocrine disorders. By imaging, fibrous dysplasia of the skull base can be divided into sclerotic or compact forms with ground-glass appearance on CT (50% of cases), lytic disease with an egg-shell appearance (15% of cases), or mixed or pseudo-pagetoid disease (35% of cases). The lytic and mixed forms can be more aggressive clinically and sometimes grow rapidly during the teenage years [33]. The natural history of fibrous dysplasia is variable, but many patients experience stabilization after age 25 or 30 years. The risk of malignant degeneration is low but is increased significantly by radiation (an ineffective therapy).

Fibrous dysplasia may present as cranial-facial deformity, exophthalmos, or vision disturbance. The goals of treatment are generally mitigation of cosmetic deformity or neurologic symptoms, but extensive lesions of the skull base often cannot be removed completely. Surgery for symptomatic extensive skull base fibrous dysplasia usually involves a bifrontal craniotomy; sacrifice of olfaction when reaching the sphenoid and orbital apex is necessary for optic nerve decompression. The skull base is reconstructed in the same setting. More anterior disease presenting as cosmetic deformity is usually approached transfacially with sublabial or Weber–Ferguson incisions [34]. Depending on the location and extent of the lesion, surgeons are increasingly using transnasal endoscopic approaches for symptomatic patients with the goal of reducing surgical morbidity [35,36].

Case 5

A 17-year-old female presented with a history of progressive proptosis and visual loss starting at age 11 years. She had undergone five previous transnasal endoscopic procedures at another institution for subtotal excision of a skull base lesion consistent with fibrous dysplasia with areas of aneurysmal bone cyst. Previous procedures had been complicated by CSF leak and major blood loss, and visual loss had progressed to almost total blindness. Her principle complaint at this presentation was unremitting, disabling headache. Imaging demonstrated mass effect involving ethmoid, orbital, and sphenoid bone extending posteriorly to the clivus with compression of both optic canals (Fig. 7), which was progressing when compared with prior views. After consultation with plastic and neurosurgery members of the craniofacial team, she underwent excision using a bifrontal craniotomy and facial splitting (Weber–Ferguson) approach.

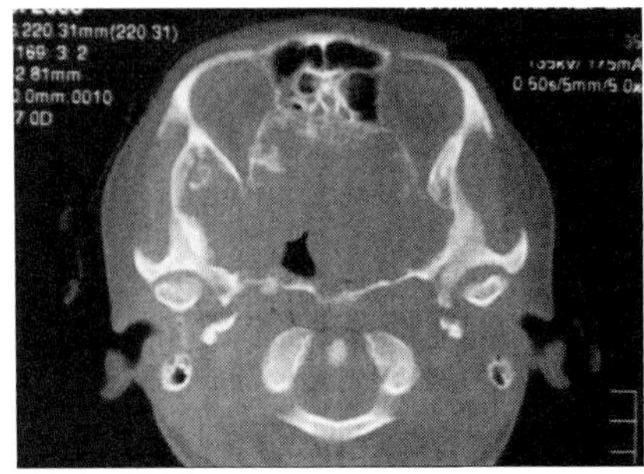

Fig. 7. Large anterior and middle cranial fossa skull base fibrous dysplasia/aneurysmal bone cyst.

The surgery was complicated by a CSF leak at the most posterior limit of dissection (clivus), and reconstruction was accomplished with split calvarial bone grafts, a temporalis muscle graft, and a large pericranium graft. She experienced postoperative transient gait disturbance presumably caused by brainstem ischemia. Visual acuity did not improve, but headache symptoms have remained much diminished at 18 months after surgery. Follow-up imaging demonstrates residual disease at resection margins.

Meningiomas are rare in children and are usually associated with a history of radiation therapy or with neurofibromatosis type 2 [37]. They are more common in females and often involve the sphenoid bone. Management of pediatric meningiomas is complicated by the reluctance to expose young patients to the long-term effects of radiation therapy; therefore, complete surgical excision is the goal when possible.

Case 6

A previously reported [37] 4-year-old girl presented with nasal obstruction and progressive left-sided proptosis. Imaging was consistent with a massive anterior planum sphenoidale meningioma with orbital and sinonasal involvement. She underwent a 16-hour combined neurosurgery, plastic craniofacial, and otolaryngology excision by bifrontal craniotomy (with two-piece excision including removal of the fronto-orbital band), and facial split with Weber–Ferguson incision (Fig. 8). The tumor appearance varied from soft, lobulated, mass lesions within sinus and orbit to indistinct, soft, thickened skull base bone. Reconstruction of skull base and orbit was accomplished with split calvarial grafts. The patient experienced clinical recurrence 2 years later with mostly right-sided proptosis and underwent re-excision using the same approach. This time the pathology was principally of intraosseus meningioma with grossly indistinct margins extending to the posterior cranial fossa. She is doing well clinically with no neurologic symptoms, but plans are underway for radiation therapy.

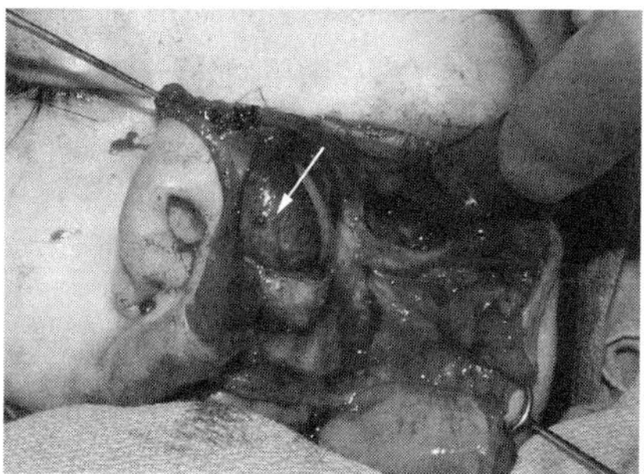

Fig. 8. Modified Weber–Ferguson incision (combined with frontal craniotomy) for exposure of large anterior skull base meningioma. Arrow points to tumor within ethmoid sinus.

Pituitary lesions

As first described by Cushing in 1914, the sublabial transseptal hypophysectomy has been the most common approach to midline pituitary lesions. This technique also is used commonly for other midline lesions of the sphenoid and clivus, such as mucoceles and clivus chordomas. Experience with endoscopic sinus surgery techniques, however, has led to a rapid shift in many centers to a purely transnasal endoscopic approach for pituitary lesions such as microadenomas. A leap of faith is required initially in the shift from the microscope with binocular vision to endoscopes with less depth of field but the ability to look around corners. Also, the bulky C-arm is replaced by increasingly sophisticated image guidance systems. Authors report significantly reduced morbidity and sometimes improved outcomes with endoscopic versus traditional techniques in series of adult patients.

White et al [38] compared 50 adult sublabial transeptal hypohysectomies with 50 endoscopic hypohysectomies and found a lower rate of nasal complications and CSF leak with the endoscopic technique. Similarly, Casler et al [39] recently found less postoperative pain, shorter hospitalization, and less blood loss with purely endoscopic approaches. No exclusively pediatric series have yet been reported, but lessons learned in adult patients are increasingly being applied to younger patients.

Techniques for endoscopic approaches vary but share many similarities. An image guidance system must be used. The instruments used must maximize efficiency in a tight space (eg, straight instead of bayonet designed curettes, narrow malleable bipolar cautery devices, low-profile rongeurs, narrow tapered drills, microscissors, and endoscopic speculum holders) [40–42]. Most authors begin by removing a portion of the middle turbinate (at least on the side of the endoscope, usually the side of the surgeon's nondominant hand) and then creating bilateral sphenoidotomies with rongeurs or a drill. The sphenoid rostrum is then removed, creating a common opening in the posterior septum for visualization or instrumentation from either side. The straight or angled telescopes can be held manually by an assistant (the otolaryngologist during the neurosurgical portion of the procedure) or by a speculum-holding device. The neurosurgeon then creates a wide exposure over the sella with drills and rongeurs, using image guidance appropriately for demarcation of carotid arteries, optic nerves, and cavernous sinuses. Unlike the practice during sublabial exposure, in which the otolaryngologist leaves the room after the sphenoidotomy and returns for closure, a team approach is key to success with endoscopic approaches. The otolaryngologist's job is to ensure that the neurosurgeon has adequate visualization of the relevant skull base (usually with everyone looking at the monitor positioned past the head of the patient), and all parties need expertise in skull base anatomy and terminology.

Pediatric patients with sphenoid or pituitary pathologies present special challenges because of smaller nasal size, less sphenoid pneumatization, and variable location of the sphenoid sinus in relation to the sella. Neurosurgeons generally prefer MRI for evaluation of pituitary lesions, but axial and coronal CT is ideal for assessing sphenoid pneumatization and feasibility of endoscopic approaches. With the most common set-up, namely the endoscope and suction in one nostril (the patient's right for right-handed surgeons) and neurosurgical instrument in the opposite nostril, space can be gained by positioning the suction superiorly and looking "up" with an angled telescope positioned inferiorly. In a tight pediatric nose, additional space can also be gained by partially drilling off the pterygoid process.

Cerebrospinal fluid leaks

The ability to manage CSF leaks is fundamental to surgical approaches to skull base lesions. There is nothing unique to the pediatric age group in this regard, other than perhaps a lower overall incidence of leaks after head trauma [42]. As mentioned previously, improved techniques (usually endoscopic) for managing CSF leaks from the nasal side has lead to a shift from craniotomy to endoscopic nasal approaches for many pediatric entities such as congenital basal encephalocele.

When a CSF leak is suspected in cases such as meningitis with a history of previous head trauma, the usual initial diagnostic procedure is high-resolution coronal head CT with contrast. High-flow leaks and skull base defects are easily demonstrated, although the clinician must be aware that anterior leaks may result in pooling of contrast more posteriorly, such as in the sphenoid sinus. For low-flow, intermittent leaks, pledget studies are sensitive but are poorly localizing. Similarly, beta-2 transferrin studies can be useful to confirm high-flow leaks but are less useful in low-flow, intermittent leak situations. Magnetic resonance cisternography requires no lumber puncture and can be helpful for leaks involving abnormalities in brain parenchyma such as encephaloceles. Intrathecal fluorescein is not approved for use in the United States but is sometimes used (with informed consent) in low concentrations (a few drops of 10% intravenous fluorescein in 5 mL CSF reinjected over 5 minutes through lumbar puncture) by some surgeons [43].

After diagnosis and localization, the key to successful endoscopic management of CSF leaks is wide exposure. In pediatric patients with leaks in the areas of the ethmoid roof or cribiform, at least partial excision of the middle turbinate may be necessary for adequate visualization. The middle turbinate also can be an excellent source for a free mucosal graft. Small skull base defects (<1.25-cm diameter) can be repaired with free mucosal or commercial collagen grafts alone after careful removal of mucosa from surrounding boney margins (such as with a 2.9-mm angled diamond burr microdebrider). Moderate sized defects, 1.3 to 2.5 cm, are usually repaired with cartilage (conchal bowl or septum) or bone (mastoid cortex) sized to fit precisely within the defect. Most authors also apply a hemostatic agent such as bovine collagen to the defect, and many use tissue glue (although some surgeons believe that glue applied to dura can interfere with healing). Short-term lumber drains are usually used except for very small defects.

Case 7

A 12-year-old boy presented with meningitis 1 year after sustaining a left frontal sinus and medial orbital blowout fracture in a motor vehicle accident. The patient had a history of initial CSF rhinorrhea at the time of injury that resolved with conservative management. High-resolution CT with contrast revealed an area of anterior ethmoid opacification but no definite leak. An endoscopic left total ethmoidectomy was performed with findings of inflamed mucosa in the frontal recess cells. After exposure of the fovea, a small CSF leak was apparent through a fracture line with the patient in Trendelenberg's position. The adjacent area of anterior middle turbinate was removed flush with the skull base, and the edges of the fracture line were drilled clean with a diamond burr. A lumber drain was placed and opened by the neurosurgical service. The defect was repaired with a free mucosal graft from the middle turbinate, and the patient has remained well at 1-year follow-up.

Summary

Advances in management of adult skull base pathologies are increasingly being applied in children. Pediatric patients present special challenges because of their smaller anatomy, but potential gains in reduced morbidity make improvements in skull base approaches well worth pursuing.

References

[1] Gruber DP, Brockmeyer D. Pediatric skull base surgery. Embryology and developmental anatomy. Pediatr Neurosurg 2003;38:2–8.

[2] Brockmeyer D, Gruber DP, Haller J, et al. Pediatric skull base surgery. Experience and outcomes in 55 patients. Pediatr Neurosurg 2003;38:9–15.

[3] Teo C, Dornhoffer J, Hanna E, et al. Application of skull base techniques to pediatric neurosurgery. Childs Nerv Syst 1999;15:103–9.

[4] Hug EB, Sweeney RA, Nurre PM, et al. Proton radiotherapy in management of pediatric base of skull tumors. Int J Radiat Oncol Biol Phys 2002;52:1017–24.

[5] Meazza C, Ferrari A, Casanova M, et al. Evolving treatment strategies for parameningeal rhabdomyosarcoma: the experience of the Instituto Nazioanle Fumari of Milan. Head Neck 2005;27:49–57.

[6] Brown OE, Pownell P, Manning SC. Choanal atresia: a new anatomic classification and clinical management applications. Laryngoscope 1996;106:97–101.
[7] Schoem SR. Transnasal endoscopic repair of choanal atresia: why stent? Otolaryngol Head Neck Surg 2004;131:362–6.
[8] Samadi D, Shah U, Handler S. Choanal atresia: a twenty-year review of medical comorbidities and surgical outcomes. Laryngoscope 2003;113:254–8.
[9] Kubba H, Bennett A, Bailey CM. An update on choanal atresia surgery at Great Ormond Street Hospital for Children: preliminary results with mitomycin-C and the KTP laser. Int J Pediatr Otorhinolaryngol 2004;68:939–45.
[10] Schlosser RJ, Faust RA, Phillips CD, et al. Three-dimensional computed tomography of congenital nasal anomalies. Int J Pediatr Otorhinolaryngol 2002;65:125–31.
[11] Mankarious LA, Smith RJH. External rhinoplasty approach for extirpation and immediate reconstruction of congenital midline nasal dermoids. Ann Otol Rhinol Laryngol 1998;107: 786–9.
[12] Penner CR, Thompson L. Nasal glial heterotopia: a clinicopathologic and immunophenotypic analysis of 10 cases with a review of the literature. Ann Diagn Pathol 2003;7: 354–9.
[13] Yokoyama M, Inouye N, Mizuno F. Endoscopic management of nasal glioma in infancy. Int J Pediatr Otorhinolaryngol 1999;51:51–4.
[14] Rahbar R, Resto VA, Robson CD, et al. Nasal glioma and encephalocele: diagnosis and management. Laryngoscope 2003;113:2069–77.
[15] Agirdir BV, Derin AT, Ozbilim G, et al. Endoscopic management of the intranasal glioma. J Pediatr Surg 2004;39:1571–3.
[16] Woodworth BA, Schlosser RJ, Faust RA, et al. Evolutions in the management of congenital intranasal skull base defects. Arch Otolaryngol Head Neck Surg 2004;130:1283–8.
[17] Marxhall AH, Jones NS, Robertson IJ. Endoscopic repair of basal encephaloceles. J Laryngol Otol 2001;115:545–7.
[18] Coppit GL, Perkins JA, Manning SC. Nasopharyngeal teratomas and dermoids: a review of the literature and case series. Int J Pediatr Otorhinolaryngol 2000;30:219–21.
[19] Kingdom TT, Delgaudio JM. Endoscopic approach to lesions of the sphenoid sinus, orbital apex, and clivus. Am J Otolaryngol 2003;24:317–22.
[20] Benlyazid A, Lescanne E, Robier MA, et al. Teratoma of the rhinopharynx and the infratemporal fossa in neonates: report of 3 cases (French). Ann Otolaryngol Chir Cerviofac 2001;118:54–60 [in French].
[21] Rotenberg B, El-Hakim H, Lodha A, et al. Nasopharyngeal teratocarcinosarcoma. Int J Pediatr Otorhinolaryngol 2002;62:159–64.
[22] Grant GH, Ellenbogen RG, Manning SC. Diagnosis and management of juvenile angiofibromas. In: Winn HR, editor. Youman's neurological surgery, vol 1. 5th edition. Philadelphia (PA): Elsevier; 2004. p. 1351–9.
[23] Radkowski D, McGill T, Healy GB, et al. Angiofibroma: changes in staging and treatment. Arch Otolaryngol Head Neck Surg 1996;122:122–9.
[24] Lewark TM, Allen GC, Chowdhury K, et al. Le Fort 1 osteotomy and skull base tumors—a pediatric experience. Arch Otolaryngol Head Neck Surg 2000;126:1004–8.
[25] Newlands SD, Weymuller EA Jr. Endoscopic treatment of juvenile nasopharyngeal tumors. Am J Rhinol 1999;13:213–8.
[26] Wormald PJ, Hasselt AV. Endoscopic removal of juvenile angiofibromas. Otolaryngol Head Neck Surg 2003;129:684–91.
[27] Onerci TM, Yucel OT, Ogretmemoglu O. Endonasal surgery in treatment of juvenile nasopharyngeal angiofibroma. Int J Pediatr Otorhinolaryngol 2003;67:1219–25.
[28] Mair EA, Battiata A, Casler JD. Endoscopic laser-assisted excision of juvenile nasopharyngeal angiofibromas. Arch Otolaryngol Head Neck Surg 2003;129:454–9.
[29] Roger G, Tran Ba Huy P, Froehlich P, et al. Exclusively endoscopic removal of juvenile nasopharyngeal angiofibroma. Arch Otolaryngol Head Neck Surg 2002;128:928–35.

[30] El-Banhawy OA, El-Hafiz Shehab El-Dien A, et al. Endoscopic-assisted midfacial degloving approach for type 3 juvenile angiofibroma. Int J Pediatr Otorhinolarygnol 2004;68:21–8.
[31] Hartnick CJ, Myseros JS, Myer CM. Endoscopic access to the infratemporal fossa. A cadaveric study. Arch Otolaryngol Head Neck Surg 2001;127:1325–7.
[32] Chen C, Selva D, Wormald PJ. Endoscopic modified Lothrop procedure: an alternative for frontal osteoma excision. Rhinology 2004;42:239–43.
[33] Itshayek E, Spector S, Gomori M, et al. Fibrous dysplasia in combination with aneurismal bone cyst of the occipital bone and the clivus: case report and review of the literature. Neurosurg 2002;51:815–7.
[34] Anastassov YC, Anastassov GE, Lumerman HS, et al. Craniofacial fibrous dysplasia: conservative surgical management. Review of the literature and report of a case. Folia Med (Plovdiv) 2004;46:56–61.
[35] de Minteguiaga C, Portier F, Guichard JP, et al. Aneurysmal bone cyst in the sphenoid bone: treatment with minimally invasive surgery. Ann Otol Rhinol Laryngol 2001;110:331–4.
[36] Post G, Kountakis SE. Endoscopic resection of large sinonasal ossifying fibroma. Am J Otolaryngol 2003;26:54056.
[37] Mohit A, Grant G, Stevenson K, et al. A large planum sphenoidale meningioma with sinonasal extension in a child. Case report and review of the literature. Pediatr Neurosurg 2003;39:270–4.
[38] White DR, Sonnenburg RE, Ewend MG, et al. Safety of minimally invasive pituitary surgery (MIPS) compared with a traditional approach. Laryngoscope 2004;114:1945–8.
[39] Casler JD, Doolittle AM, Mair EA. Endoscopic surgery of the anterior skull base. Laryngoscope 2005;115:16–24.
[40] Thomas RF, Monacci WT, Mair EA. Endoscopic image-guided transethmoid pituitary surgery. Otolaryngol Head Neck Surg 2002;127:409–16.
[41] Couldwell WT, Weiss MH, Rabb C, et al. Variations on the standard transsphenoidal approach to the sellar region, with emphasis on the extended approaches and parasellar approaches: surgical experience in 105 cases. Neurosurg 2004;55:539–50.
[42] Lacatelli D, Castelnuovo P, Santi L, et al. Endoscopic approaches to the cranial base: perspectives and realities. Childs Nerv Syst 2000;16:686–91.
[43] Schlosser RJ, Bolger WE. Nasal cerebrospinal fluid leaks. J Otolaryngol 2002;31(Suppl 1):S28.

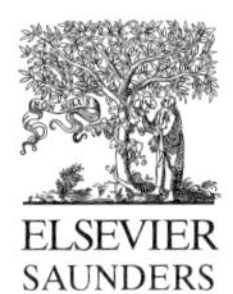

ELSEVIER
SAUNDERS

Otolaryngol Clin N Am
38 (2005) 795–808

OTOLARYNGOLOGIC
CLINICS
OF NORTH AMERICA

Avoiding Pitfalls in Surgery of the Neck, Parapharyngeal Space, and Infratemporal Fossa

Pramod K. Sharma, MD, FACS*,
Becky L. Massey, MD

Division of Otolaryngology–Head and Neck Surgery, Department of Surgery, University of Utah, 50 North Medical Drive, Salt Lake City, Utah 84132, USA

Surgical treatment of lesions of the skull base has advanced dramatically in the last 25 years. Multiple surgical approaches have been developed to address lesions that were previously designated as unresectable. These procedures, however, are often complex and can lead to a variety of sequela or complications. Ideally, preoperative evaluation and planning minimize the morbidity patients face. This article attempts to describe some of the problems that are encountered in surgical procedures of the neck, parapharyngeal space, and infratemporal fossa.

Multiple paragangliomas

Paragangliomas are rare neoplasms of neural crest origin. These lesions often present as asymptomatic neck masses. Diagnosis is commonly made by imaging studies (Figs. 1 and 2). Head and neck paragangliomas most commonly consist of carotid body tumors, glomus jugulare, glomus vagale, and glomus tympanicum. These lesions can present in the neck, parapharyngeal space, and infratemporal fossa. Multiple paragangliomas occur in 10% of patients with sporadic paragangliomas and in approximately 30% to 40% of patients with familial paragangliomas. All patients should undergo MRI of the head and neck to evaluate the presenting lesion and to identify possible multiple paragangliomas (Fig. 3). Particular attention must be paid to patients with a familial history of paragangliomas. Multiple lesions can alter the treatment approach because of the possible cumulative

* Corresponding author.
E-mail address: pramod.sharma@hsc.utah.edu (P.K. Sharma).

doi:10.1016/j.otc.2005.03.003

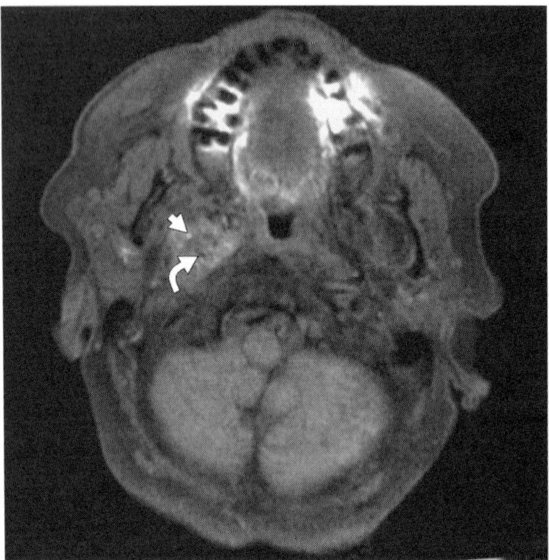

Fig. 1. The axial precontrast T1-weighted MRI with fat saturation shows a lesion within the right carotid space, with some heterogeneous signal and with internal foci of both bright (*arrow*) and dark (*curved arrow*) signal consistent with the salt-and-pepper appearance of a paraganglioma. (Courtesy of Pramod K. Sharma, MD, Salt Lake City, UT.)

sequelae of multiple surgical approaches. Observation or radiation therapy may be more appropriate in some patients. The identification of multiple paragangliomas should also alert the clinician to evaluate for possible familial paraganglioma.

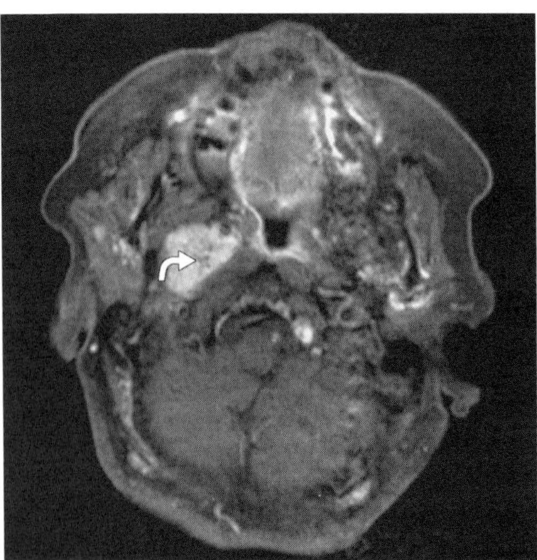

Fig. 2. The corresponding axial postcontrast T1-weighted MRI with fat saturation shows the avid enhancement of the right carotid space lesion, with internal flow voids (*curved arrow*) consistent with a paraganglioma. (Courtesy of Pramod K. Sharma, MD, Salt Lake City, UT.)

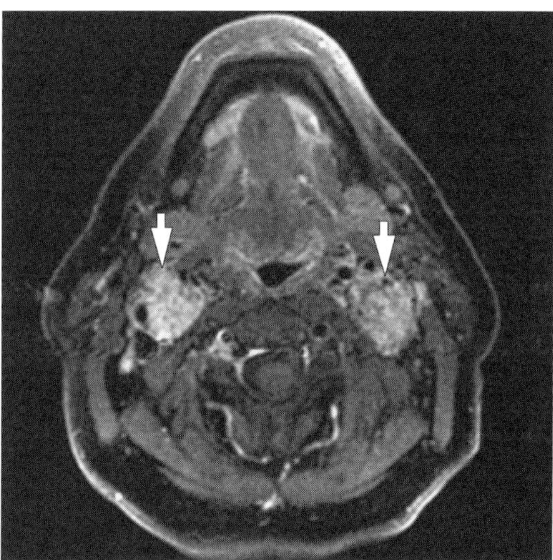

Fig. 3. An axial T1-weighted MRI with fat saturation at the level of the carotid bifurcations shows the bilateral heterogeneous enhancing lesions (*arrows*) with characteristic splaying of the carotid vessels, consistent with bilateral carotid body tumors. (Courtesy of Pramod K. Sharma, MD, Salt Lake City, UT.)

Catecholamine secreting tumors

Inappropriate catecholamine secretion may occur from paragangliomas. The most common secreting paragangliomas are adrenal in origin, commonly referred to as pheochromocytomas. Less than 1% of head and neck paragangliomas secrete catecholamines. Symptoms of inappropriate catecholamine secretion include labile blood pressure, headaches, cardiac arrhythmias, weight loss, and unusual flushing or sweating. Patients suspected of having head and neck paragangliomas should be questioned directly regarding these symptoms. If symptoms are present, preoperative medical work-up is required. In asymptomatic patients, routine work-up is not recommended.

Evaluation of plasma levels of free metanephrines is a highly sensitive and cost-effective test [1]. Confirmatory biochemical testing is performed only if plasma levels are elevated. If these tests are also positive, conventional anatomic imaging (CT or MRI) and functional imaging ([^{123}I]metaiodobezylguanidine) should be performed to localize the lesion. If a pheochromocytoma is identified, it should be treated before addressing the head and neck paraganglioma. If systemic work-up fails to identify a non–head and neck source of catecholamine production, one must suspect the head and neck paraganglioma as the source. Preoperative adrenergic blockade must be optimized. Typical treatment includes alpha-adrenergic blockade (phenoxybenzamine) and beta blockade (propranolol). A multi-disciplinary approach (anesthesia and internal medicine/endocrinology) should be used in the preoperative preparation of the patient for surgery. Patients with pheochromocytoma or secreting head and neck paragangliomas should be identified by obtaining appropriate history and medical work-up. Failure to identify these rare situations can lead to intraoperative crises with potentially fatal outcomes.

Nerve injury

Multiple cranial nerves and sensory nerves are at risk during surgical procedures of the neck, parapharyngeal space, and infratemporal fossa. Ideally, all cranial nerves would be preserved during surgical procedures. Cranial nerves V, VII, VIII, IX, X, XI, and XII are most commonly at risk. The surgical approach and tumor type determine the risk of injury to these nerves.

Cranial nerve V

The trigeminal nerve is most at risk for injury in the type B and C infratemporal fossa approaches in which more anterior and medial exposure is obtained. The trigeminal ganglion is located near the precavernous petrous internal carotid artery. Branches may be injured in approaching the clivus, nasopharynx, or cavernous sinus. The ophthalmic division may be sacrificed for tumors involving the superior orbital fissure or cavernous sinus. When the ophthalmic nerve is sacrificed, the most significant deficit is loss of corneal sensation. Ophthalmic drops, ointments, and protective moisture chambers decrease risk of exposure keratitis. With concomitant facial nerve injury, surgical protection of the cornea with temporary tarsorraphy or early gold weight implantation may be necessary. In the type C infratemporal fossa approach, sacrifice of the maxillary nerve results in loss of midface and intraoral sensation. Stretch injury to the maxillary nerve should be avoided, because it has been shown to be more susceptible than the other two branches to developing postoperative neuralgia after manipulation [2]. In the type B infratemporal fossa approach, sacrifice of the mandibular nerve causes subsequent weakness of muscles of mastication, mandibular drift, and temporomandibular joint discomfort. Permanent malocclusion and trismus can be prevented with jaw-opening exercises or dental appliances.

Cranial nerve VII

The facial nerve is at risk for injury during resection of superior neck lesions and deep-lobe parotid neoplasms presenting as parapharyngeal space tumors. Identification and isolation of the facial nerve for a cervico-parotid approach minimizes iatrogenic injury.

In the classic Fisch type A infratemporal fossa approach, the facial nerve is mobilized in the middle ear and mastoid before it is transposed anteriorly to allow improved anterior visualization. Manipulation of the nerve and compromise of its blood supply may lead to temporary and sometimes permanent facial nerve weakness. Unless lesions involve the jugular foramen, facial nerve transposition may not be necessary in type B, C, or D approaches. The extent and location of a skull base lesion determine the treatment of the facial nerve. Facial nerve trauma is minimized during mobilization by assuring adequate removal of bone around the fallopian canal, avoiding dehydration of the tissues, and limiting tension or pressure on the nerve.

If transposition of the nerve is necessary, modifications have been described that are thought to decrease rates of facial nerve paresis. Brackmann [3] described a modification in which the dissection of the facial nerve out of the stylomastoid foramen includes mobilizing all of the soft tissue of the stylomastoid foramen with the nerve enclosed in periosteum. Less nerve trauma and less disruption of blood supply is credited with better immediate and long-term facial nerve results. Pensak [4] has described an intact fallopian bridge technique in which the vertical segment of the facial nerve is skeletonized to the level of the second genu. Infralabyrinthine and retrofacial air cells are exenterated, leaving the bone-covered facial nerve bridging the space. The need to work around the bridge may increase the operative time, but the facial nerve results are desirable.

The benefits of continuous facial nerve monitoring in acoustic neuroma surgery have been clearly established in multiple series. Monitoring of the facial nerve in skull base surgery with facial nerve transposition has been associated with improved outcomes [5]. Facial nerve monitoring has also been shown to be associated with improved facial nerve function following parotidectomy [6]. Continuous facial and lower cranial nerve monitoring is recommended, especially when anatomy is distorted by pathology or previous treatment.

Cranial nerve VIII

Conductive hearing loss is an expected outcome of surgery when the external auditory canal is closed and the middle ear obliterated. Modifications of the classic Fisch approaches may spare exenteration of the middle ear and external auditory canal when tumor location is amenable. Sensorineural hearing loss may occur secondary to labyrinthine trauma or inadvertent drill entry.

Cranial nerve IX

The glossopharyngeal nerve exits the anterior part of the jugular foramen and descends between the internal carotid artery and internal jugular vein. The nerve travels medially and forward to the pharyngeal plexus. The majority of the fibers are sensory. The glossopharyngeal nerve is at risk for injury high in the neck/parapharyngeal space. Injury results in decreased sensation and paresis of the ipsilateral pharynx. Isolated cranial nerve IX injuries rarely lead to clinically significant sequelae, but associated multiple cranial neuropathies (cranial nerve X and cranial nerve XII) can result in significant dysphagia.

Cranial nerve X

The vagus is easily identifiable in the carotid sheath. Proximal and distal isolation from the tumor optimizes preservation attempts. Certain lesions do not allow preservation, and the patient should be counseled preoperatively regarding the potential outcome. Neurofibromas cannot be resected without resecting the nerve because of the interdigitation of the neoplasm with the nerve fibers. Small paragangliomas and neurilemoma (schwannomas) can allow anatomic preservation of the nerve, although functional outcome may vary. Large paragangliomas and neurilemomas typically result in permanent dysfunction with resection of the nerve.

Resection results in varying levels of dysphonia, dysphagia, and aspiration. Patients with preoperative paresis often have already compensated and have less difficulty postoperatively. Older patients and those with multiple cranial neuropathies typically have more difficulties postoperatively. Patients should be prepared for dysphonia and dysphagia and a possible need for enteral feeding by nasogastric tube or gastrostomy tube. Speech and swallowing therapists can be beneficial in rehabilitation. Ideally, the patient is evaluated preoperatively and postoperatively to optimize rehabilitation. Some patients do not require intervention after cranial nerve X resection. Others benefit from vocal cord medialization or arytenoid adduction. Typically, the decision to perform an intervention and the ideal method are determined within 3 to 6 months postoperatively.

Cranial nerve XI

The spinal accessory nerve is usually easily identified. It travels through the jugular foramen and typically is found on the lateral surface of the jugular vein near the skull base. It continues laterally and gives branches to the sternocleidomastoid muscle. The nerve can be identified as the sternocleidomastoid muscle is retracted laterally. Primary tumors of the spinal accessory nerve are rare. Thus resection of the spinal accessory nerve is uncommon. The nerve may require dissection to separate it from neoplasms in the neck or parapharyngeal space.

Injury to the spinal accessory nerve results in denervation of the sternocleidomastoid muscle and trapezius. The sternocleidomastoid muscle dysfunction rarely results in clinically significant problems. Trapezius weakness results in the shoulder syndrome. Findings include shoulder pain, limitations of abduction, shoulder droop, and scapular winging. Physical therapy should be initiated early to maintain range of motion and to strengthen compensatory muscles. Additionally, shoulder dysfunction may be improved by progressive resistance exercise training [7].

Cranial nerve XII

The hypoglossal nerve may need to be dissected from tumors of the neck and parapharyngeal space. Careful dissection allows preservation of the nerve, but paresis is common. Paresis typically resolves over a 6-month period, but some permanent dysfunction is usual. Symptoms vary from mild dysarthria to severe dysphagia. Severity of symptoms is influenced by the condition of the other lower cranial nerves. The combination of cranial nerve X and XII dysfunction can lead to significant dysphagia.

Sympathetic plexus

Injury to the sympathetic plexus results in an ipsilateral Horner syndrome characterized by miosis and anhidrosis and upper lid ptosis. Ptosis repair should be considered if a visual field defect is present.

Vessel injury

The internal carotid artery, external carotid artery, vertebral artery, and jugular vein are at risk during surgical procedures of the neck, parapharyngeal space, and infratemporal fossa. Preoperative evaluation is critical in preventing complications. Imaging studies can help to determine the relationship of the tumor and the surrounding vasculature. MRI evaluation can provide anatomic detail. A visualized fat plane between the mass and vessel indicates an easy plane of surgical dissection. The amount of circumferential involvement by a tumor should also be noted. It is common to find a carotid artery surrounded partially or completely by a carotid body tumor. This benign tumor usually can be dissected from the artery with partial effacement (Shamblin stage I or II). Large lesions, however, can completely surround the internal or external carotid artery (Shamblin stage III) (Fig. 4). There is increased chance for the need of a carotid artery resection in these situations. With a malignant lesion, a 270° or greater effacement is often associated with vascular invasion (Fig. 5).

Carotid artery resection must be considered if there is suspicion of vascular invasion. Interruption of the carotid artery blood flow may result in symptoms ranging from no neurologic changes to severe hemispheric strokes. Collateral circulation through the circle of Willis may allow adequate blood flow and prevent neurologic sequelae after occlusion of an internal carotid artery. A variety of methods have been proposed to assess the adequacy of collateral blood circulation. They include temporary balloon occlusion with clinical neurologic evaluation or continuous

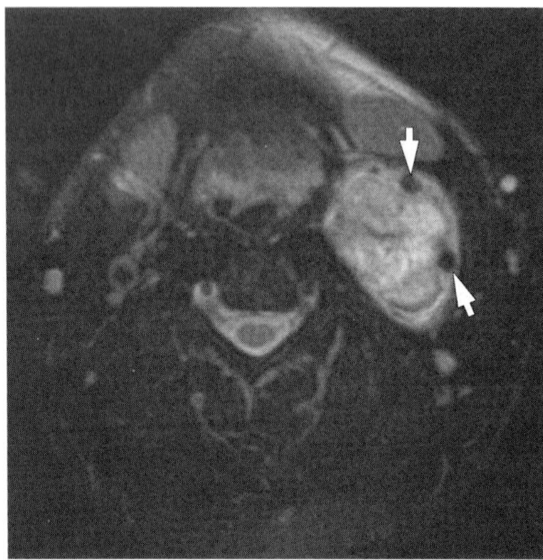

Fig. 4. An axial T2-weighted MRI with fat saturation demonstrates a heterogeneously bright lesion within the left carotid space, located near the carotid bifurcation, with lateral displacement and apparent encasement of the carotid vessels (*arrows*). This lesion was found to be a carotid body tumor on pathology. (Courtesy of Pramod K. Sharma, MD, Salt Lake City, UT.)

electroencephalogram, temporary balloon occlusion with Xenon-enhanced CT imaging, and temporary balloon occlusion with transcranial Doppler ultrasonography measurement of collateral blood flow. No method is foolproof, and patients with borderline collateral flow may not be identified. A recent study did show improved negative and positive predictive values when temporary balloon occlusion of the internal carotid artery was performed, Xenon-133 was injected within the carotid artery, and cortical cerebral blood flow was measured by scintillation detectors [8]. Ideally, all patients undergoing elective carotid artery resection undergo immediate carotid flow shunting and vascular bypass reconstruction to minimize neurologic deficits from inadequate collateral blood flow.

Patients with lesions that do not allow carotid resection should also undergo collateral blood flow testing. If flow is adequate, a permanent balloon occlusion can be performed. If collateral blood flow is inadequate, other methods of treatment should be investigated.

The vertebral artery can, rarely, be within the surgical field in management of lesions of the neck. The vertebral artery arises from the first portion of the subclavian artery. It travels superiorly in the neck within the foramen of the transverse processes of the cervical vertebrae. The vessel usually enters the foramen at C6, although it can enter at C5 or C4. The artery then pierces the atlantooccipital membrane and joins with the contralateral vertebral artery to form the basilar artery [9]. Injury may occur

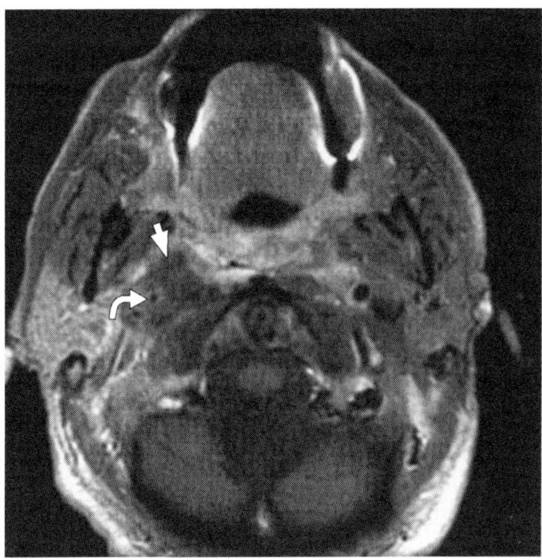

Fig. 5. An axial postcontrast T1-weighted MRI with fat saturation shows a lesion within the right carotid space (*arrow*), without significant enhancement, which is encasing the right internal carotid artery (*curved arrow*) instead of displacing the vasculature. This lesion was found to be a malignant peripheral nerve sheath tumor on pathology. (Courtesy of Pramod K. Sharma, MD, Salt Lake City, UT.)

when resecting lesions in the posterior neck. Occlusion may result in vertebral basilar insufficiency. Blood clot may also propagate and lead to ischemic strokes. Patients with lesions that extend to the vertebral artery should be assessed further by angiography or MR angiography to determine the entire course of the artery. Intraoperative care must be taken to avoid injuring the vertebral artery.

Injury to the jugular vein rarely causes sequelae. Deliberate isolation, ligation, and division can often improve surgical exposure to lesions in the high neck or parapharyngeal space.

Complications of the mandibular osteotomy site

Exposure of the high neck and parapharyngeal space often is limited by the mandible, which lies lateral to this region. Mandibular osteotomy has been advocated as a method of improving surgical access to large tumors or tumors high in the parapharyngeal space. A variety of osteotomy sites have been advocated (Fig. 6).

Mandibular osteotomy and mobilization provides excellent exposure to the parapharyngeal space, but a variety of complications may arise. Early descriptions of osteotomy approaches often required division of the inferior alveolar nerve within the mandibular bony canal, resulting in lip numbness.

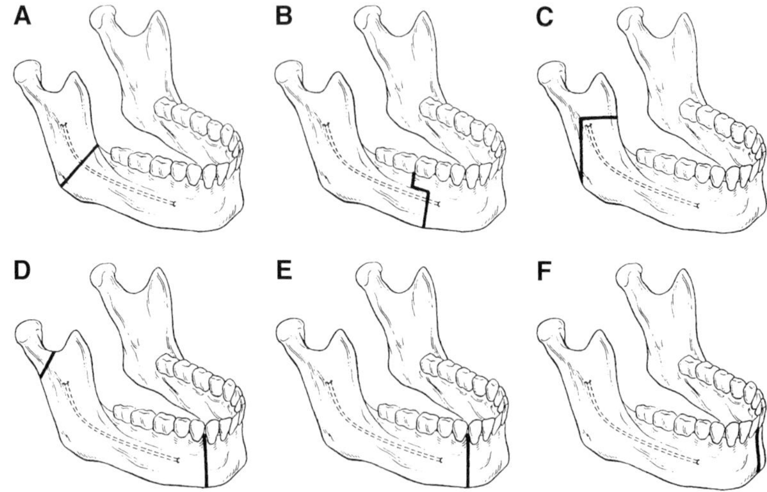

Fig. 6. A variety of osteotomies have been described to improve access to the parapharyngeal space. (*A*) Angle osteotomy. (*B*) Lateral stair-step osteotomy. (*C*) Inverted L osteotomy. (*D*) Double osteotomy. (*E*) Parasymphyseal osteotomy. (*F*) Symphyseal osteotomy. (Courtesy of Pramod K. Sharma, MD, Salt Lake City, UT.)

Osteotomy anterior to the mental foramen, where the inferior alveolar nerve exits, or posterior to the mandibular foramen, where the inferior alveolar nerve enters the mandible, preserves lip sensation.

Anterior osteotomies are typically performed by a lip- and chin-splitting incision. This incision results in a facial scar. It also requires a tracheostomy because of the oral cavity edema and feeding tube placement during the initial healing phase. An alternative approach that avoids the lip and chin incision has been described [10,11]. In this approach, osteotomies are performed through a neck incision with elevation of the soft tissue from the mandible without a lip and chin incision. The bony osteotomy is performed without dividing any additional soft tissue. The oral cavity is not violated, thus avoiding a tracheostomy or feeding tube.

Malunion or non-union is a potential complication for all osteotomy sites. Surgical technique is the main factor, although patient variables (diabetes, prior radiation, steroid use) can also play a significant role. Ideally, a thin blade is used initially to perform a partial osteotomy to mark the site definitively. This step is followed by appropriate bending of a rigid fixation plate. A minimum of two holes are drilled on each side of the osteotomy site. The plate is then removed, and the osteotomy is completed. After tumor removal, the plate is reapplied to provide rigid fixation. Poor technique can lead to poor fixation and eventual motion, resulting in malunion or non-union. Many different types and locations of osteotomies have been described. The stair-step or chevron osteotomy was used to decrease motion of the fragments after fixation. Fixation was typically performed with wires.

With modern fixation plates, there is no significant advantage to these osteotomies. A straight mandibulotomy provides a simple, reproducible, and effective osteotomy with few complications postoperatively [12].

Tooth loss can occur because of planned extraction to allow for osteotomy or from inadvertent loss caused by damage to the tooth root. Tooth extraction is not necessary to create space for an osteotomy. Modern oscillating saws with thin blades can be used to create accurate osteotomies between teeth in most patients.

An alternative surgical approach to a lesion high in the parapharyngeal space is a lateral approach, which avoids a mandibular osteotomy and its inherent complications. This method involves disconnecting the sternocleidomastoid muscle from the mastoid tip and removing the mastoid (Fig. 7). In addition to improved exposure of the skull base, this approach allows lesions with intracranial extension to be addressed. This approach has been used successfully at the University of Utah School of Medicine as an alternative to mandibulotomy approaches.

Cerebrospinal fluid leak

In the infratemporal fossa approaches, the most common serious complication is cerebrospinal fluid (CSF) leak. CSF leak may present with leakage through the scalp incision, the neck incision, the external auditory canal, or through the nose through the eustachian tube. Watertight dural closure is often difficult to obtain with large skull base defects, but careful repair of any dural opening and obliteration of the surgical cavity with a free

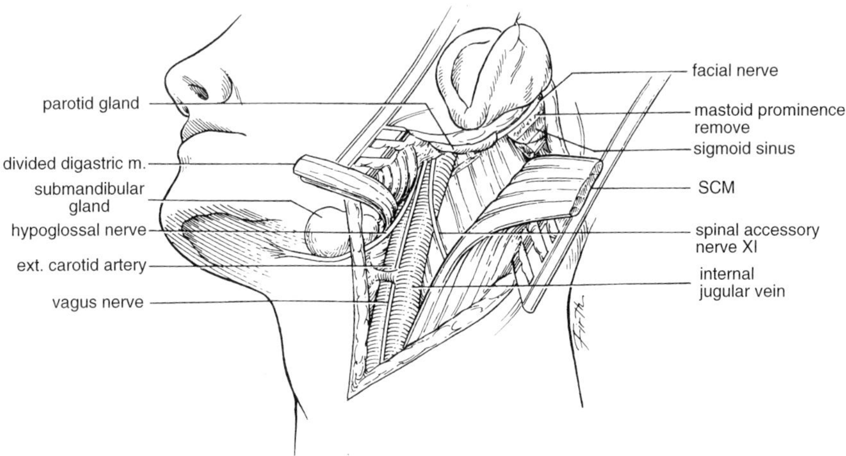

Fig. 7. Lateral approach to the parapharyngeal space provides exposure to the high parapharyngeal space without a mandibular osteotomy. (Courtesy of Pramod K. Sharma, MD, Salt Lake City, UT.)

fat graft minimizes the risk of CSF leak. Closure of the external auditory canal and obliteration of the eustachian tube decreases potential routes for CSF to communicate with the exterior. If dura is resected, it should be replaced with a carefully sutured graft. A lumbar drain and pressure dressing may facilitate sealing of defect when dural defects remain or the repair is tenuous. Support of the graft with soft tissue or bone flaps may help prevent leaks. Failure to reconstruct large skull base defects can lead to encephaloceles or pseudomeningoceles. A temporalis flap is adequate for obliterating small dead spaces and small bony defects if the vascular supply is maintained. Closure of large defects with vascularized tissue reduces healing time and morbidity. Avoidance of suction drains or positioning them away from dural defects minimizes drawing CSF into the wound. A high degree of suspicion for CSF leak must be maintained to allow early treatment and prevention of meningitis.

Salivary gland complications

When manipulation or mobilization of the parotid is necessary to obtain access to the parapharyngeal space or infratemporal fossa, any of the complications associated with parotidectomy may occur. Sialocele occurs because of salivary leakage from the cut surface of the parotid gland. Management includes needle aspiration and the application of a pressure dressing. Injection of Botox after aspiration will decrease secretion and may avoid the need for repeat aspirations [13]. Gustatory sweating of the cheek region (Frey's syndrome) may occur after parotid surgery. Frey's syndrome occurs from aberrant regeneration of the postganglionic secretomotor parasympathetic nerve fibers into cutaneous sweat glands. Gustatory stimulation then causes sweat gland activity. The incidence of Frey's syndrome may be reduced by raising a thick skin flap in a plane deep to the superficial musculoaponeurotic system (SMAS) rather than a subcutaneous plane [14,15]. Interposition of an acellular dermis graft between the parotid bed and skin flap has also been shown to reduce the rate of Frey's syndrome [16].

First-bite syndrome

Surgeries of the neck and parapharyngeal space may lead to postoperative parotid pain and cheek sweating from gustatory stimuli. This phenomenon has been described as first-bite syndrome. Patients describe an intense pain that is most severe with the first bite of food at a meal. This syndrome may result from surgical interruption of autonomic fibers to the parotid gland. The level of pain can vary from mild discomfort to debilitating. The severity of the symptoms tends to diminish over time. This complication is probably underreported by patients.

Temporomandibular joint dysfunction

Mobilization and division of the temporomandibular joint in the type B infratemporal fossa approach can result in dysfunction and malocclusion of the temporomandibular joint. Denervation of the muscles of mastication by resection of the mandibular nerve also contributes to occlusive abnormalities. Avoiding excessive lateral distraction of the jaw, incision into the joint capsule, and prolonged immobilization minimizes prolonged symptoms.

Summary

The region of the upper neck, parapharyngeal space, and infratemporal fossa contains many vital structures in a confined area. Access is often limited, making surgical treatment challenging. Preoperative assessment is critical in determining the optimal surgical approach. In spite of improvements in preoperative evaluation and surgical techniques, sequelae from surgical therapy are sometimes unavoidable. Awareness of the potential problems is necessary to counsel patients appropriately regarding treatment options and all potential risks.

References

[1] Goldstein DG, Eisenhofer G, Flynn JA, et al. Diagnosis and localization of pheochromocytoma. Hypertension 2004;43(5):907–10.
[2] Niparko JK, Mattox DE. Complications of lateral skull base surgery. In: Eisele DW, editor. Complications in head & neck surgery. St. Louis (MO): Mosby; 1993. p. 613–23.
[3] Brackmann DE. The facial nerve in the infratemporal approach. Otolaryngol Head Neck Surg 1987;97(1):15–7.
[4] Pensak ML, Jackler RK. Removal of jugular foramen tumors: the fallopian bridge technique. Otolaryngol Head Neck Surg 1997;117(6):586–91.
[5] Leonetti JP, Brackmann DE, Prass RL. Improved preservation of facial nerve function in the infratemporal approach to the skull base. Otolaryngol Head Neck Surg 1989;101(1):74–8.
[6] Terrell JE, Kileny PR, Yian C, et al. Clinical outcome of continuous facial nerve monitoring during primary parotidectomy. Arch Otolaryngol Head Neck Surg 1997; 123(10):1081–7.
[7] McNeely ML, Parliament M, Courneya KS, et al. A pilot study of a randomized controlled trial to evaluate the effects of progressive resistance exercise training on shoulder dysfunction caused by spinal accessory neurapraxia/neurectomy in head and neck cancer survivors. Head Neck 2004;26(6):518–30.
[8] Marshall RS, Lazar RM, Young WL, et al. Clinical utility of quantitative cerebral blood flow measurements during internal carotid artery test occlusions. Neurosurgery 2002;50(5): 996–1004 [discussion: 1004–5].

[9] Hollinshead WH. Anatomy for surgeons: the head and neck. 3rd edition. Philadelphia (PA): JB Lippincott, 1982. p. 453–5.
[10] Seward GR. Nodular enlargements of the salivary glands. In: Moore JR, editor. Surgery of the mouth and jaws. Oxford (UK): Blackwell Scientific Publications; 1985. p. 694.
[11] Teng MS, Genden EM, Buchbinder D, et al. Subcutaneous mandibulotomy: a new surgical access for large tumors of the parapharyngeal space. Laryngoscope 2003; 113(11):1893–7.
[12] Amin MR, Deschler DG, Hayden RE. Straight midline mandibulotomy revisited. Laryngoscope 1999;109(9):1402–5.
[13] Vargas H, Galati LT, Parnes SM. A pilot study evaluating the treatment of postparotidectomy sialoceles with botulinum toxin type A. Arch Otolaryngol Head Neck Surg 2000; 126(3):421–4.
[14] Singleton GT, Cassisi NJ. Frey's syndrome: incidence related to skin flap thickness in parotidectomy. Laryngoscope 1980;90(10 Pt 1):1636–9.
[15] Taylor SM, Yoo J, Matthews TW, et al. Frey's syndrome and parotidectomy flaps: a retrospective cohort study. Otolaryngol Head Neck Surg 2000;122(2):201–3.
[16] Govindaraj S, Cohen M, Genden EM, et al. The use of acellular dermis in the prevention of Frey's syndrome. Laryngoscope 2001;111(11 Pt 1):1993–8.

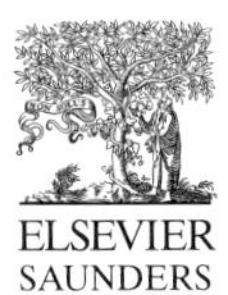
ELSEVIER
SAUNDERS

Otolaryngol Clin N Am
38 (2005) 809–817

OTOLARYNGOLOGIC
CLINICS
OF NORTH AMERICA

Treatment of Dysphagia and Dysphonia Following Skull Base Surgery

K. Linnea Peterson, MD, FACS*,
Joanne Fenn, CCC-SLP

Voice and Swallowing Clinic, Department of Otolaryngology/Head and Neck Surgery, Virginia Mason Medical Center, 1100 Ninth Avenue, P.O. Box 900, Seattle, WA 98111, USA

Given the complexity of skull base anatomy, lesions involving the skull base can result in a multitude of symptoms. Understanding the anatomic relationships, particularly of the lower cranial nerves, facilitates understanding the potential deficits that can result from the tumor and subsequent treatment. This article provides an overview of considerations in the evaluation and treatment of lower cranial nerve deficits, specifically in cranial nerves IX, X, and XII, in the context of skull base tumors and their treatment.

Glossopharyngeal nerve

The glossopharyngeal nerve is a mixed sensory and motor nerve. The first branch of the glossopharyngeal nerve is the tympanic nerve, also known as Jacobson's nerve, supplying sensation to the middle ear and parasympathetic fibers to the parotid gland. The pharyngeal branches of the glossopharyngeal nerve include a branch that innervates the stylopharyngeus muscle and sensory fibers to the tonsils and anterior and posterior tonsillar pillars and provides taste and sensation for the posterior tongue. Functionally, glossopharyngeal nerve deficits impact swallowing sensation.

Vagus nerve

Vagus nerve injuries result in dysphagia and dysphonia. The site of the deficit affects the overall symptoms but does not necessarily determine the final resting position of the true vocal cord [1]. A unilateral deficit results in

* Corresponding author.
E-mail address: otoklp@vmmc.org (K.L. Peterson).

doi:10.1016/j.otc.2005.01.008 **oto.theclinics.com**

a weak, breathy voice, difficulty with maintaining a normal length of voicing, loss of voice with attempts at projection, and difficulty in swallowing with risk of aspiration. Because of the difficulty in adjusting laryngeal resistance with incomplete glottic closure, patients often feel short of breath. A high vagal lesion results in more significant symptoms than a recurrent laryngeal nerve (RLN) deficit. The vagus nerve has several branches: the pharyngeal branches supply motor function to the pharynx and palate with the exception of the tensor veli palatini; the superior laryngeal nerve (SLN) branch has both internal and external branches. The internal branch of the SLN supplies sensory and parasympathetic fibers to the epiglottis, tongue base, aryepiglottic folds, and the larynx to the level of the glottis. The external branch of the SLN is a motor branch, innervating the cricothyroid muscle and inferior pharyngeal constrictors and participating significantly in pitch control and swallowing. These combined sensory and motor deficits result in a higher likelihood of aspiration and more complex phonatory problems. The vagus also communicates with the intercarotid plexus, monitoring carbon dioxide and oxygen tensions.

Hypoglossal nerve

Hypoglossal nerve involvement by a skull base lesion results in dysarthria and oral-phase dysphagia. As an isolated deficit, hypoglossal loss may be compensated with swallowing and articulatory therapy. In combination with other nerve deficits, however, hypoglossal nerve injury increases functional loss and affects rehabilitation.

Evaluation

Initial diagnosis of a skull base tumor may follow presentation with one or more cranial nerve deficits. Treatment planning includes anticipation of further nerve deficits. Careful attention should be paid to time of onset (preexisting or after treatment), voicing symptoms (weak voice, raspy quality, hypernasality, and so forth), extent of dysphagia (oral, pharyngeal, and hypopharyngeal phases), previous surgeries, cognitive status, and goals of rehabilitation. Assessment by the skull base surgeon, laryngologist, and speech pathologist early in the course of diagnosis and treatment helps facilitate a comprehensive, coordinated approach.

Vagus nerve

With findings of a vocal cord paralysis, clinical assessment should include examination of palatal movement, assessment of vallecular or pyriform sinus pooling, and subjective evaluation of voice quality, vocal range, and maximum phonation time (MPT). MPT varies significantly, but a range below 12 seconds typically is associated with a breathy voice with difficulty sustaining phrasing with connected speech. Pharyngeal or palatal weakness or decreased sensitivity should be suspected with significant pooling of secretions. The oculocardiac reflex can be tested as part of the clinical evaluation. This testing involves placing pressure on the eye on the side of the lesion and monitoring the pulse. The pulse will become slower if the site of the lesion is distal to the communication of the vagus nerve with the intercarotid plexus (proximal to the takeoff of both the SLN and the RLN). Full assessment of dysphagia is important in determining an appropriate treatment plan. High vagal lesions typically result in failure of coordination of the oral and pharyngeal phases of swallowing, with poor coordination of the relaxation of the upper esophageal sphincter, and with pooling and overflow into the larynx [2].

Diagnostic studies may include static (CT, MRI), or dynamic (modified barium swallow [MBS]) radiographic studies; dynamic clinical examinations (functional endoscopic evaluation of swallow [FEES] or FEES with sensory testing [FEESST]) [3], videolaryngoscopy/videostroboscopy, electromyography (EMG), manometry, aerodynamic/airflow measures, and other evaluations of voicing.

CT scanning or MRI is done as part of the initial assessment of the skull base tumor. Their subsequent role in treatment planning is more limited.

A MBS study is useful to assess and document dysphagia. Sensory deficits and nasopharyngeal reflux may be more apparent on a MBS than on visual inspection alone. The MBS examines oral, pharyngeal, and esophageal function. It identifies the cause of aspiration (ie, when and how the event occurs during the swallow hierarchy) and also allows assessment of the efficacy of treatment and management strategies.

Functional endoscopic evaluation of swallow and functional endoscopic evaluation of swallow with sensory testing

FEES [4] and FEESST can be done in clinic to assess the degree of dysphagia and sensory deficit. A screening FEES test can be performed easily by using a flexible nasopharyngoscope and monitoring velar closure, pooling, and aspiration while a patient swallows blue-colored water. Topical anesthetics must be avoided in this examination to avoid bias. A more sophisticated evaluation can be done with puffs of air through a dedicated scope, assessing sensation throughout the hypopharynx and larynx (FEESST).

Additionally, but less often, ultrasound and manometry may be used to evaluate specific components of the swallow such as lateral pharyngeal wall motion or tongue base to posterior pharyngeal wall pressures.

Videolaryngoscopy/videostroboscopy

Videostroboscopy is a key portion of the clinical examination. A rigid 70° or 90° scope can allow assessment of mucosal wave, amplitude of vibration, glottal gap, mucosal lesions, and pooling. A flexible scope examination adds significantly to the assessment of vocal cord motion and may reveal subtle deficits or asymmetry. Patients can phonate more freely with a nasopharyngoscope, and various vocal tasks can be assessed. Glottic closure should be evaluated including any evidence of atrophy or scar. The position of the vocal processes and motion with pitch change should be determined.

Voicing measures

Voicing is assessed by subjective analysis and by a voice handicap index. Measurements of voicing intensity and MPT are benchmarks to use as an estimate of glottal resistance [5]. MPT is a measure that is easy to acquire and can be readily assessed at various points during treatment to monitor progress. MPT is measured with the patient in a sitting or standing position, sustaining a vowel sound at a comfortable pitch and loudness level, for as long as possible on one breath. It can be measured in a supine position, as an intraoperative assessment during a medialization procedure, although the MPT is shorter in this position [6]. Formal assessment by a speech language pathologist (SLP) can help in assessing the level of symptoms for an individual and to evaluate for any compensatory maneuvers.

Electromyography

If there is question about the prognosis for recovery, serial EMG studies may help guide treatment. The availability of laryngeal EMGs varies, and the interpretation and application are subject to debate. An initial EMG should be done at least 2 weeks after injury. A second EMG done 6 weeks later allows additional assessment of recovery. If there is no evidence of reinnervation, and the patient is sufficiently symptomatic and motivated, an early permanent medialization is appropriate.

Treatment of vagus nerve deficits

Treatment options include voice or swallowing therapy; amplification devices, injectable substances to improve glottic closure, surgical medialization, treatment of velopharyngeal incompetence, and treatment of cricopharyngeal hypertonicity or dysfunction.

Considerations in voice and swallowing therapy are discussed in more detail later in this article. Voice or swallowing therapy should be considered a complementary treatment regardless of any other interventions.

Temporizing approaches that help to improve glottic closure include injection of fat, Gelfoam (Pharmacia Upjohn, Kalamazoo, MI) [7], fascia [8], collagen [9] (bovine or human [10]), hyaluronic acid [11], or hydroxyapatite [12]. Other implants have been and continue to be studied [13–15].

Collagen can be injected into the vocal cord under direct visualization transorally or transcutaneously in a clinic setting based upon the comfort and experience of the clinician. Bovine collagen has been used most extensively in this setting. There is risk of a delayed hypersensitivity reaction (hypersensitivity ranges from 1.2%–3%) [16]; therefore, skin testing is required before injection. Resorption does occur. Human collagen (Cymetra, Lifecell, Branchburg, NJ) can be injected without testing for allergy/sensitivity. Cymetra is an acellular dermis that is converted into micronized particles. Because it is processed from human skin, there is some theoretical risk of transmission of human pathogens. Injection of Cymetra requires the use of a larger-gauge needle (18- to 21-gauge) than bovine collagen (27-gauge). Injection of fat, which must be harvested first, is generally performed under a general anesthetic. Hyaluronic acid can be injected in the clinic with a small-gauge needle. There is some risk of an allergic reaction, depending on the form of hyaluronic acid used. Hyaluronic acid holds great promise because of its viscoelastic properties, which closely approximate vocal fold mucosa [17].

Teflon (Dupont, USA) can be injected into the larynx and true vocal cord but requires precise placement, and is unforgiving. Teflon injection is best done under a general anesthetic to allow direct visualization and magnification with microscopic guidance. Improper placement of Teflon results in poor voice quality with a stiff true vocal cord and potential for granuloma formation. Removal of Teflon is challenging in the best of circumstances.

Surgical procedures

Type I thyroplasty is the workhorse of the laryngologist. This procedure allows positioning of an immobile vocal cord to allow complete glottic closure with phonation and swallow. A variety of implants and implant materials are available. These include Silastic, (Dow Corning, Midland, MI) hydroxyapatite, and expanded polytetrafluoroethylene (Gore-tex; W.L. Gore, Inc., Newark, Deleware) [18].

Arytenoid adduction may be done as a stand-alone procedure or in conjunction with a type I thyroplasty. An arytenoid adduction is done by placing a suture in the arytenoid, rotating the muscular process posteromedially, allowing for glottic closure and improving posterior closure. Vocal cord medialization improves glottic closure and decreases dynamic aspiration risk, but poor coordination of swallow and weakness with resultant pooling still result in significant symptoms. Despite immediate medialization for vagal paralysis, most skull base patients remain dependent on enteral methods of nutritional support for up to 1 year or permanently, despite improvement in voicing [19].

Arytenoid adduction can be combined with a type I thyroplasty if sufficient posterior closure is not obtained with an implant alone. Conversely, a type I thyroplasty can be done secondarily if arytenoid adduction does not result in adequate anterior glottic closure. A medialization procedure (injection, implantation, or arytenoid adduction) can be combined with a reinnervation procedure with the goal of improving or maintaining tone. There are various methods of reinnervation, including direct anastomosis and nerve-muscle pedicles. Reinnervation can give long-term improvement, but results are delayed [20], taking up to 1 year for full recovery.

Treatment of velopharyngeal incompetence can improve speech and swallowing in skull base patients. This treatment may involve working with an SLP or use of a palatal prosthesis. In addition, surgical options such as a palatal adhesion technique may be useful for this unilateral deficit [21].

Cricopharyngeal hypertonicity can be treated by myotomy or botulinum toxin (Botox; Allergan, Inc., Irvine, California) injection. Botox injection, with temporary results, may be useful if prognosis is uncertain, or if the patient is not stable enough for a more invasive procedure.

Hypoglossal nerve

Tongue atrophy results in oral-phase dysphagia and dysarthria. Clinical assessment should include evaluation by an SLP. Tongue atrophy from a hypoglossal nerve deficit is treated primarily by articulatory therapy. Injecting a bulking agent has also been reported to improve symptoms [22].

Decision for and timing of treatment depends upon level of symptoms, risk for aspiration, prognosis for recovery, and the patient's motivation and wishes.

Speech and swallowing therapy

The SLP plays a vital role in the evaluation, treatment, and management of temporary or permanent neuropathies often associated with skull base tumors and their resection. These cranial nerve deficits, involving one or more of cranial nerves IX, X, XI, and XII, have a varying impact on speech, mastication, and swallowing. Deficits can be relatively mild and temporary or devastating in their disfigurement and disability. Many patients benefit from consultation with an SLP in both the pre- and postoperative phases of their treatment. There may be benefit in delaying surgical reconstruction and rehabilitation procedures while assessing the nature and severity of the deficit [23].

Speech, voice, and swallowing deficits following skull base surgeries typically are related to altered function in the velopharyngeal mechanism and lingual musculature and to vocal cord paralysis. The procedures and methods used in evaluation, management, and treatment of these deficits vary according to the type and severity f the deficits.

Management practices can be distinguished as behavioral or nonbehavioral and as compensatory or rehabilitative. Behavioral practices, such as pharyngeal strengthening exercises, involve active participation of the patient, typically over a long period. Nonbehavioral interventions (eg, palatal prosthesis) are more medically based and may alter physiology. Compensatory strategies typically provide an immediate but transient effect on function, such as the use of a chin tuck during swallowing. Rehabilitative interventions, such as breathing or vocal fold adduction exercises, are thought to result in permanent changes in physiologic substrates when provided over time [24]. The following discussion provides a broad overview of the SLP's role in the evaluation, management, and treatment of swallowing, speech, and voice following skull base surgery.

Swallowing

There are multiple methods used to evaluate swallowing safety and efficiency. Methods can be categorized as screening procedures used to identify the dysphagic patient, such as a noninstrumental, bedside evaluation, and procedures that identify the component of disordered anatomy or physiology in the swallow.

Typically, the most common diagnostic procedure used with patients who have had skull base surgery is fluoroscopy or the MBS. Screening procedures include the noninstrumental bedside evaluation, the use of endoscopy (FEES, FEESST), cervical auscultation, blue dye test for patients with a tracheotomy, the rapid water test, and the laryngeal cough reflex test [25]. Additional instrumental procedures are used to measure swallow activity, such as surface EMG, which quantifies timing and degree of muscle activity and can be used for biofeedback of timing and laryngeal elevation.

Treatment may involve a nonbehavioral approach such as a palatal prosthesis for palatal defect. Ideally, the SLP works closely with the prosthodontist to determine appropriate candidacy, assess the contour of augmentation, provide speech and swallow exercises, and to perform fluoroscopic re-evaluation of the swallow. Palatal augmentation prostheses have been demonstrated to result in improvement in multiple aspects of disordered swallow function [26].

With respect to behavioral swallowing interventions, compensatory strategies are selected with attention to the underlying physiologic abnormality. A chin tuck may be used for delayed onset of pharyngeal swallow, neck extension is commonly used for improved oral transit of the bolus, and head rotation (toward the side of weakness) may help reduce aspiration risk in the patient with unilateral true vocal cord paralysis. Additional behavioral strategies include the supraglottic and super-supraglottic swallow for improved airway protection, the dry swallow, cyclic ingestion of solids/liquids, the use of thickened liquids or modified solid textures, lingual sweep, thermal gustatory stimulation, and modifications in the route of intake to circumvent the oral phase of swallow (such as a catheter tip syringe) [27,28].

Rehabilitative swallowing treatment is intended to result in changes in the physiology of the swallow through muscle strengthening or retraining. Treatment includes oral motor exercises, vocal adduction exercises, modified Valsalva (effortful) swallow (Logemann), Mendelsohn maneuver (Mendelsohn), and Masako maneuver (Fujiu).

Voice and speech

The SLP can assist the otolaryngologist or in some cases can perform a videostroboscopic evaluation of the vocal fold function. In cases of suspected dysphagia, FEES or FEEST screening can be obtained along with laryngeal sensitivity testing. During the transnasal, flexible laryngeal examination, the SLP is able to introduce relaxation and therapeutic techniques to assess potential for improvement in vocal quality. Voice therapy often plays an important role in the general treatment of vocal fold paralysis. Patients may develop hyperfunctional behaviors in an attempt to compensate for glottic insufficiency. These behaviors may contribute to overall deterioration in vocal quality and endurance, and they may persist following surgical treatment. An initial voice evaluation by the SLP may include acoustic and aerodynamic measures to serve as a baseline and for objective monitoring of improvement. Therapeutic or facilitative techniques are used during videostroboscopy and the initial voice evaluation to determine the patient's potential for improvement in vocal quality. Examples of potentially helpful facilitating approaches include digital manipulation, head positioning, or training the patient to say fewer words per expiration or to inspire more often [28]. The SLP can assist the patient, when appropriate, in selecting an appropriate personal voice amplification device for improved voice projection and intelligibility. In cases of unilateral vocal fold paralysis, the goal of voice therapy is to promote the best voice possible, enhance vocal endurance, and prevent maladaptive compensatory behaviors.

Rehabilitation of voice and swallowing requires a team approach, combining the expertise of various health care providers with the needs and goals of the patient. Preoperative assessment and anticipation of deficits can help greatly to facilitate rehabilitation and recovery, optimizing outcome.

References

[1] Woodson GE. Configuration of the glottis in laryngeal paralysis. I: clinical study. Laryngoscope 1993;103:1227–34.

[2] Jennings KS, Siroky D, Jackson CG. Swallowing problems after excision of tumors of the skull base: diagnosis and management in 12 patients. Dysphagia 1992;7:40–4.

[3] Aviv JE, Martin JH, Keen MS, et al. Air pulse quantification of supraglottic and pharyngeal sensation: a new technique. Ann Otol Rhinol Laryngol 1993;102:777–80.

[4] Perie S, Toubeau B, St. Guily JL. Laryngeal paralysis: distinguishing Xth nerve from recurrent laryngeal nerve paralysis through videoendoscopic swallowing study (VESS). Dysphagia 2003;18:276–83.

[5] Benninger MS, Crumley RL, Ford CN, et al. Evaluation and treatment of the unilateral paralyzed vocal fold. Otolaryngol Head Neck Surg 1994;111:497–508.

[6] Lundy DS, Casiano RR, Xue JW. Can maximum phonation time predict voice outcome after thyroplasty type I? Laryngoscope 2004;114:1447–54.

[7] Schramm VL, May M, Lavorato AS. Gelfoam paste injection for vocal cord paralysis: temporary rehabilitation of glottic incompetence. Laryngoscope 1978;88:1268–73.

[8] Rihkanen J. Vocal fold augmentation by injection of autologous fascia. Laryngoscope 1998; 108:51–4.

[9] Ford CN, Martin DW, Warner TF. Injectable collagen in laryngeal rehabilitation. Laryngoscope 1984;94:513–8.

[10] Pearl AW, Woo P, Ostrowski R, et al. A preliminary report on micronized AlloDerm injection laryngoplasty. Laryngoscope 2002;112:990–6.
[11] Hertegard S, Hallen L, Laurent C, et al. Cross-linked hyaluronan used as augmentation substance for treatment of glottal insufficiency: safety aspects and vocal fold function. Laryngoscope 2002;112:2211–9.
[12] Rosen CA, Thekdi AA. Vocal fold augmentation with injectable calcium hydoxylapatite: short-term results. J Voice 2004;18:387–91.
[13] Lee B-J, Wang S-G, Goh E-K, et al. Intracordal injection of autologous auricular cartilage in the paralyzed canine vocal fold. Otolaryngol Head Neck Surg 2004;131(1):34–43.
[14] Sittel C, Thumfart WF, Potoschinig C, et al. Textured polydimethylsiloxane elastomers in the human larynx: safety and efficacy of use. J Biomed Mater Res 2000;53:646–50.
[15] Alves CB, Loughran S, MacGregor FB, et al. Bioplastique medialization therapy improves the quality of life in terminally ill patients with vocal cord palsy. Clin Otolaryngol 2002;27: 387–91.
[16] Cooperman L, Michaeli D. The immunogenicity of injectable collagen. J Am Acad Dermatol 1984;10:638–46.
[17] Klemuk SA, Titze IR. Viscoelastic properties of three vocal-fold injectable biomaterials at low audio frequencies. Laryngoscope 2004;114(9):1597–603.
[18] Hoffman HT, McCulloch TM. Medialization laryngoplasty with Gore-Tex. Operative Techniques in Otolaryngology-Head and Neck Surgery 1999;10(1):6–8.
[19] Bielamowicz S, Gupta A, Sekhar LN. Early arytenoid adduction for vagal paralysis after skull base surgery. Laryngoscope 2000;110:346–51.
[20] Crumley RL. Update: ansa cervicalis to recurrent laryngeal nerve anastomosis for unilateral laryngeal paralysis. Laryngoscope 1991;101:384–8.
[21] Netterville JL, Fortune S, Stanziale S, et al. Palatal adhesion: the treatment of unilateral palatal paralysis after high vagus nerve injury. Head Neck 2002;24:721–30.
[22] Burres S. Intralingual injection of particulate fascia for tongue paralysis. Laryngoscope 2004;114:1204–5.
[23] Day TA, Davis BK. Skull base reconstruction and rehabilitation. Otolaryngol Clin North Am 2001;34:1241–57.
[24] Huckabee ML. Beyond compensatory strategies: an interactive forum on dysphagia rehabilitation. Presented at Conferences for Learning by Speech Language and Learning Services, Seattle, WA. January 16–17, 1998.
[25] Lazarus C. Management of speech, voice and swallowing disorders in head and neck cancer patients. Presented at the continuing education seminar by Northern Speech Services, Inc., San Francisco, CA. November 1–2, 2003.
[26] Davis JW, Lazarus C, Longeman JA, et al. Effect of a maxillary glossectomy prosthesis on articulation and swallowing. J Prosthet Dent 1987;57:715–20.
[27] Logemann JA. Treatment for aspiration related to dysphagia: an overview. Dysphagia 1986; 1:34–8.
[28] Logemann JA. Management of the patient with disordered oral feeding. In: Logemann JA, editor. Evaluation and treatment of swallowing disorders. San Diego (CA): College Hill Press; 1983.

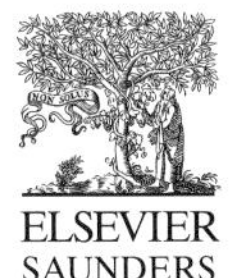

ELSEVIER
SAUNDERS

Otolaryngol Clin N Am
38 (2005) 819–824

OTOLARYNGOLOGIC
CLINICS
OF NORTH AMERICA

Index

Note: Page numbers of article titles are in **boldface** type.

A

doi:10.1016/S0030-6665(05)00080-0 *oto.theclinics.com*

D

E

F

G

H

Changing Your Address?

Make sure your subscription changes too! When you notify us of your new address, you can help make our job easier by including an exact copy of your Clinics label number with your old address (see illustration below.) This number identifies you to our computer system and will speed the processing of your address change. Please be sure this label number accompanies your old address and your corrected address—you can send an old Clinics label with your number on it or just copy it exactly and send it to the address listed below.

We appreciate your help in our attempt to give you continuous coverage. Thank you.

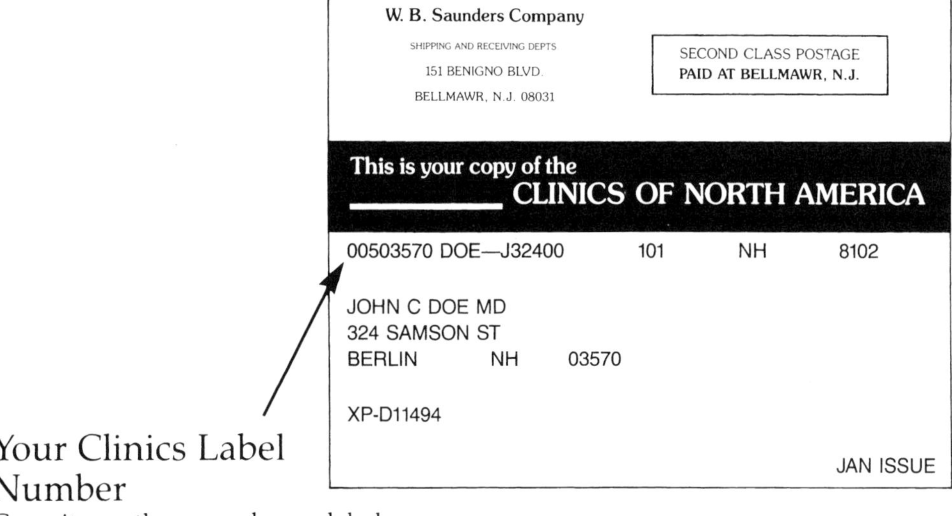

Your Clinics Label Number

Copy it exactly or send your label along with your address to:
W.B. Saunders Company, Customer Service
Orlando, FL 32887-4800
Call Toll Free 1-800-654-2452

Please allow four to six weeks for delivery of new subscriptions and for processing address changes.

Order your subscription today. Simply complete and detach this card and drop it in the mail to receive the best clinical information in your field.

YES! Please start my subscription to the **CLINICS** checked below with the ❑ first issue of the calendar year or ❑ current issues. If not completely satisfied with my first issue, I may write "cancel" on the invoice and return it within 30 days at no further obligation.

Please Print:

Name ____________________

Address ____________________

City ____________ State ____________ ZIP ____________

Method of Payment

❑ Check (payable to **Elsevier**; add the applicable sales tax for your area)

❑ VISA ❑ MasterCard ❑ AmEx ❑ Bill me

Card number ____________ Exp. date ____________

Signature ____________________

Staple this to your purchase order to expedite delivery

❑ **Adolescent Medicine Clinics**
- ❑ Individual $95
- ❑ Institutions $133
- ❑ *In-training $48

❑ **Anesthesiology**
- ❑ Individual $175
- ❑ Institutions $270
- ❑ *In-training $88

❑ **Cardiology**
- ❑ Individual $170
- ❑ Institutions $266
- ❑ *In-training $85

❑ **Chest Medicine**
- ❑ Individual $185
- ❑ Institutions $285

❑ **Child and Adolescent Psychiatry**
- ❑ Individual $175
- ❑ Institutions $265
- ❑ *In-training $88

❑ **Critical Care**
- ❑ Individual $165
- ❑ Institutions $266
- ❑ *In-training $83

❑ **Dental**
- ❑ Individual $150
- ❑ Institutions $242

❑ **Emergency Medicine**
- ❑ Individual $170
- ❑ Institutions $263
- ❑ *In-training $85
- ❑ Send CME info

❑ **Facial Plastic Surgery**
- ❑ Individual $199
- ❑ Institutions $300

❑ **Foot and Ankle**
- Individual $160
- Institutions $232

❑ **Gastroenterology**
- ❑ Individual $190
- ❑ Institutions $276

❑ **Gastrointestinal Endoscopy**
- ❑ Individual $190
- ❑ Institutions $276

❑ **Hand**
- ❑ Individual $205
- ❑ Institutions $319

❑ **Heart Failure (NEW in 2005!)**
- ❑ Individual $99
- ❑ Institutions $149
- ❑ *In-training $49

❑ **Hematology/ Oncology**
- ❑ Individual $210
- ❑ Institutions $315

❑ **Immunology & Allergy**
- ❑ Individual $165
- ❑ Institutions $266

❑ **Infectious Disease**
- ❑ Individual $165
- ❑ Institutions $272

❑ **Clinics in Liver Disease**
- ❑ Individual $165
- ❑ Institutions $234

❑ **Medical**
- ❑ Individual $140
- ❑ Institutions $244
- ❑ *In-training $70
- ❑ Send CME info

❑ **MRI**
- ❑ Individual $190
- ❑ Institutions $290
- ❑ *In-training $95
- ❑ Send CME info

❑ **Neuroimaging**
- ❑ Individual $190
- ❑ Institutions $290
- ❑ *In-training $95
- ❑ Send CME inf0

❑ **Neurologic**
- ❑ Individual $175
- ❑ Institutions $275

❑ **Obstetrics & Gynecology**
- ❑ Individual $175
- ❑ Institutions $288

❑ **Occupational and Environmental Medicine**
- ❑ Individual $120
- ❑ Institutions $166
- ❑ *In-training $60

❑ **Ophthalmology**
- ❑ Individual $190
- ❑ Institutions $325

❑ **Oral & Maxillofacial Surgery**
- ❑ Individual $180
- ❑ Institutions $280
- ❑ *In-training $90

❑ **Orthopedic**
- ❑ Individual $180
- ❑ Institutions $295
- ❑ *In-training $90

❑ **Otolaryngologic**
- ❑ Individual $199
- ❑ Institutions $350

❑ **Pediatric**
- ❑ Individual $135
- ❑ Institutions $246
- ❑ *In-training $68
- ❑ Send CME info

❑ **Perinatology**
- ❑ Individual $155
- ❑ Institutions $237
- ❑ *In-training $78
- ❑ Send CME inf0

❑ **Plastic Surgery**
- ❑ Individual $245
- ❑ Institutions $370

❑ **Podiatric Medicine & Surgery**
- ❑ Individual $170
- ❑ Institutions $266

❑ **Primary Care**
- ❑ Individual $135
- ❑ Institutions $223

❑ **Psychiatric**
- ❑ Individual $170
- ❑ Institutions $288

❑ **Radiologic**
- ❑ Individual $220
- ❑ Institutions $331
- ❑ *In-training $110
- ❑ Send CME info

❑ **Sports Medicine**
- ❑ Individual $180
- ❑ Institutions $277

❑ **Surgical**
- ❑ Individual $190
- ❑ Institutions $299
- ❑ *In-training $95

❑ **Thoracic Surgery (formerly Chest Surgery)**
- ❑ Individual $175
- ❑ Institutions $255
- ❑ *In-training $88

❑ **Urologic**
- ❑ Individual $195
- ❑ Institutions $307
- ❑ *In-training $98
- ❑ Send CME info

*To receive in-training rate, orders must be accompanied by the name of affiliated institution, dates of residency and signature of coordinator on institution letterhead. Orders will be billed at the individual rate until proof of resident status is received.

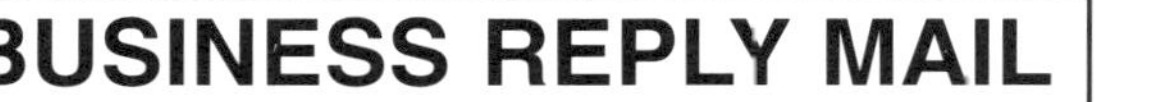

NO POSTAGE
NECESSARY
IF MAILED
IN THE
UNITED STATES

BUSINESS REPLY MAIL

FIRST-CLASS MAIL PERMIT NO 7135 ORLANDO FL

POSTAGE WILL BE PAID BY ADDRESSEE

PERIODICALS ORDER FULFILLMENT DEPT
ELSEVIER
6277 SEA HARBOR DR
ORLANDO FL 32821-9816